WEEK LO

NURSES IN NAZI GERMANY

Bronwyn Rebekah McFarland-Icke

Nurses in Nazi Germany

MORAL CHOICE
IN HISTORY

Princeton University Press, Princeton, New Jersey

Copyright © 1999 by Princeton University Press
Published by Princeton University Press, 41 William Street,
Princeton, New Jersey 08540
In the United Kingdom: Princeton University Press,
Chichester, West Sussex

Library of Congress Cataloging-in-Publication Data

McFarland-Icke, Bronwyn Rebekah, 1965–
Nurses in Nazi Germany : moral choice in history /
Bronwyn Rebekah McFarland-Icke.
p.   cm.
Includes bibliographical references and index.
ISBN 0-691-00665-2 (cl. : alk. paper)
1. Psychiatric nursing—Moral and ethical aspects—Germany—
History—20th century. 2. Nursing ethics—Germany—
History—20th century. 3. Medical policy—
Germany—History—20th century. 4. National socialism
and medicine—Germany. 5. World War, 1939–1945—Atrocities.
6. Euthanasia—Germany—History—20th century.
7. Medical ethics—Germany—History—20th century.
I. Title.
RC440.M325   1999
610.73′0943′0904—dc21   99-18151

This book has been composed in Palatino

The paper used in this publication meets
the minimum requirements of
ANSI/NISO Z39.48-1992 (R1997)
(Permanence of Paper)

http://pup.princeton.edu

Printed in the United States of America

10 9 8 7 6 5 4 3 2

Contents

Preface

THE FOLLOWING study is the product of a long-standing interest in how people make moral choices. In the context of National Socialism, this becomes a volatile, and indeed central, issue, since the cumulative choices of millions of people in a modernizing and seemingly "civilized" society added up to genocide—genocide that was unprecedented in its terrifying mix of brutality and bureaucratic efficiency. How could this happen? How could traditional networks of human solidarity—political parties, the Church, local and professional organizations, personal relationships—prove in the end to be so fragile?

Over the last fifty years, it has been customary for historians to discuss morality under National Socialism in terms of resistance and collaboration.[1] To a large extent, the resulting literature implicitly or explicitly defined resisters as those who conformed to *our* expectations of heroic virtue by firmly, vocally, and completely renouncing National Socialism. There are, to be sure, numerous examples of people who resisted the regime and its policies in precisely this fashion and, in many instances, paid with their lives. Their stories should be written and remembered. Yet this approach failed to address adequately the central issue, which is not how Germans under National Socialism measure up against our moral yardstick, but rather how and why they behaved as they did in a time of moral crisis—what *mobilized* or *immobilized* them—and how their choices, regarded collectively, produced institutionalized barbarism.

Over the years, historians have indeed developed more nuanced accounts of the motives of resisters and collaborators, and they have broadened their scope beyond organized resistance to include people who acted individually, spontaneously, or clandestinely in opposition. Even so, I cannot not help but think that the resistance-collaboration paradigm itself tends to pro-

duce a polarized and unrealistic view not only of people's behavior but also of the choices they faced. Although psychologically appealing insofar as it neatly divides historical protagonists according to their alliance with the forces of either good
or evil,[2] it risks romanticizing history to the point of overlooking
situations where the available choices could not possibly have
been described in terms of choosing "good" over "evil." As Hannah Arendt wrote, "When a man is faced with the alternative
of betraying and thus murdering his friends or of sending his
wife and children, for whom he is in every sense responsible—
to their death; when even suicide would mean the immediate
murder of his own family—how is he to decide? The alternative
is no longer between good and evil, but between murder and
murder."[3]

Even if most Germans were spared this particular kind of
limit situation, there is a great deal to suggest that people's
choices in daily life did not, and could not, reflect a complete
acceptance or rejection of National Socialism as a coherent entity
representing a set of coherent principles. The inconsistencies between thought and action are legion: the widespread denunciations that kept the Gestapo so busy often had nothing to do with
support for the Reich or any particular aspect of it; rather, in
many instances people denounced for personal reasons such as
a desire for retaliation.[4] Peasants in Bavaria opposed the Jewish
boycott for largely economic reasons;[5] and a number of cases of
Christian rescue of Jews in Poland were unplanned and
prompted simply by confrontation with a despondent Jew.[6]

Particularly in cases of rescue attempts, an *intention* to undermine National Socialism *as such* did not always lend itself to
clear articulation, and one can even question the extent to which
a spirit of opposition to the regime existed.[7] Although ethical,
religious, or political motives were no doubt consciously present
in many cases of rescue, often such actions were based on more
parochial sentiments such as "he is my neighbor."[8] Yet such rescuers are just as important to an understanding of moral deliberation under National Socialism as are better-known resisters
such as Hans and Sophie Scholl. Unwilling to hide behind a wall

of indifference, such "spontaneous" rescuers expressed compassion for the regime's victims when the exclusion of such people was not only desired but insisted upon by a terrorist dictatorship. Their example points to severe inadequacies in the traditional resistance-collaboration paradigm as a tool for grasping moral choice under National Socialism as a historical and sociological phenomenon.

This methodological concern underlies the following study of psychiatric nurses. It goes without saying, in this light, that I have sought not only to fill a historiographical gap (for nurses remain a relatively understudied group in the history of medicine) but also to develop a perspective that returns moral choice to its historical context and examines it in all its complexity. In this study, psychiatric nurses under National Socialism are of interest first and foremost as a group of men and women who faced, indeed *lived*, a moral contradiction of monumental proportions: alongside their function of participating in racially motivated compulsory sterilization and "euthanasia" policies (not to mention presiding over deplorable institutional conditions), they remained subject to an ethical imperative to heal and promote life in a spirit of charity—that is, irrespective of the identity of the person in question. From our perspective today, these seem fundamentally irreconcilable; yet on some level they *must* have been reconcilable in order for National Socialist racial policy to radicalize in the midst of daily life. My point of departure, quite simply, is "How did this happen?"

In developing a research strategy, I found it useful to separate moral principles from moral deliberation. It would not be enough to study professional ethics without understanding their relevance, or lack thereof, for the nurses themselves; nor would it suffice to study their everyday lives without understanding the demands, both moral and administrative, that were being made on them. I decided, therefore, to divide my attention between the theoretical and practical aspects of psychiatric nursing. On the one hand, analysis of nursing periodicals and textbooks could provide a "window" on the (evolving) moral status of patients and rules governing their treatment. Institutional administrative and personnel records would, I hoped, provide insights into their implementation (or lack thereof) in daily institutional life. In particular, I was interested in exploring which circumstances favored the manifestation of these ethics, and which militated against it.

To this end, I studied a variety of published materials for the instruction of psychiatric nurses. The most useful source turned out to be a monthly journal devoted to this purpose, founded in 1896 and entitled *Die Irrenpflege: Monatschrift für Irrenpflege und Krankenpflege zur Belehrung und Fortbildung des Pflegepersonals an den Heil- und Pflegeanstalten und zur Hebung seines Standes.* (In an attempt to overcome psychiatry's long-standing association with detention, the editors changed the name to the more medically up-to-date *Geisteskrankenpflege* in 1930. Although both titles could be roughly translated as *Psychiatric Nursing,* the new German title indicated a change of perspective: nurses were caring for people who were considered "mentally ill" [*geisteskrank*] rather then "insane" or "crazy" [*irre*].) Its authors came from the ranks of professionals in whose purview the mentally ill fell: psychiatrists, nurses, social welfare workers, and clergy. Each issue consisted of several fairly short articles followed by book reviews and brief reports from everyday institutional life: conferences, memorial days, directorial changes, obituaries, statistics, organizational information, and union news.

This journal was important, in part, because it informed me about nurses' technical responsibilities in the context of hospital maintenance, patient care, and therapies. In addition, it helped me to place nurses in the context of a more general problem that persisted from the nineteenth century clear through the period to be studied and left its mark on their professional development: low morale among psychiatric nurses, high staff turnover, and a poor reputation among the public. In hopes of generating professional self-esteem, the journal proffered an image of psychiatric nursing as a respectable, challenging profession full of important responsibilities. Articles that celebrated the scientific advances and humanization of psychiatry during the nineteenth century, and those which described institutional psychiatry in other countries, such as England and America, provided nurses with historical and geographic context that would heighten their sense of belonging and, it was undoubtedly hoped, their professional allegiance.

Ultimately, however, the journal was most useful—indeed, indispensable—because it discussed the moral status of patients explicitly and went into such minute detail about how they should be treated. Articles advised nurses on the importance of their tone and choice of words, their manner and way of walking. Attempting to help nurses cope with the grim realities of daily life, contributors did not limit themselves to rehearsing restraint methods for violent patients; they also explained the logic behind them. Armed with a rudimentary background in mental illnesses and their symptoms, nurses, it was hoped, would understand *why* the patient had become violent, and would thus be able to control the impulse to requite violence with violence. *Die Irrenpflege/Geisteskrankenpflege* was thus potentially an important medium for shaping the attitudes of nurses toward patients and the relationship that emerged between them. Moreover, since I had access to monthly issues for the two decades under consideration in this study, the journal provided a means for tracing subtle developments in ethical orientation that were ultimately of great significance in illuminating how the aims of psychiatric nursing were rendered compatible with the aims of National Socialism.

Investigating the relevance of these prescriptive texts in daily life was a considerably more daunting prospect because, especially during the years of National Socialist dictatorship, the occasions when nurses sat down to pen critical or self-reflective commentaries on contemporary developments are not likely to have been numerous. In addition, as I began to make written inquiries to German archives in search of relevant material, I came to realize the great extent to which institutional records were destroyed or otherwise disappeared after the war. Things did not look terribly promising until I contacted Christina Härtel of Berlin's Karl-Bonhoeffer-Nervenklinik (hereafter KBoN), who offered to let me use what remained of their records for the

Wittenauer Heilstätten, as this institution was called from 1924 to 1957.

This was in the spring of 1993; had I made my request a dozen years earlier, I learned, the answer would very likely have been different. During investigations in connection with legal proceedings against doctors and nursing personnel in the 1960s, the clinic's administration had reported that all administrative and patient records from the 1933–1945 period had been burned by the invading Red Army. Although the personnel records of doctors and all administrative records from the 1933–1945 period have indeed disappeared, Dr. Bernd-Michael Becker and interested KBoN staff formed a research team in the mid-1980s which discovered that the institution housed not only personnel and patient records from the NS-period but also many dating back to the institution's founding. "The recovery of the materials in the archive," the team proceeded to write in its first book, "was more a problem of wanting to look."[9]

The archive to which I was led, a dark basement in the administration building, reflected these decades of neglect. The dusty personnel files lay stacked in pigeonholes, and I was permitted to bring armloads of records up to a vacant office. (One year later I would work under similar arrangements at the Eichberg institution, in what is today the federal state of Hesse.) That these tattered, "official" records would offer relatively vivid glimpses into the lives and minds of the people who created them was far from obvious. Documents of varying shapes and sizes were assembled more or less chronologically in each file, facilitating my ability to follow bureaucratic proceedings, but the need to decipher a considerable number of handwritten documents and marginal scrawl made the analysis of such files a time-consuming process. It was time well spent, however, because some files were several hundred pages long and filled with the details of long and (for my purposes) interesting careers, and some shorter ones offered equally interesting, if less substantial, anecdotal information.

Although I visited a number of archives, this is how I spent most of my time during the research phase of this study: reading personnel records on institutional grounds. This proved to be an immensely rewarding arrangement, since a number of buildings at KBoN and Eichberg still resemble photographs from the 1920s and 1930s. Working "on location," among today's institutional staff and patients, gave the dramas about which I read a vividness that would have been unattainable in a traditional archive setting. As it turned out, my journey to the Eichberg institution entailed leaving the train in Eltville-am-Rhein and then riding a shuttle bus through a few Rhein valley villages up to Eichberg. While this would have been an unexceptional experience under other circumstances, at the time it offered even more visual reinforcement for the task at hand: a glimpse of the fields in which patients worked, the routes nurses traveled in their private time, the wine country as it appeared to patients through the window of a bus as they were transported to their deaths.

Since finding useful material was very much a hit-or-miss affair, a word of caution is in order. The most useful personnel records were useful precisely because they dwelled less on "everyday life" than on the *exceptional*, or at least what should have been exceptional: that is, the nurse in question had somehow deviated from prescribed norms and thereby generated a mountain of paperwork. The vast majority who performed their jobs without incident exist in the administrative record mainly in the form of personal data and a few absentee slips. Although administrative dealings with deviant nurses provide insight into everyday administrative politics and, by extension, nurses' experience, the circumstances under which these records were generated must be kept in mind. At best, administrative and personnel records illuminate moral choice only indirectly. They are most useful in enabling the researcher to construct a picture of the *atmosphere* administrative policy may have created and its implications for moral deliberation among individuals.

The last major category of source materials used in this study, and the most substantive, consists of postwar trial testimonies of nurses who were accused of participating in, or otherwise had knowledge of, the "euthanasia" measures that claimed the lives of 100,000–200,000 institutionalized patients between 1939 and

1945.[10] Here, too, methodological difficulties cannot be avoided, insofar as the testimonies were generally given many years after the events took place, and thus are of questionable utility, in terms of both factual accuracy and degree of self-critical reflection. This must be kept in mind. As chapter 8 will make clear, however, I have tried to circumvent this problem by reading the records not as a source of factual information but rather as documents that give us hints about how these nurses understood their choices and why they may have behaved as they did. Chapter 8 is therefore in many ways a study of subtexts.

In the course of my research, I was permitted access to archival sources containing unpublished personal information under the proviso that I refrain from disclosing the identity of the persons in question. I have therefore turned the initials of all nurses (except authors of articles) into pseudonyms throughout the book in the interests of readability. The names of doctors and administrators that have been published in secondary literature have been left in their original forms. Unless otherwise noted, all translations are my own.

The dissertation on which this book is based was begun at the University of Chicago but written and revised after I had "emigrated" to a provincial German town. Many people provided support that enabled me to complete it under these somewhat unconventional circumstances. Michael Geyer, John W. Boyer, Jan Goldstein, and Leora Auslander followed the progress of my research from its beginnings in the early 1990s and offered helpful critical feedback on the resulting dissertation. Professor Geyer, in particular, offered encouragement, useful suggestions, and practical assistance that helped me complete the dissertation so far away from the U of C. That this study has, under the circumstances, reached a wider audience is in large part thanks to him.

During the research phase of this study, Christina Härtel of the Karl-Bonhoeffer-Nervenklinik and Christina Vanja of the Landeswohlfahrtsverband Hessen provided not only assistance in gaining me access to materials I needed but also encouragement through their ongoing interest in what I was doing with them. Hilde Steppe, Liselotte Katscher, Alf Lüdtke, and Hans-Joseph Wollasch, among many others, listened with interest to my ideas and provided useful research tips. Thanks are due to the many archivists and archival and library staff who assisted me along the way, and especially to Herr Grün and Frau Schultz of the Stadtbücherei Idar-Oberstein, who processed dozens of interlibrary loan requests. My research was assisted by a grant from the Berlin Program for Advanced German and European Studies of the Free University of Berlin and the Social Science Research Council with funds provided by the Volkswagen Foundation.

I also wish to thank Brigitta van Rheinberg at Princeton University Press, who not only offered expert advice on how to turn a dissertation into a book but also cheerfully accommodated such inconveniences as my lack of e-mail. Thanks are also due to the readers who recommended the publication of my dissertation and offered useful suggestions on ways to improve the manuscript, and to Lauren Lepow for her thorough and insightful copyediting. Grateful as I am to them and to all who have helped me along the way, I alone am responsible for any errors of fact or interpretation.

Over the last six years, my parents, Rodney and Sandra McFarland, periodically came to my rescue by running assorted stateside errands for me—sometimes, as these things go, without much warning. For this, and for the far more meaningful support they have always provided as loving parents, I thank them. Finally, and above all, Norbert Icke has been my "true companion" for the duration of this study, offering the love, humor, patience, and practical support that I needed to complete it. His presence has been a constant source of happiness; and even if he had very little to do with the actual writing of this book, my greatest indebtedness is to him.

Abbreviations

BBG	Berufsbeamtengesetz (short form of Gesetz zur Wiederherrstellung des Berufsbeamtentums, or Law for the Restoration of the Professional Civil Service)
DI	*Die Irrenpflege*
GVeN	Gesetz zur Verhütung erbkranken Nachwuchses (Law for the Prevention of Hereditarily Diseased Progeny)
HGA	Hauptgesundheitsamt (Main Health Office)
HHSAW	Hessisches Hauptstaatsarchiv Wiesbaden
KBoN	Karl-Bonhoeffer-Nervenklinik
KPD	Kommunistische Partei Deutschlands (German Communist Party)
LA Berlin	Landesarchiv Berlin
LWV-Eichberg	Archiv des Landeswohlfahrtsverbandes Hessen, Eichberg branch
MO	Meseritz-Obrawalde trial records, file no. 112 Ks 2/64
NSBO	Nationalsozialistische Betriebszellenorganisation (National Socialist Cell Organization)
NSDAP	Nationalsozialistische Deutsche Arbeiterpartei (National Socialist German Workers' Party)
NSV	Nationalsozialistische Volkswohlfahrt (National Socialist Public Welfare)
PF	Personnel File
PNW	*Psychiatrisch-Neurologische Wochenschrift*
RGO	Revolutionäre Gewerkschafts-Opposition (Revolutionary Trade Union Opposition)
SPD	Sozialdemokratische Partei Deutschlands (German Social Democratic Party)

NURSES IN NAZI GERMANY

1

Introduction
Ordinary Germans Revisited:
Nurses, Psychiatry, and Morality
in Historical Context

I maintained at the time, and had always maintained,
that a human being may not kill a living being of his
or her own accord. I also considered the psychiatric
patients . . . in Obrawalde to be human beings. On these
grounds I regarded the killing of psychiatric patients as
an injustice.[1]

Nurse Kremer

THIS POSITION, taken by a former Meseritz-Obra-
walde nurse in 1962, did not stop her from transporting patients
into the institution's so-called killing room during the war years,
where they received lethal doses of sedatives in the course of
"euthanasia" measures. It suggests, among other things, that
nurses could participate in National Socialism's exterminatory
policies without sacrificing their sense of right and wrong—that
they could remain masters of their own hearts. It raises obvious
and crucial questions that apply not only to nurses but to all
perpetrators under National Socialism and to German society as
a whole: What was the relevance of a person's attitude toward
a victimized group—for example, antisemitism, or the idea that
handicapped people are "unworthy of living"—in securing his
or her participation in, or tolerance of, murder? Did such beliefs
play a central role, or were other factors involved?

These questions have been thrown into relief in recent years as historians have turned their attention to "ordinary Germans" at the bottom of institutional hierarchies, who did not make rules or generate policies but rather implemented those policies in the course of their working lives. For them in particular, the kind of virulent hatred espoused by National Socialism's ideological exponents and embodied in their sordid policies is often difficult to detect. What was going on in the minds of these people? Did the victims cease to be objects of moral concern, and if so, how did that happen? If moral concern was not extinguished, how did perpetrators reconcile their feelings with their activity?

Daniel Jonah Goldhagen brought this debate to an unprecedented level of intensity in the area of Holocaust history when, in *Hitler's Willing Executioners*, he tarred "ordinary Germans" with an "eliminationist" antisemitism traditionally attributed to the Nazi leadership. The overwhelming majority of Germans, he argued, believed the extermination of the Jews to be just, and this in turn explains the readiness—indeed eagerness—of reserve policemen to engage in veritable killing sprees in the East. "Masters of their hearts" indeed, they killed because they *wanted* to do so. This thesis was in part a critique of Christopher R. Browning's earlier work on Reserve Police Battalion 101, which had pointed to a variety of circumstantial factors that seem to have influenced the men's willingness to kill. While it would be wrong to conclude that the men were compelled to behave contrary to their innermost beliefs, he suggested, their participation may not always have been a direct and willful expression of their beliefs either. While murder was the result of the "unleashing" of the men's innate, eliminationist antisemitism for Goldhagen, in Browning's view it was largely the result of their adaptation to genocidal circumstances.[2]

While both authors claimed to be telling us about the experience of "ordinary Germans," Goldhagen's account was marred by, among other things, his failure to separate the *impulse* for exterminatory policies from the question of their *viability*. The two are obviously related but, particularly if we are speaking of "ordinary" Germans, are not interchangeable. While no one

would dispute the widespread and increasingly radical character of German antisemitism in the 1930s, historical scholarship
has placed clear limitations on antisemitism as a tool for explaining the behavior of those outside the sphere of Nazi policy
making. Identifying the pervasiveness of cultural antisemitism
cannot substitute for an analysis "from the bottom up." It is on
this point that the strength of Browning's approach manifested
itself. Fully aware of the policemen's cultural background, and
of the licentious brutality that they visited upon their victims,
Browning looked below the surface, so to speak, and discovered
potentially significant circumstantial factors that seem to shed
light on the complicity of individual men.[3] Browning did not
marshal these factors to call the brutality of these men into question, or to suggest that they were indeed morally intact but
simply could not resist being drawn along. Rather, Browning
discovered that the men availed themselves of the ample opportunities to accommodate themselves psychologically to what
they were doing.[4] Obviously, a great many of these men did not
need this kind of help—both Browning and Goldhagen point
out that there were always enough volunteers—but Browning's
work sheds light on how and why the less enthusiastic members
may have joined in, and, by extension, helps us begin to understand how this kind of hands-on mass murder could become not
only conceivable but viable.

A similar perspective is currently lacking in the historiography of psychiatry under National Socialism, and as a result
we confront statements from "ordinary Germans" like Nurse
Kremer with little explanatory ammunition. Until recently,
scholars have tended to focus on psychiatrists, National Socialist
bureaucrats, and other ideological exponents of the eugenics
movement who provided the impulses for radicalization and extermination while leaving the experience of the vast majority of
participants—and thus the ultimate viability of these policies—
unexamined. At one end of the spectrum, so-called modernizing
theories have explained the radicalization of psychiatry as the
result of scientific opportunism that knew no bounds and had
no patience for unresponsive cases.[5] Other studies have sug-

gested that psychiatrists appropriated sterilization and aggressive therapies more as a response to professional crises than out of medical conviction—and when those proved unable to boost statistics on therapeutic success, they became increasingly receptive to the idea of killing those patients who did not respond.[6] Insecurity and ineffectiveness, in short, generated a desire to try different, increasingly radical recipes for professional "success." More recently, Michael Burleigh has rejected "modernizing" theories as suitable explanations for the cruelty of psychiatry's leading personalities under National Socialism, their grotesque medical experiments, and the "medieval" institutional living conditions that they deliberately created.[7]

Wherever one stands on this spectrum, contempt for psychiatric patients, appropriated to varying degrees, appears to have supplanted medical ethics and hardened personnel to the fate of their charges. They no longer saw individual, suffering patients, but only hopeless cases for whom they could do little and who appeared more and more as "useless eaters." Pressure from official propaganda and cost-slashing bureaucrats only increased the temptation to accept and deploy radical solutions. Killing these patients simply followed as a matter of course; it was "mass murder without a guilty conscience."[8] But this is not the end of the story, because scientific enthusiasm or political sympathy with Nazi ideals did not always imply support for murder. There is evidence that some psychiatrists complied with National Socialist policy only sluggishly, which is of interest even if the meaning of this behavior is subject to a variety of interpretations.[9] (Dr. Karsten Jasperson, for example, attempted to complete paperwork in connection with the T4 "euthanasia" program in a way that would favor patients' survival, despite being a member of the Nazi "Old Guard.")[10] Likewise, as we shall see, some nurses also opposed such policies and refused to participate in their implementation. In any case, conscience did not disappear entirely—even if on a collective level it appears that way—and this fact poses the additional question of how we are to understand the complicity of those who participated in mass murder *with* or *in spite of* a guilty conscience. This requires a different perspective, namely, one that approaches the history of psychiatry from the bottom up, through the eyes of "ordinary Germans."

It is especially timely to extend Browning's analytical perspective to psychiatry, since the links between the Holocaust and the extermination of the mentally and physically handicapped are a subject of growing scholarly interest.[11] It is now well known, for example, that the murder techniques deployed in the extermination of the Jews were first "tested" on Germany's mentally and physically handicapped in the context of the T4 program, in the course of which over 70,000 patients were killed in gas chambers followed by tens of thousands more in the program's decentralized, "medicalized," second phase. Between the spring of 1941 and spring 1943, T4 personnel collaborated with the SS in killing concentration camp inmates,[12] and after the gas chambers were closed in the summer of 1941, 96 out of around 400 T4 personnel were redeployed in the East in the service of the "Final Solution."[13] There are even parallels to be found in everyday strategies of psychological relief, such as the distribution of alcohol to the perpetrators of mass shootings of Jews as well as to the stokers of T4's gas ovens.[14] In light of the numerous ideological, technical and bureaucratic links between mass murder of the handicapped and of the Jews, Sinti and Roma ("Gypsies"), and other persecuted groups, Henry Friedlander has argued that "euthanasia was not simply a prologue but the first chapter of Nazi genocide."[15] This begs the question of whether the experience of ordinary Germans enlisted in the murder of the handicapped shared similarities with that of other perpetrators.

One thing is certain: although "euthanasia" programs had plenty of ideologically committed people in their service, the regime seems to have been aware that the idea of "lives unworthy of living" was not sufficient to guarantee peace of mind to everyone else involved in the killing process, nor would it pacify the even greater number of relatives and onlookers. If Hitler and his cohort could not take the acceptance of such policies for granted, however, they could at least try to ensure their tolerance. Just as they were aware that close relations with Jews could interfere with exclusionary and eventually exterminatory policies, they realized that "euthanasia" would be viable only if people were permitted to maintain a safe physical and psychological distance from it; and they adapted their implementational strategies accordingly.[16]

This insight was partially the result of a survey that had been conducted in 1920 after the publication of Karl Binding and Alfred Hoche's *Über die Freigabe der Vernichtung lebensunwerten Lebens*, which promoted the termination of "unworthy" life as an act of mercy and an expression of economic, social, and political wisdom. A critic of the tract who was himself wondering about the potential public reception of such an idea, Chief Medical Officer Ewald Meltzer, distributed a questionnaire on the subject to the parents of two hundred children at the Katharinenhof Institution for Ineducable and Feebleminded Children at Großhennersdorf. He discovered, probably to his astonishment, that it was acceptable to debate the issue, and that the practice might even be tolerable; but asking them to *agree* to this was too much. In the event of the implementation of a "euthanasia" policy, it would be better if they were not told the true story of what had happened. Knowledge implied a degree of responsibility that they preferred to avoid.[17] As Meltzer himself summarized, "One would like to free oneself, and perhaps also the child, from the burden, but one wants to have peace of mind [*Gewissensruhe*]."[18] Hitler's personal doctor Theo Morell studied Meltzer's findings and very likely concluded that *agreeing* was different from *not objecting*, and that one might be able to exploit people's willingness not to object.

It followed from this that "euthanasia" needed to be edged out of public discourse. To be sure, Hitler's *Reichskanzlei* drew up a "euthanasia" law in October 1940; but, significantly, it was never implemented. Instead, Götz Aly has argued, its existence in the *minds* of the program's organizers and assistants gave the *idea* and, eventually, the *practice* of "euthanasia" a degree of moral legitimacy—if not legality—that enabled them to "sleep peacefully."[19] At the same time, by stopping one step before the law's actual implementation, the National Socialists kept the practice of "euthanasia" out of the realm of "official" public knowledge and secured its—at least temporary—tolerance. Aly writes: "It was a question of informally legitimating the institutional killings and simultaneously delegating them through propaganda and speech-regulation to an absolutely private matter, a controversial 'problem,' before which each person is alone. In order to carry it out, there could be precisely no *public* confrontation with 'euthanasia.'"[20] One year later, the regime appointed a plenipotentiary ("Reichsbeauftragte für Heil- und Pflegeanstalten") who was charged with the "economization" of institutions and empowered to take unspecified—and implicitly *unlimited*—"necessary steps" in the process. A paragraph to this effect was published in the *Reichsgesetzblatt* on October 27, 1941. To be sure, the meaning of various camouflaged terms such as "economization measures" (*planwirtschaftliche Maßnahmen*) had meanwhile become abundantly clear to Reich administrative officials, the Church, health insurance companies, and the *Deutscher Gemeindetag* (which played an advisory and mediational role in communal administration).[21] Direct language was not only unnecessary; it would have contradicted the entire logic behind the regime's handling of the issue. The point was to move the killings a step closer to formal legality without jeopardizing the (in its view) psychologically favorable effects of keeping them outside of official discourse. "Euthanasia" thus retained its ambivalent, morally sedative character, at once painfully *real* and yet discursively, "officially," *unreal*.

Having left "ordinary Germans" without clear statements of policy, and thus free to react—or not react—to rumors as they saw fit, the regime attempted to eliminate uncomfortable reminders about the truth. That is, just as in the case of the Jews, it went to great lengths to cultivate the public's physical and psychological distance from the victims of mass murder. This was not altogether successful during the first organized phase of the killings up to the summer of 1941, when even layover institutions and deliberate attempts to obscure the fate of patients did not suffice to keep the spread of knowledge and disquiet under control. The regime did, however, learn a good lesson.

When its "euthanasia" planning commission suggested a complete institutional separation of curable and incurable patients in 1942, Robert Müller vigorously protested. Heaven forbid that word get around about the existence of institutions for dying! No, one of the fundamental requirements of the program was that it be discreet. "Euthanasia" should take place in *normal* institutional surroundings and not differ in its appearance from natural death.[22]

The results of the Meltzer survey, the quasi-legalization of the killings, and organizational strategies all suggest a keen awareness among the regime's "euthanasia" enthusiasts that subscribing to the killings *in practice* was bound up with a process of moral deliberation that went beyond forming a personal opinion on the measure in question. They suggest that the translation of ideas into widespread social practice was not simply a matter of distributing propaganda; it required certain bureaucratic and institutional structures that channeled human deliberations in certain directions and encouraged people to *internalize* a certain way of thinking about their place—and individual power—in the world. Sometimes this involved terror, but apparently it also could involve nothing more than exploiting people's desire for normalcy and emotional security, and anesthetizing those moral impulses which might generate solidarity with the victims and prompt them to take risks on their behalf.

These insights are of great importance, because they remind us that Germans' complicity in, or tolerance of, exterminatory policies was a far more complicated affair than theories of anti-semitism or eugenic radicalization would suggest. We are reminded that an ideological impulse for mass murder cannot substitute for an explanation of its historical possibility and *viability*. This, in turn, means that, just as one cannot fully explain the motives of reserve policemen with reference to cultural anti-semitism, one cannot fully explain the complicity of psychiatric staff by pointing to a general tendency to speak of patients as "lives unworthy of living." This is particularly so in psychiatry because institutional staff were not only subject to propaganda but also (at least theoretically) bound by medical ethics that ran counter to such propaganda; moreover, they confronted patients' relatives on a regular basis. Something was going on, in short, that cannot be grasped with reference to ideological currents alone. In order to understand how psychiatric staff dealt with this internal tension, we must suspend the idea of "radicalization," which has connotations of an inexorable linear progression, and concentrate on the contradictions within psychiatry whose confrontation and resolution by individuals culminated in moral disaster.

The following chapters seek to contribute to this end by holding a magnifying glass over those at the bottom of the institutional hierarchy, who had the most intimate contact with the victims of National Socialist policies against the handicapped. Nurses, it seems, faced a contradiction of monumental proportions: alongside their function in implementing National Socialist policies against their patients, they remained subject to a moral imperative to care for all patients regardless of their (racial) identity. Instructional texts for nurses throughout the period under study claimed that institutional psychiatry had an essentially humanitarian agenda to fulfill. We are not speaking here of a pseudo-Christian moralization of murder as "deliverance" from suffering hastily conceived in the early 1940s to soothe consciences but rather of a discursive trait with roots extending back to the mid–nineteenth century. In light of this, how could nurses—men and women with ethical training to the contrary, precious little to gain from their involvement, and nothing to lose in case of refusal—turn around and become murderers?

This has not been regarded as a particularly mystifying question up to this point, since postwar trial records and general characteristics of the profession seem to suggest that obedience to authority supplanted any competing imperatives nurses may have confronted. In 1965, a Munich court described the fourteen Meseritz-Obrawalde nurses facing charges of being an accessory to murder as people "who on the basis of their education and activity had developed limitless trust in the doctors and also, on account of their mental rigidity, were equipped with only a below-average critical capacity."[23] More recent accounts have generally echoed the sentiments of the Munich court, insofar as they explain (although they do not necessarily excuse) nurses' complicity in "euthanasia" measures with reference to a long-standing pattern of professional socialization that dictated obedience, practical and intellectual subordination to doctors, and a fundamentally reactive, adaptive mode of professional performance.[24] While there is obviously some truth to this explanation, it comes close to turning an effect into a cause. It cannot explain the persistence of traditional medical ethics in the midst of public propaganda about "lives unworthy of living," nor does it explain why "euthanasia" planners deemed a division of labor and official secrecy to be desirable. Moreover, by suggesting that nurses blindly accepted orders to perpetrate or tolerate murder just as they would any other order, it implies a widespread ideological sympathy with the killings among nurses that has yet to be demonstrated.

This book has two areas of focus that are examined in the course of a chronological narrative: nurses' professional morality and the realities of institutional life. After a brief discussion of the professionalization of psychiatric nursing in chapter 2, chapters 3 and 6 look closely at nursing literature as a "window" on professional ethics and proceed to work out how psychiatrists and other contributors made room for the expression of moral impulses in institutional life at the same time as they encouraged nurses to distance themselves emotionally from their patients. The persistence of nursing literature's ethical orientation was no accident, nor was it a cynical gesture; it was ultimately of great potential importance in securing psychological adaptation to murderous activities. Chapters 4, 5, and 7 examine the realities of everyday institutional life with special attention to how hierarchical arrangements, disciplinary policy, and political sea changes affected, and in many instances subverted, the realization of professional imperatives. In chapter 8, nurses' reflections on their complicity in murder reveal not only the psychological "preparation" of the preceding years but also the effect of specific bureaucratic and institutional organizational strategies that facilitated murder.

Throughout, I have tried as much as sources permitted to recover the moral agency of nurses, which has so often been obscured by their status as order-takers. They made choices, and
their choices added up to the betrayal of thousands of people
who were utterly dependent on them. This study explicitly
problematizes what is at stake in the debate over "ordinary Germans," namely, our understanding of how people made sense
of events that were unfolding around them, and more generally,
our understanding of the genesis and expression of moral feeling in a setting that militates against it.

Neither Riffraff nor Saints:
The Ambivalent Professionalization
of the Psychiatric Nurse

Around the turn of the nineteenth century, an observer described the inmates of the Berlin Insane Asylum as "complete maniacs . . . each alone, as long as the senseless fury lasts, locked up unclothed in narrow containers or crates . . . where one gives them their food and drink through holes, in copper basins fastened with chains."[1] Their caretakers, known as attendants, almost always took up the job as a temporary measure, sometimes simply to have a roof over their heads during the winter.[2] They came not only from the destitute population at large, but also from the ranks of former soldiers, prisoners, and patients themselves—a situation that raised its own set of image and disciplinary problems.[3] The situation drove Ernst Horn, the first head of the psychiatric department at Berlin's Charité Hospital, to exasperation; in 1818 he complained that the attendant's body size and defiant appearance were all that mattered, and that the worst riffraff in Berlin could not be worse than they.[4]

Such was institutional life at the beginning of the century that would witness psychiatry's birth as a medical science.[5] Not surprisingly, in this light, "care" for the earliest attendants (up to around 1840) meant little more than ensuring that the occupants of an institution remained alive, orderly, and (if the institution doubled as a workhouse)[6] productive. But change was on the horizon: in the wake of the French Revolution and the Enlightenment, scientists and intellectuals began to see the insane as people worthy of humane treatment. Following in the footsteps of Pinel, nineteenth-century German psychiatrists increasingly rejected physical coercion of the insane and opted instead for a "therapeutic" approach based on the nonviolent reintegration of the patient into the world of the sane. The increasing popularity of a "therapeutic" approach in Germany is generally attributed to the work of Wilhelm Griesinger (1817–1868), who defined mental illness as an "illness of the brain" that could be treated just as corporeal illnesses could. The insane person began to acquire the status of a *patient*. "Treatments" involving mechanical force, such as straitjackets, were increasingly avoided, banned, or at the very least applied discreetly, behind closed doors.[7]

THE WORLD OF THE PSYCHIATRIC ATTENDANT

This last comment brings us to the fact that reality fell far short of the ideas articulated in this humanitarian discourse. Nineteenth-century political and socioeconomic crises increased the numbers of criminals, alcoholics, prostitutes, and destitute—that is, those people who were grouped together in poorhouses and insane asylums. Although the latter half of the century witnessed the expansion of provincial, municipal, and private institutions to accommodate them, sedatives were not widely available and overcrowding was often severe.[8] Compelled to attend in the first instance to detention and order, and barely able to do that, psychiatrists could only hope to popularize the *idea* of insanity as a medical problem in the nineteenth century.[9] As Griesinger himself conceded, "it is difficult to introduce the no-restraint treatment in overcrowded institutions and it works [only] with great effort."[10]

Part of the reason for this sorry state of affairs is that, especially in the early and mid–nineteenth century, many psychiatric institutions were simply improvised—that is, local administrations converted castles or cloisters into facilities for the insane. In the Duchy of Nassau, for example, such initiatives date back to 1805, when administrators turned the Eberbach Abbey into a prison and, in 1815, added facilities for the accommodation of approximately 50 insane people.[11] By 1837, space was already becoming scarce, with six attendants struggling to keep up with 88 asylum occupants. Plans to separate the detentional and psychiatric functions of the Eberbach asylum came to fruition in 1849, when the Eichberg psychiatric institution was founded on a plot of land not far away.[12] Although midcentury calculations had suggested that building the Eichberg institution with a capacity for 220 patients was sensible, the patient population grew steadily, and by 1863 crowding and the resulting disorder compelled administrators to have bars installed to separate attendants' beds from those of the patients.[13] By the early 1870s the patient population had topped 300, prompting the construction and use of a temporary psychiatric branch at Eberbach until 1884.[14] In the meantime, expansion and technical improvement proceeded apace, and by the mid-1880s Eichberg could accommodate 450 patients.[15]

Institutionalization initiatives became less improvisational in the course of time, and the latter half of the century witnessed a blossoming of architectural innovation that waxed and waned as finances, demographic pressures, and therapeutic strategies dictated.[16] While the Eichberg institution was serving as home to a mentally ill princess with her own quarters and her own servants in the second half of the nineteenth century, for example,[17] Berlin officials were busy planning the construction of the Dalldorf institution (after 1924 named Wittenauer Heilstätten) in response to the century's classic urban problems: poverty and destitution. Berlin's existing Municipal Institution for the Care of the Insane, established in 1862, had proved incapable of meeting the growing demand for publicly financed care.[18] Constructed on the outskirts of the city in a woodsy setting, Dalldorf was designed to offer the approximately 1,000 patients a degree of peace and quiet while simultaneously making them invisible to the public.[19] Three more municipal institutions were soon to follow: in 1893, both the Herzberge institution, with a projected capacity of 1,200, and the Wuhlgarten institution for 1,150 epileptics were opened. In 1906, the Berlin-Buch psychiatric institution was opened for 1,500 patients.[20]

Although institutions varied in structure and composition according to location and therapeutic focus (if any), they generally included buildings for administration, maintenance, and staff housing. Separate patient pavilions were maintained for various observational and therapeutic activities, with a strict separation of the sexes among patients and staff. Nurses in the observation room tended to patients who were potentially violent or otherwise posed a danger to themselves or others. Special fortified stations for potential escapees required especially experienced nurses for adequate supervision. Patients with corporeal illnesses were treated in wards designed to isolate them from other patients and to facilitate the kind of care that would be offered in a hospital. In large institutions, separate stations were maintained for new patients who underwent several days of initial observation before being classified and moved to an appropriate station.[21] The Obrawalde institution, completed in 1904 near the town of Meseritz in the former province of Posen, even supplemented its facilities for the mentally ill with a convalescent home, a home for children, a maternity hospital, and a facility for the physically handicapped. Constructed at a time of great concern for psychiatry's public image, the institution's buildings resembled villas more than facilities of a medical institution.[22]

In addition to the basic arrangements for patient treatment, most institutions gradually acquired their own pharmacies, mortuaries, laboratories, butchers, carpenters, libraries, leisure programs, and facilities for religious services, and they grew some of their own food in fields and greenhouses. A considerable contribution to institutional self-sufficiency was made by patients themselves; they were occupied with sewing, knitting, weaving, preliminary food preparation (such as peeling potatoes), carpentry, harvesting, garden work, and a variety of other community-sustaining tasks. In this context, nurses accompanied patients' movements on institutional grounds and supervised leisure activities such as pool, playing musical instruments, and card playing. Also, from time to time walks, singing, small concerts, and dancing events were organized and supervised by nurses. Most important, they had to perform all of the above duties with an eye for individual patients' tastes and capabilities, and to follow any special doctor's orders restricting specific patients from specific activities.[23]

The increasingly multifunctional character of institutions meant that nurses' responsibilities expanded into virtually every area of institutional activity. They not only woke, dressed, and bathed patients; they supervised them at mealtimes and in the course of their daily activities. However, prevailing therapeutic techniques, namely, "bed therapy" and long-term baths (*Dauerbäder*), generated a far less stimulating daily agenda for nurses who had to supervise them. An awkward compromise between medical aspirations and the desperate need to maintain order, these "therapies" entailed confining patients to their beds or a bathtub for many hours (fourteen–sixteen hours at Berlin's Dalldorf Asylum). Essentially sedation techniques, they facilitated discipline and order, and they gave institutions the appearance of a hospital rather than of a prison. In addition, they permitted simultaneous supervision of a number of patients by one nurse—an important administrative benefit.[24]

Lack of privacy—and indeed, of private *life*—was perhaps the most salient feature of life as a psychiatric nurse. Ideally, psychiatrists maintained, nurses should place themselves entirely at the disposal of the institution's patients and administration. In many institutions, they were required to take their meals in the same rooms as patients and (until around the turn of the century) sleep in the same rooms with patients. Psychiatrists generally supported marriage bans for all nurses, even if they admitted that enforcing this demand was not always feasible.[25] Institutional residents and staff, it was hoped, would *substitute* for the family of a nurse. The doctor, in this scheme, functioned as the institutional patriarch, and the nurses and patients were akin to his children.[26] In this respect, nurses in psychiatry confronted the same expectations as their colleagues in general medicine: they were to be present around the clock, attending to routine needs and supervising leisure. The doctor made his rounds only once a day and was in any case concerned with the

treatment of an illness; the nurse, by way of contrast, was to perform a more imprecise art: to learn and attend to the needs of
the patient as a person. In an era that witnessed the bureaucrati-
zation of medical care, the nurse was delegated the task of preserving an aura of humanity in the midst of, as it were, modern
anonymity.

The Attendant Question

This, it is worth repeating, was the *goal* of state and institutional administrators. In fact, from the beginnings of post-En-
lightenment psychiatry well into the twentieth century, they
struggled to bring reality into line with this ideal. The so-called
attendant question was formally raised for the first time in 1842,
when the *Leipziger Zeitung* invited its readers to compete for the
best essay on the following topic: "How can compassionate
(*menschenliebende*) attendants and supervisors be acquired for
insane asylums?" From this point into the early decades of the
twentieth century, doctors and administrators at professional
conferences would periodically discuss possibilities for making
the profession attractive to more desirable candidates. Although
disagreement was rife, they repeatedly returned to the observation that they would never acquire a steady supply of qualified,
reliable nursing staff without two initiatives: they would need
to limit access to the job—that is, make some kind of training
a pre- or corequisite for formal employment—and, once they
had acquired suitable candidates, to retain them with competi-
tive pay, the introduction of benefits, and some kind of public
recognition.[27]

These initiatives were only slowly forthcoming for a number
of reasons. First, there was resistance within the ranks of the profession: a number of psychiatrists feared that such improvements would weaken the doctor's patriarchal authority in institutional life and, even worse, give the nurse the feeling that he
or she was superior to the patient(!). It was better, in their view,
to hire nurses for periods of five or six years and to keep them
firmly under the doctor's thumb by banning marriage, civil ser-

vant status, and social security in old age. As one director commented in 1895, "I have to be in a position to set aside my tool when it no longer performs satisfactorily."[28]

Second, reform-minded psychiatrists confronted an ongoing tension between the requirements of a long-term solution and the needs of the present. As badly as institutions wanted qualified personnel for the sake of their patients, of psychiatry's reputation, and of administrative efficiency, they also needed people—any people—simply to maintain order and keep the institution running. Suitable applicants were not easy to find: in the first half of the nineteenth century, institutions competed with expanding industries for labor; and in the second half, social democracy's achievements in improving working conditions in other occupations made psychiatric nursing even less attractive. There were limitations to how serious administrators could be about establishing selection criteria.[29]

Be this as it may, in the late nineteenth century many institutions took small steps to make the profession more attractive and keep current employees satisfied. In order to attract more men, for example, they organized special housing for them and their families. (Before the First World War, female nurses were generally forced to quit once they married.)[30] They attempted to boost nurses' professional egos by formally designating them as nurses (*Krankenpflegepersonal*) rather than attendants (*Wartepersonal*), and some introduced vacation time. Thus they strove to combat a poor public image, low employee morale, and staff shortages with a minimum of state intervention.

The Conservatism of Progressives: Early-Twentieth-Century Organizational Initiatives

Equally crippling to the acquisition of various employee rights was the timidity and uncertainty of nurses themselves. Until the 1920s they had no formal wage contract, no legal regulation of work time, no accident insurance, and no retirement benefits.[31] Yet when the above-mentioned superficial improvements in their lives and reputations were slowly made, gratitude for isolated improvements seems to have confused the struggle for legal rights initiated by unions. One male nurse writing for *Die Irrenpflege* in 1906, for example, was decidedly conservative on the subject of social change because, apparently, he perceived state and psychiatric administrators as essentially benevolent agents who required patience and gentle prodding; aggressive or destructive action was as ungracious as it was counterproductive.[32] To be sure, he acknowledged that nurses' demands for better working conditions were not "superfluous," but contended that "in our case it is not a question of an 'emergency' which would justify a stampede."[33] As in everyday professional life, nurses should assert themselves in matters political with moderation and a spirit of cooperation.

This attitude was, of course, a boon for a medical establishment keenly interested in keeping its supply of exploitable labor in check, and it was by no means accidental or unique: nursing ethics had already been tailored to this purpose in the course of the previous centuries. The more caretaking strayed from its Christian institutional and ethical basis after the Reformation, and the more it became a source of a living wage, the more loudly nursing was trumpeted as charitable activity that demanded the purest character and selfless devotion to those who suffered—even in the face of long hours, low public esteem, low pay, and poor working conditions. The ethic of charity, in short, became a convenient rhetorical tool for minimizing self-assertion among nurses and maintaining work discipline. Transforming a lack of adequate professional compensation into a source of dignity, those involved in recruitment, training, and supervision fostered an ambivalence among nurses that ultimately rendered them ill-equipped to claim compensatory rights for themselves among the ranks of the employed.[34]

To be sure, some psychiatric nursing associations did come into being on a local or regional basis, but they remained uninfluential. The Regional Association of Nurses in Hesse, for example, prepared in 1910 to strike for better wages, better working conditions, and an end to the marriage ban. The necessary solidarity for such a move could not be generated, however; a medical corps had been assembled and was ready to assume nurses' positions in the event of a strike. Generally speaking, psychiatric nursing advocates who supported organizational activity at the turn of the century agreed that a major stumbling block in the acquisition of employee rights was widespread indifference of their colleagues on social questions.[35]

These advocates themselves may have contributed to the problem insofar as they were decidedly hostile to socialism and were careful to couch their demands in terms that would not allow this to be misunderstood.[36] Their refusal to cooperate with the workers' movement undoubtedly prevented them from exploiting its political power and its momentum. Perhaps more important in the long run, it also indicated that although nurses wanted changes, they were essentially prepared to remain loyal to doctors and administrators who accepted changes on behalf of nurses only when circumstances prevented any other choice. Although permission to marry, separate living arrangements, in-house pension schemes, and in-house training were indeed introduced in some institutions before World War I, nurses nevertheless remained dependent on the good graces of the institutional "fathers."[37]

The First World War: Thrift, Solidarity, and the Reorientation of Professional Consciousness

These feeble beginnings of professional self-assertion received an abrupt setback in 1914: for the next four years, wartime shortages would force psychiatric institutions to devote their resources and energies to the mundane issue of survival. Many male nurses were called to the front, and their stations were temporarily attended by female nurses. (This way of handling the personnel shortage was, apparently contrary to expectations, generally a success from the perspective of administrators.)[38] Personnel shortages were not as catastrophic, however, as the shortages of basic necessities like food and coal: the Hunger Blockade and a poor harvest in 1916 led to a drastic increase in sickness and death among patients, who had no chance to hoard goods when they were available and no access to the black market.[39] Detailed information about the degree of suffering during the war is scanty, but it has been estimated that the death rate among patients was roughly twice as high as in peacetime.[40] Although high death rates were registered among babies and other vulnerable and institutionalized people (such as criminals), the number of deaths among psychiatric patients has been described in comparison as "disproportionately high."[41]

At the very least, shortages produced heightened tensions in institutional daily life. In the third year of the war, for example, the lack of food in the Warstein institution became so critical that hungry patients threatened disorder on several stations. Director Schmidt told his administrative councillor that he would be forced to open the doors and let the patients go free if no potatoes were delivered by evening; the staff could not keep them in the houses any longer. A few loads were indeed delivered, and the crisis passed. But the death rate in the institution rose from a prewar figure of 4–5 percent to 30 percent during the war—a figure so high that after the war six hundred beds could be offered to undernourished and sick children.[42] Only slowly would patients physically recuperate from this catastrophe after the war; in several institutions in Baden, for example, the death rate returned to its prewar level only in 1925.[43]

Clearly, this was not an auspicious time for making demands of any kind, professional or otherwise. Nurses were reminded in the pages of *Die Irrenpflege* that they were expected to carry on "even if there is more work, vacation is cut, permission to go out cannot always be given, and other advantages have disappeared during the war."[44] As for material needs, they were told that they must tame their desires and make do with what was available. There was nothing wrong with fixing up old clothes and wearing them again; "today no reasonable person gives dirty looks to someone because he is more poorly dressed than usual." In addition to thrift, a charitable heart was expected of each and every nurse. When collection tins were being circulated, "they should not be passed on without [one's] contributing a bit, even if it is only twenty-five pfennig. Everyone has that much to spare, if they have otherwise been hanging on to their spare change."[45]

Thinking about one's own welfare was, under the circumstances, not only futile; it was also selfish and cause for shame. Food was indeed in short supply; but, nurses were reminded, *their* needs were automatically fulfilled as part of a general scheme for supplying institutions, "while families have to get what little they have from endless effort and an appreciable loss of time."[46] Certainly, everyone had to make do without certain things, one psychiatrist wrote; but "the little privations indeed weigh [on us] light as a feather in comparison to the sacrifices and the suffering that our soldiers in the trenches must endure. Everyone [should] therefore practice . . . thriftiness and consider that he is thus contributing to our final victory."[47] Whenever there was a cause for dissatisfaction, in short, nurses were reminded that others were still worse off.

Once they had their own egoistic desires under control, nurses were charged with passing their newly acquired wisdom on to hungry and unruly patients who had difficulty grasping the reasons for deteriorating institutional conditions. They needed to exercise extra patience in handling patients' crazy ideas, which at the time tended to revolve around the notion that they were being intentionally starved. "Here, personnel should have an enlightening effect on the more intelligent patients and try to awaken an understanding among the patients for the present difficult, but great, time; it should give them courage and tell them to 'endure, persevere, and be quiet' ['*Aushalten, Durchhalten und Maul halten*']."[48] If patients wanted to leave, nurses were to tell them that life on the outside was even worse; if they received no packages or visits from relatives, nurses were to explain that certain luxuries were hard to come by, and unnecessary traveling was to be avoided. At every opportunity, they were to remind patients of the widespread scarcity, of the army, and of the "invincibility of our Fatherland, [which is being] attacked by almost the entire world"; they should comfort them by reminding them of future days of peace.[49]

Nurses, in short, were charged with making patients resign themselves to their miserable plight, just as they themselves were expected to do, and to glorify that misery as a noble sacrifice and as an expression of patriotism. This was new; for according to nurses' professional moral code up to 1914, patients were ideally the primary objects of their selfless devotion. During the war, nurses would find that this moral code was redefined "from above" in a way that reimposed selflessness, but this time in the name of a different recipient: the object of nurses' untiring dedication was not the patient but rather the "Fatherland." Their moral gaze, and that of patients, was directed toward this abstract virtue, so that those on the home front would "endure, persevere, and be quiet."

REVOLUTION AND REFORMISM

The November Revolution brought with it the renewed prospect of initiating all German nurses into the sphere of professionals with not only better pay but also its accompanying social security and public esteem. The struggle for recognition and compensation was spearheaded by union leaders and sympathetic nursing advocates, whose main publication, *Die Sanitätswarte*, greeted the revolution in 1919 with palpable optimism: "The revolution brought only political liberation as citizens first. At the same time, however, the path to liberation from economic exploitation and repression has been cleared. . . ."[50] In the course of the following dozen years, their efforts would bring about the first widespread implementation of wage contracts in nursing (1919–1921), the legal restriction of work time to a ten-hour-day, sixty-hour week (1924), the introduction of accident insurance (1928) and social security, and a gradual expansion of training and certification programs.[51] This falls far short of what they demanded, namely, an eight- (not ten-) hour day, paid vacations, and equal pay for men and women (which would not come about until the 1950s).[52] Although exhaustively discussed, training and certification procedures remained a source of continued controversies over scope, financing, and organization. The implementation of legal reforms remained unregulated, uneven, and, particularly in the case of work time, in many cases unenforced.[53] Many nurses in fact worked far more than sixty hours a week.[54]

Ideological differences among female professional organizations, unionized nurses, and Church-sponsored nursing representatives in large part account for this legislative shortfall on a national level.[55] Within psychiatry, an additional major stumbling block was the resistance of psychiatrists. To be sure, the labor secretary considered salaried nurses in public institutions subject to inclusion in work-time regulation.[56] His view was shared by at least fourteen psychiatric institutions (including Dalldorf) that had instituted the forty-eight-hour week for nurses by May 1920.[57] Even so, the prevailing sentiment among psychiatrists was decidedly negative. Speaking for many of his colleagues, Dr. Gustav Kolb argued that the eight-hour workday would not only generate the need for more nurses and, thus, more financial outlays in already lean times; it would also create serious management problems. The rapid turnover of personnel would make tracing mistakes in patient care difficult; proper supervision of personnel would be impossible; and nurses would invariably "miss work or report to work not well rested, but rather overtired from work or pleasure, inebriated, sexually infected, [or] in a serious condition."[58]

Moreover, Kolb argued, nursing was by definition a service to patients whose numbers and conditions were always in flux; and as such it resisted prearranged temporal boundaries. Patients' needs and nurses' rights were, indeed, fundamentally incompatible: "Rights must end where higher duties toward patients begin."[59] By joining the ranks of professionals, nurses entered a world where the "laws" of giving and receiving transcended the sterile preoccupation with hours and pay. The charitable imperative thus provided a powerful rhetorical strategy for checking the political power of nurses, strengthening their allegiances to the psychiatric enterprise, and providing a psychological bulwark against the appeal of the workers' movement.[60]

Clearly, the clash of traditional and progressive forces reflected a continuing and fundamental disagreement about what nursing was. Psychiatrists (among many others) sought to uphold the sacrificial nature of nursing; unionized nurses and their advocates, in contrast, sought to popularize the image of nurses as professionals who were entitled to corresponding compensation and legal protection. The supreme injustice of prevailing arrangements, in their view, lay precisely in the constant accountability of nurses *as* nurses and the absence not only of temporal but also of psychological and physical "space" in which they might live as private individuals.

For the purposes of argument, however, they privileged the language of pragmatism over that of moral indignation, focusing on the often hushed-up fact that overworked nurses suffered from physical and emotional exhaustion. They urged their opponents to look at confessional nursing, which did not observe the ten-hour-day, sixty-hour work week implemented in 1924 and instead maintained a fourteen–sixteen hour workday with hardly any free days or vacations. Precisely in this subgroup, tuberculosis and other infectious diseases afflicted nurses at an extraordinarily disproportionate rate.[61]

Nervous exhaustion tended to victimize primarily female nurses and psychiatric nurses.[62] Georg Streiter, member of the Reich Health Committee and chairman of the German Association of Nurses, cited a report from Frankfurt-am-Main which stated that "the nurses stand out mostly on account of their bad appearance and depressed nature. They complain of sleeplessness and complete lack of appetite, feelings of great tiredness and inefficiency." Such a sorry state of affairs often led to tragedy, as the February 1928 suicide attempt of a Goddelau nurse demonstrates. The nurse in question had thrown herself into the Altrhein and was saved at the last minute by a colleague. It was later determined that she was suffering from "carnival psychosis." It should not come as a surprise, *Die Sanitätswarte* maintained, that she had temporarily forgotten the seriousness of her profession and given herself over to the pleasures of life: "To do one's responsible duty day after day in the oppressive atmosphere of a psychiatric institution, always to confront the poorest of the poor with an even temper, patiently and gently—there, even a young nurse craves a distraction from time to time."[63] In the city, of course, nurses could avail themselves of theater, films, and other diversions without public or administrative scrutiny. In rural areas, however, the personal freedom afforded by urban anonymity vanished, rendering leisure stressful, if not impossible. Administrators had little sympathy for their nurses' need for pleasurable diversion and expected nurses to devote the entire range of their emotional resources to their patients. When a nurse temporarily abandoned this emotional "base" and took part in carnival festivities, *Die Sanitätswarte* bitterly remarked, the result was "dismissal—desperation—suicide!"

The author was quick to note that unionized nursing personnel in no way supported or tolerated behavior in private life that damaged the reputation of their profession. On the other hand, "one should not try to wrap us in the monastic cloak of renunciation," as the local professional nursing organization wanted. "It is preposterous to want to keep a female nurse from eighteen to twenty-five years old constantly behind the walls of a psychiatric institution without giving her the possibility of enjoying something in a worldly connection." Nurses were not superhuman but rather human beings with human needs, one of which was the opportunity to escape periodically from the shadow of daily responsibilities.

This had implications for the ordering of the spaces in which nurses worked and lived. "The work in a psychiatric institution," J. Lerrsen wrote, "makes great psychological and physical demands on the nurse. Compensation in [one's] free time is absolutely necessary." Living out-of-house, he felt, offered nurses the most advantages in this respect. He did, of course, appreciate the fact that the institution was responsible for around-the-clock care and thus required that some nurses live in-house; but the common practice of assigning several nurses to one room denied them privacy and adequate opportunities for rest. "A badly rested person cannot, by day, do his or her work cheerfully and attentively." On a psychological level, it was detrimental to staff morale: "Precisely the single working people who live outside of the family miss [having] a place that they can decorate according to their taste with flowers, pictures, and so forth; a room in which they can, undisturbed, be alone, rest, read, do handwork, ... make music—in short, a small kingdom for leisure time."[64] The provision of private space, then, was demanded not as a "right" (a strategy likely to fail in the midst of accusations of egoism) but rather as an administratively sensible arrangement.

Sensible or not, however, this kind of pragmatism often fell on deaf ears. In the face of continued shortages of funds, government officials pursued plans throughout the late 1920s to "rationalize" health care (i.e., save money) by, among other things, instituting strict personnel-patient ratios in medical institutions. Nurse Josef Koch, speaking at the 1930 conference of the German Association for Professional Nursing and Social Work, maintained that, while he sympathized with the desire to avoid unnecessary outlays of governmental funds, implementing nurse-patient ratios was a profoundly misguided attempt to control spending. Schematizing the employment of doctors and nurses according to abstract calculations ran counter to the inherent contingency of staff requirements in their profession. Doctors and nurses were not only "technicians" but also "experts" who needed a broad familiarity with mental illness as well as the ability to deploy that knowledge in everyday situations. Health care was not an operation where a "conveyor belt" mentality was justified. Rather, it required a certain degree of administrative flexibility and imagination to succeed. Thus, as Koch told his colleagues, "We may not be reduced to a number."[65]

It went without saying, in this light, that unionized nursing's advocates looked with increasing frustration on the protracted stalemate over the introduction of nationwide certification and training procedures for psychiatric nurses.[66] To be sure, psychiatrists and many government officials could generally agree that some kind of regulation was desirable. Negotiations, however, were repeatedly bogged down by the protests of participants at various levels of government who could not agree on the logistics, feasibility, and necessity of such regulation. Initiatives were also stymied by the fear that the introduction of professional prerequisites would chase away potential applicants.[67] In the end, a variety of training schemes took shape on a regional basis over the course of the Weimar years and persisted through the Second World War, in-house training remaining the most common.

Emil Kandzia, secretary of the union-affiliated German Association for Professional Nursing and Social Work, claimed to represent the standpoint of nursing personnel on this issue and contributed a number of articles to *Die Irrenpflege* during the Weimar years. His rhetorical point of departure was a goal that no one could possibly dispute: public health (*Volksgesundheit*). Nurses, he reminded his readers, were not mere *supervisors* of patients but rather *observers* whose reports to a doctor were the basis of diagnosis. They bore partial responsibility, if only indirectly, for a patient's treatment—a fact that rendered their training a serious matter indeed.[68] If psychiatrists and the public at large were sincerely interested in individual and public health, they should be able to agree that providing nurses with only a rudimentary background in mental illness, and none whatsoever in general nursing, was an irresponsible breach of public trust.

Moreover, anyone interested in efficient, reliable health care should be able to understand that well-trained nurses had to be retained. This was not only a matter of paying them well and offering them attractive insurance and pension programs; it was also a matter of emotional compensation through public recognition. "Nursing personnel," Klaus Uenzen lamented, "still do not enjoy the respect and esteem that are due to them on account of their self-sacrificing and important activity in the service of the sick person, the 'body' of the nation [*Volkskörper*]."[69]

The best way to bestow such recognition, Kandzia argued, was to cease treating psychiatric nurses like prison guards and, rather, replace this antiquated imagery with one identifying them as health care professionals. The first step in this direction was to rethink the wisdom of training and certifying psychiatric nurses separately from general nurses; for in this scenario, psychiatric nurses would be doomed to the status of "second-class" nurses.[70] It would be better, in his view, to introduce an exam in psychiatric nursing that would not be a less-esteemed *replacement* for state certification in general nursing but rather a preliminary, officially recognized step toward that goal.[71] Although other nurses were willing to accept separate training and certification procedures as preferable to the present chaotic state of affairs, it was agreed that some kind of nationwide, publicly recognized procedure was necessary "because the assessment of our profession from a societal ... perspective absolutely depends on it."[72]

It is tempting to interpret unionized nursing's efforts as a humanitarian campaign for the creation and protection of a private sphere for nurses, on the one hand, and emotional compensation for their hard work, on the other. We have seen, however, that nurses' welfare as human beings was not a rhetorical point of departure but rather a self-evident component of a larger program with public health as its goal. We, they told their opponents, have exactly the same goals as you do, namely, therapeutic success and public health (achieved, of course, as economically as possible). The best way to meet that goal on all levels was to treat nursing not as an act of charity but rather as professional activity. It was on the basis of this principle (again, rhetorically speaking) that they militated for improved working conditions and social benefits. Working their way backward from a universally shared goal, they sought to demonstrate the economic and administrative prudence in granting nurses benefits that, in their own circles, were undisputed rights.

We will never know what might have become of these movements, since by the summer of 1933, the National Socialists had destroyed the unions along with publications like *Die Sanitätswarte*. Even up to that point, however, it is noteworthy that nurses and their advocates did not seem prepared to question the priorities set by psychiatrists, administrators, and the state;

they formulated their demands in a way that took those priorities as a given. Granted that they confronted the daunting task
of turning a well-rooted and still prevalent conception of nursing on its head, their rhetorical strategy may well have been politically necessary for them to have had even a remote chance of
success. It may ultimately have been to their detriment, however, that they consistently subordinated the moral legitimacy of
their proposals to their compatibility with the interests of the
health care enterprise as a whole.

Hence the concept of *exploitation*, and the sense of moral violation it implies, did not play a central role in their brief reformist
era. They had no interest in challenging the logic of bureaucratic
rationality, only a desire to use it to their own advantage. Even
before the National Socialists took power, deference to administrative authority (which we encountered among pre–World War
I nurses) dovetailed with the kind of uncritical acceptance of
the moral authority of groups that was encouraged during wartime. This did not bode well for the next decade; for if nurses
were unable to manifest their will in the political arena on their
own behalf, they were not likely to do so later on behalf of their
patients.

Educating Nurses in the Spirit of the Times: Weimar Psychiatry in Theory and Practice

THE WINDS of change that psychiatric nursing advocates welcomed in 1918 were a psychiatrist's nightmare. From the war's end through 1923, their profession would experience a crisis of legitimacy[1] caused by dwindling institutionalization rates, shortages of funds, and threatening political and legal developments. Hunger and disease during the war years, as we have seen, had decimated institutional populations. In addition, economic depression severely limited the ability of families and communities to support psychiatric care, and authorities tended to channel potential patients into forms of treatment cheaper than institutionalization.[2] At the same time, psychiatrists found themselves confronted with a new democratic government that regarded their institutions as monarchist leftovers in need of consolidation and reform. They were uncertain whether the new state would recognize their former financial and social status and unsettled by deliberations about the "socializing" of the health care profession.[3] To make matters worse, state bureaucrats took initiatives to marginalize psychiatric opinion in institutionalization decisions; and finally, as we have seen, some nurses began to challenge the charitable imperative and thereby, if only implicitly, psychiatrists' administrative authority.

Psychiatrists responded to these developments by playing up their profession's indispensability as a haven of medical expertise and insisting that such expertise could flourish only if the integrity of medical and administrative judgment were preserved. Out of this profoundly defensive posture, as we shall see, evolved a peculiar scientific and humanitarian enthusiasm that would extend into the area of therapeutic innovations, guide their instruction of nurses, and persist long after the Weimar Republic had been consigned to history: psychiatry was useful, insofar as it rehabilitated potential workers and family members, and it was guided by a profoundly moral purpose— helping the helpless.

From a logical point of view, utility and morality are sometimes incompatible and beg the assignment of priority: either one pursues the dictates of utility and lets the chips fall where they may, morally speaking; or one decides to prioritize the welfare of human beings and support them above and, at times, against a potentially more efficient course of action. This sense of contingency and logical tension was absent from psychiatry's campaign of self-promotion of the 1920s. Morality was not problematized but rather smoothly incorporated into various all-embracing "solutions" to the perceived challenges posed by revolution and democracy. While this would leave an indelible mark on nursing ethics, we will see in chapter 4 how evasive stellar professional performance would remain.

The Crisis of Legitimacy and Its Aftermath

Confronted in the immediate postwar years and again at the end of the twenties with decreasing institutionalization rates and economic crisis, psychiatrists spent much of the Weimar years attempting to demonstrate that their work with a highly stigmatized group of people was useful and important, and should continue to be financed. This entailed addressing vexing moral questions concerning who deserves what in times of economic hardship: How are we to handle conditions of scarcity? Would we be fair in granting the sick only as much the population at large, knowing as we do that their lack of personal freedom places them at a disadvantage? Would it be justified, perhaps even morally imperative, for us to give them more?

These kinds of debates, it is often pointed out, did *not* have a formal precedent in the far more urgent conditions of scarcity during the war years. Patient deaths had skyrocketed during the war; but during the November Revolution and the period of Soviet experimentation in Bavaria the following year, leading psychiatrists such as Emil Kraepelin busied themselves with the diagnosis—quite literally—of the social-psychological problems plaguing the masses and leaders of immediate postwar Germany.[4] Those who turned their attention to institutional psychiatry compiled medical evaluations of the effects of hunger on body weight.[5] Other common themes were the increase in alcohol consumption and the treatment of veterans' war neuroses. Those who did mention the starvation were unapologetic: Director Ilberg of the Sonnenstein institution, for example, stated in 1922 that "if one surveys the higher death rate among the mentally ill in psychiatric institutions during the war, the great sacrifice of death that our innocent patients had to offer is naturally painfully regrettable. . . . At any rate, it was not possible and not justified to give the mentally ill more food than the healthy."[6]

On a purely psychological level, it is certainly possible that, after presiding over four years of escalating disease and death in institutions, psychiatrists "processed" this experience in the same way as they had processed the experience of confronting war neuroses, which left them medically helpless, intellectually humiliated, and prone to patient abuse.[7] "Embarrassing experiences," Heinz Faulstich has observed, "are . . . only seldom an occasion for self-critical reflection; they are much sooner repressed or warded off in such a way that in the end the flaw becomes attached to the source."[8] They are especially not occasions for self-critical reflection when one's professional survival is at stake.

The most often cited reason, however, is that psychiatrists, the progeny of Germany's nascent eugenics movement, simply did not perceive a moral dilemma. Criticism of Binding and Hoche's *Über die Freigabe der Vernichtung lebensunwerten Lebens* in the medical press was relatively isolated—almost, according to one account, as if the tract "had [already] been firmly anchored in the realm of the thinkable."[9] The silence of psychiatrists on the subject of starvation coupled with their increasing boldness in the assessment of human worth, it has been argued, reflect a latent consensus concerning the validity of social Darwinist principles. Rather than departing from the basic right to life of all human beings, even in war, they discerned varying degrees of human "worth" based on an individual's potential contribution to the social whole. Their willingness to sacrifice the weak for the benefit of the strong in wartime is regarded as psychological groundwork for the extermination of psychiatric patients as "unworthy life" twenty years later.[10]

While there is a great deal of truth to this, one need not deduce ideological sympathy from "silence." Instead, we can look to psychiatrists' attempts to maintain the flow of funds to their institutions during the Weimar years, which constitute an *indirect* discourse on the moral implications of scarcity. The problem, as Dr. Adolf Groß put it, was that although everyone could agree on "humanitarian" grounds that spending money on the mentally ill was necessary, such expenditures were regarded as "socially unproductive"—and thus as a luxury that the "new Germany" could not afford.[11] The logic of utility, to return to the paradigm introduced at the outset of this chapter, was at odds with the logic of morality. The postwar economic crisis coincided with debates about their relative priority.

Psychiatrists' strategy, with few exceptions,[12] was to dodge the issue of priority and argue that psychiatric institutions *were* indeed socially productive: they treated illnesses and were crucial to the maintenance of public security. Moreover, they also pushed forward the frontiers of scientific progress.[13] No one would dream of cutting the financial base from cancer or tuberculosis treatment centers if such cuts would hinder doctors' scientific or therapeutic activities, and if it weren't for widespread prejudice and superstition, no one would do so in the case of psychiatric institutions either.[14] There was, in short, no intrinsic conflict between morality and utility: psychiatric institutions *were* useful, they fulfilled a humane purpose, and they should thus not be closed, consolidated, or grossly underfunded.

Throughout these debates, psychiatrists took great pains to avoid the impression that they were demanding special status or above-average provisions for their institutions. To the contrary: they would of course have to adapt to economic crisis just as everyone else did. As Dr. Groß conceded, "If all of our national comrades must live under more confined, less comfortable conditions, then it may not seem unfair if the mentally ill also take part in this economization[;] and [when held] to a certain degree that may not be exceeded, this will also be possible without negative consequences for their health."[15] Writing for *Die Irrenpflege*, Dr. Erich Friedlaender likewise instructed nurses that they would have to relinquish aspirations to provide their patients with the highest quality care and instead resign themselves to "being satisfied if it is possible to maintain reasonably adequate care of the sick."[16] Heeding dictates of "humanity" under these circumstances meant little more than seeing to it that hygienic standards and food provision were satisfactory for survival. Through a curious twist of logic, the humanist idea that "patients had the same rights as everyone else" meant alternatively—even preferably—that *patients were not entitled to any material advantages that the healthy population did not enjoy.* A concept of "rights" that under most circumstances is invoked by those seeking to acquire more of something for ailing or disadvantaged people was deployed to justify less.

One wonders, in this light, what "treatment" was to entail in the minds of these psychiatrists. Surely, it made no sense simply to replicate the circumstances that had led to a person's institutionalization in the first place. Yet, with their backs to the wall, they were apparently prepared to undermine their potential medical effectiveness by equating the needs—or at least entitlements—of patients with those of the population at large. In addition, and more significant in the long run, they accepted the terms of the debate: rather than trying to defend a helpless and stigmatized group of people against the ravages of economic crisis, they entangled themselves in a war of words over whether the public coffers were half full or half empty and, in the process, lost the necessary moral leverage for resisting deprivation when it was no longer temporary but rather a matter of policy. This capitulation would begin to bear bitter fruit well before the Weimar Republic came to an end.

BE THIS as it may, psychiatrists recognized the need for alternative strategies for keeping their institutions financially viable and therapeutically useful. The most promising strategy, they quickly began to realize,[17] was to support the development of various forms of outpatient care. This, it was hoped, would at once preserve psychiatry's function and, by shortening patients' length of stay, placate cost-slashing bureaucrats. These forms, to be sure, were not new; family care programs and relief organizations for financial and general support (*Irrenhilfsvereine*) had existed since the nineteenth century as "bridges" between institutional and "normal" life. Counseling centers for those whose condition did not require institutionalization had also existed since the prewar years under the auspices, or in any case ultimate control, of community and city administrations. Weimar psychiatrists wanted to reorganize such outpatient care from an institutional, rather than governmental, base.[18]

Toward middecade, psychiatrists' concern with outpatient care developed into much more than a way to remain useful during lean years. This is due partially to the government's passage of a welfare law (*Reichsfürsorgegesetz*) in 1924 that lessened the financial burden for institutionalization borne by families and communities, and partially to a variety of social and political reasons. Institutionalization rates sharply increased thereafter and psychiatrists found themselves confronted with an entirely new set of problems.[19] Institutional population pressures presented a backdrop against which Weimar psychiatrists redefined the professional aims of their enterprise.

The main problem, of course, was how to accommodate such large numbers of patients in a way that was medically and economically acceptable. Because of limited institutional capacity, they could not simply continue bed treatment, baths, and other prewar therapeutic schemes; they would need to release higher numbers of patients, regardless of psychiatry's actual therapeutic effectiveness. The expansion of outpatient care enabled psychiatrists to market institutions as a kind of "filter" for Germany's mentally ill. The patient was increasingly seen not as a sick person but rather as a "possible case for discharge."[20]

It is thus more than a coincidence that the crisis of the mid-1920s was accompanied by the growing popularity of *Erziehung* as a guiding therapeutic principle. The term translates roughly into "education" or "socialization" and is generally used in describing parent-child, teacher-student, or other relationships in which one person offers not only knowledge but also experience and wisdom to another. No longer able to house patients for long periods of time, Weimar psychiatrists drew on this concept to redefine their medical and social task as one of "raising" patients back to health.

The means to this end, psychiatrists believed, was activity. Adopting the ideas of Henry Simon,[21] they took as their starting point the understanding that there existed "healthy" parts of the mentally ill mind which responded to a variety of external influences. In addition to creating an institutional environment in which order and calm prevailed, institutional staff could work wonders by engaging patients in activities ranging from field and garden work to handicrafts, cleaning patients' rooms, sewing, ironing, washing clothes, and assisting in the kitchen.[22] The therapeutic value of activity derived from its ability (1) to maintain or restore patients' "connection with life," (2) to divert them from their crazy ideas or unhappy thoughts, and (3) to channel their energy into "useful" tasks.[23] As such, it could cure the curable and slow down mental deterioration among the incurable.[24] To be sure, the assignment of work to patients in and around the institution was a practice as old as institutions themselves, and psychiatrists had previously "recognized" its therapeutic benefits. Weimar psychiatrists, however, went even farther: they made work the foundation of therapy itself, extended it to all patients, and thus rendered it a norm of institutional life.[25]

Objectively speaking, work therapy's appeal was in large part derived from its ability to bring some semblance of peace and quiet to institutional wards—which, in light of days gone by, was alone an indication of medical progress. In addition, however, publishing psychiatrists did not miss the opportunity to highlight its nontherapeutic benefits, such as its favorable impact on the *economy*: the more patients were drawn into useful activity, the more self-sufficient institutions made themselves, the less money the state would have to provide, and the larger the probability became that institutions could stay financially afloat.[26]

In nursing texts, however, psychiatrists attempted to downplay the economic value of the work itself and emphasize, instead, its therapeutic value.[27] (Indeed, for this reason some psychiatrists preferred to speak of "occupational" rather than "work" therapy.)[28] The kind of work assigned was to be determined not by cost-effectiveness but rather by the abilities, inclinations, and medical condition of the patient.[29] *Purposeful* activity was indeed deemed most medically effective, but "purposeful" could refer to activities that in the outside world would not necessarily be considered remunerative labor. Thus harvesting tomatoes during the week and doing needlepoint on a Sunday were both potentially effective therapeutic measures.[30]

Up to this point, the agenda seems relatively clear: work therapy was to be deployed primarily because of its potential to cure; it also, incidentally, had economic benefits. But this prioritization of therapeutic over economic value was complicated by a third factor, the *symbolic* value of work therapy. The occupation of patients, they noted, would help eliminate the reputation of institutions as expensive residences for so-called individuals unworthy of life (*lebensunwerte Individuen*).[31] It justified, in short, the financial and human resources devoted to patient care. This symbolic value was relevant not only with respect to public image, however; psychiatrists *themselves* subscribed to the linkage of industriousness, social and economic utility, and human worth. For example, Dr. Möckel declared that "our present purpose must be to accustom the patients to work as quickly as possible in order to be able to discharge them again soon, or when discharge is for some reason not possible, to raise the patients into productive and thus valuable members of human society, or to maintain them as such."[32] Work was therapeutically effective—and therefore "good"—because it oriented patients toward the world to which it was hoped that they would soon return—a world in which work was the criterion of utility, and utility the criterion of human worth. However, we see here that psychiatrists applied the norms of that world even to those who had no hope of returning, which calls into question the priority of therapeutic benefits. Work was not only a *means* to therapeutic success but also an expression, in and of itself, of human worth. Work could offer all patients a source of redemption; and psychiatry, whether it cured or not, preserved its social function. Priorities, in this discourse, seem to have been deemed unnecessary—or if not unnecessary, at least nearly impossible to discern with certainty.

It is beyond the scope of the current discussion to evaluate the degree to which this linkage of the "good" and utility was a technocratic adaptation to postwar pressures, and the degree to which it reflects sincere ideological changes.[33] The very least which can be said is that work therapy symbolized Weimar psychiatrists' attempts to bring therapeutic arrangements into line with social, political, demographic, and economic circumstances. It justified both their satisfaction and their optimism; because of it, "fresh life and movement are today making themselves felt in the treatment of psychiatric patients. We no longer confront mental illnesses with our hands tied. The successes of treatment increase and each new victory is an incentive not to despair even of the most desperate, hopeless case."[34] Weimar psychiatry sought to cast itself anew in terms that would please everyone: For the democratic-oriented, psychiatry would claim to be a clean break with the past. For those in charge of funding, psychiatry would claim efficiency. And for a suspicious public, psychiatry would claim to be friendly and humane. Nurses, as we shall now see, were subject to the simultaneous "marketing" of all three.

In Pursuit of the Ideal Nurse

In light of the previous discussion, it is not surprising that Weimar psychiatrists hailed current institutional psychiatry as "modern"—a virtual triumph of light over darkness in the treatment of the insane. Dr. Valentin Faltlhauser, one of the most prolific authors of literature for the instruction of nurses,[35] characterized pre-nineteenth-century brutality toward the insane as a manifestation of "superstition and ignorance" that only slowly, over the course of decades, was brought to an end by the "realization that the insane are sick." This piece of enlightenment was accompanied by the gradual disappearance of the "maltreatment of the poor mentally ill people" characteristic of the Middle Ages, along with the advent of attempts to heal in increasingly open, friendly institutional spaces.[36]

The glorification of those institutional spaces spearheaded Weimar psychiatrists' attempt to shed all associations with the prewar past. The "modern" insane asylum, Faltlhauser instructed nurses, was first and foremost a place where the treatable were treated and chronic cases cared for.[37] "The thoughtless public forgets this hospital-character of the institutions too easily," he bitterly observed; "they love to see solely the houses of detention of times gone by and thus completely fail to appreciate the main task of these institutions, that of healing."[38] The stigma of psychiatric institutions applied to personnel as well, making social interactions for them difficult: according to one account, many people preferred not to be greeted in public by a psychiatrist.[39]

Psychiatrists sought to eliminate this misunderstanding according to the following simple formula: "Everything possible should be avoided that runs counter to the hospital-character of the institution and calls to mind a prison."[40] The high prisonlike walls and surrounding railings of some older institutions were thus no longer acceptable; instead, the appearance of institutions should welcome, not scare away, potential patients and their families. Psychiatrists supported the construction of gathering rooms, libraries, gardens, small institutional museums, facilities for film viewing, music halls, and sports facilities not only for their therapeutic benefits but also with the perception of the public in mind.[41]

Mental Illness, Responsibility, and Charity

Psychiatrists sought to bring not only the appearance but also the theory and practice of institutional care into line with all that was medical and humane. The education of nurses in the origins and nature of mental illness was a means to that end. In articles and textbooks for nurses, psychiatrists generally avoided over-burdening their readers with scientific jargon and grouped mental disturbances according to that which was most immediate to their experience: symptoms. Disturbances of perception (hearing strange voices or seeing phantoms), of memory and time reckoning, of feeling (mania or depression), and of behavior (incomprehensible speech or bizarre movements) were listed among common illness groups.[42] These categories were the basis of specific guidelines for patient care; once nurses knew what to expect from patients with certain illnesses, they could adjust their caretaking strategy accordingly.

Categorical descriptions, however, did not exhaust psychiatrists' agenda; they seized the opportunity in these texts to eliminate any possible ignorance and superstition surrounding mental illness itself. In one account, mental illness was portrayed as a phenomenon that *sometimes* emerged among people born with a *disposition* toward mental illness in the form of some kind of weakness of the nervous system. The presence of this disposition did not guarantee that an illness would emerge; indeed, the opposite could be the case. As one psychiatrist wrote, "One must not fail to consider that very talented people, indeed a genius like Frederick the Great, have come from families predisposed in this way."[43] Very little could be done to predict the emergence of such dispositions; the most one could do was try to assure that they did not come to fruition.[44]

Conscientious child raising was the cornerstone of psychiatrists' strategy for preventing mental illness on an individual level. Attention to physical health, good schools, and attentive, caring parents all made significant contributions to this end.[45] However, even with these measures, success was hardly guaranteed and in some cases—such as with "morally insensitive psychopaths" or "born criminals"—highly unlikely.[46] In these extreme cases, even a favorable environment seems to have had no potential for therapeutic or prophylactic effectiveness.

In any case, it was impossible to control the manifold external influences on the psyche of a human being. Perhaps for this reason, psychiatrists targeted the *pool* of predisposed people for prevention strategies as well. It was possible to phase out the flow of sickly dispositions from one generation to the next by encouraging marriage abstinence among the mentally ill, epileptics, the feebleminded, and persons who in the past had been thus afflicted.[47] This does not mean that psychiatrists necessarily favored marriage bans (though some did) or involuntary sterilization. While they generally agreed that voluntary sterilization was an effective and acceptable preventive measure, they were evasive about whether the procedure should be imposed. One, for example, simply wrote that, although alluring, involuntary sterilization was currently being bogged down in America by doubts about whether such an operation against the patient's will was "permissible" (*statthaft*). For this reason, the emergence of legally imposed sterilization in Germany seemed unlikely.[48] Another psychiatrist obviously supported the idea but limited himself to the observation that forced sterilization remained illegal, wryly adding, "What the cattle breeder may do straight away, we may not do. Some say, 'Praise God, because a human being is not a beast'; the others say, 'Too bad, because then the human being would be less of a beast.' "[49]

Why was a general background in mental illness necessary for nurses? Psychiatrists had several answers to this question. On a technical level, it enabled nurses to speak the "language" of doctors—to make accurate reports on patient developments and to understand the logic of particular therapies. Such knowledge did not, to be sure, give them license to challenge existing hierarchical arrangements: diagnosis, they were told, was a complex business that often involved consideration of a variety of personal and biological factors. Since even an experienced nurse lacked the necessary insight into the workings of mental illnesses, diagnosis and treatment were the exclusive domain of doctors. Their knowledge of mental illnesses made them better assistants but nothing more.[50]

Education in mental illness also had a less direct but ultimately more important benefit: it helped nurses understand that what *appeared* as evil, perversity, hostility, or laziness among some patients was nothing more than a *symptom* of an illness. "It must be clear to [the nurse] down to the deepest conviction that he is dealing with the symptoms of an illness, that is, with unfortunate and pitiable symptoms, with expressions of a sick being, to which ultimately the absolute same meaning should be attributed as to the symptoms of corporal illnesses. . . . The mentally ill should be pitied even more, in fact the most of all patients, because they are robbed of the highest [thing] that a person possesses, the mental faculties."[51] It followed from this that, as Faltlhauser and other psychiatrists wrote with inexhaustible frequency, *a patient bore no responsibility for what he or she did*. Nurses who failed to understand this were prone to feeling degraded by their work, becoming angry with uncooperative patients, and resorting to violence. Ignorance bred feelings of moral superiority that had no place in psychiatric nursing.[52]

This point warrants emphasis, because it adds depth to the standard formulas of the charitable imperative. Nurses were expected to feel not only compassion for their patients but also a certain degree of humility. There was no basis on which to distinguish the mentally ill from the mentally healthy other than, in many cases, luck. One psychiatrist, for example, described a "large number" of psychiatric patients as "fighters" who were simply unsuccessful in overcoming life's adversities; this did not make them unworthy of the same respect that was accorded other "fighters."[53]

This call for restraint and humility in judging others was also evident in occasional comments on euthanasia. Whatever sympathy with Binding and Hoche may have existed among psychiatrists in 1920 and thereafter, nurses were clearly told that, for both ethical and professional reasons, no one in a psychiatric institution was in a position to make life-or-death decisions about patients.[54] In a particularly strongly worded article, nurses were told that nothing would be more mistaken than to view psychiatric patients as an "inferior race . . . useless beings, people who have no rights, [who] bring unhappiness and disturb and injure their fellow human beings," or as people who would perhaps be better off "if they had brought their unhappy existences to an end through an early death." Drawing on Kant's categorical imperative never to treat human beings as a means to an end, the author insisted that we have no right to place a value on other human beings according to their utility. Psychiatric patients had as much right to live as anyone else; "a living being has the right to live solely by virtue of the fact that it lives, and no one is justified in taking life from it."[55]

This was so even if one asked oneself from a humanitarian standpoint whether it might be better to allow a terminally ill patient to carry through an intended suicide. "As doctors and nurses of patients who have been entrusted to us by their families, we can never be in doubt [that] we must do everything to thwart suicidal intentions."[56] Thus even for those who sympathized with the idea of "releasing a patient from suffering," professional responsibilities overruled personal inclinations and dictated abstinence.

Technical Responsibilities and Erziehung

The behavior-as-symptom principle and the absence of patient guilt that it implied rendered the execution of technical responsibilities a far more serious matter than might initially appear to be the case. Since their patients were mentally ill and thus deemed incapable of controlling their own behavior, nurses assumed responsibility not only for the completion of tasks but also, at times, for acts of deviance that they failed to prevent.

Granted the limitless number of schemes that patients could orchestrate to escape, kill themselves, or harm others, the necessity of watching patients constantly could not be emphasized enough. Mechanical rituals of counting and searching punctuated the daily routine of nurses—rituals that were at once mundane and yet absolutely central to the preservation of order and safety. Nurses had to periodically count patients when outdoors in groups; assemble and count work tools at the end of the day; and count forks, knives, and spoons after each meal. They searched clothing and bed linens.[57] And finally, nurses had to notice everything these routines might miss. Failure to notice the smallest splinter of glass, sharp piece of iron, a forgotten knife or medication could lead to violence or suicide.[58]

It goes without saying that episodes of injury or escape severely disrupted the equilibrium of daily institutional life and created considerable problems for administrators who were ultimately responsible for the safety of all institutional residents. Nurses guilty of negligence had every reason to fear grave administrative consequences for these reasons alone. It is interesting to note in addition, however, that if a dangerous (*gemeingefährlich*) patient managed to escape, the nurse in charge could be punished with a three-month prison sentence or a fine. (*Intentionally* letting such a patient escape could lead to a prison sentence of three years.)[59]

Psychiatric nurses, then, assumed a considerable degree of responsibility for what went wrong. They were also delegated responsibility for what went *right*; that is, they were actively involved in the "healing" process. Psychiatrists were under no illusions about the huge potential of nurses to contribute to their therapeutic agenda if those nurses did so willingly and with enthusiasm. This engagement was crucial: nurses were told that passively supervising such activity was not enough. They were responsible for ensuring the participation of every single patient who was deemed capable of such activity by a doctor. "It is the chief duty of the nurse to prompt patients who do not want to occupy themselves and only sit and lie around the stations to converse, play, make music, read, look at pictures, and so forth." To arouse and maintain patients' interest, nurses were encouraged to promote the task at hand as purposeful activity, not idle or useless diversion—even if, as in the case of destructive patients, diversion was the main concern. Heeding a patient's activity preferences was also helpful in this regard.[60] Through this kind of participation in therapy, nurses saved patients from "complete mental deterioration"; even better, they channeled certain patients' destructive tendencies into useful, or at the very least harmless, activities.[61]

Nurses were also expected to lead the way in the activity in question, since "the patients will do likewise only when they see that the personnel take part in work with enthusiasm and diligence."[62] Interestingly, the power of example was not the only concern behind this rule; psychiatrists recognized shared nurse-patient activity as an ideal opportunity to bring "healthy" influences to bear on patients. In this respect, nurse-patient participation in leisure activities also bore fruit. Patients derived particular pleasure from, for example, putting on plays with nurses, and in sports a nurse's participation could work wonders; for there, one psychiatrist observed, "when institutional discipline hardly comes into view, the patient sees in the nurse not the armed 'supervisor' with the key and the 'jailer' who deprives him of his freedom. He becomes trusting, opens to him his heart, regards him as a teammate, as a comrade whom he can take into confidence."[63] As active participants in work therapy, nurses translated the theory of *Erziehung* into practice. In all areas of professional activity they were in charge of ensuring that the "good" remained useful, and what was useful remained "good."

Humane Treatment and the Ideal Nurse

Granted the innocence and limited reasoning capacity of psychiatric patients, it followed that anything resembling punishment had no place in a psychiatric institution. Nurses were continually reminded that straitjackets, other physical restraint devices, and isolation were no longer de rigueur in the treatment of patients.[64] Striking patients was of course forbidden, but nurses were instructed in the use of grips and holds to bring unruly patients under control—that is, to render them harmless without doing them harm.[65]

Psychiatrists liberally used childhood analogies to explain the logic of these "modern" innovations. In a discussion of feeble-minded people, one psychiatrist rhetorically asked, "Does a mother hit her infant? Certainly not, otherwise she would be a very irrational woman!" "Imbecilic" people, he continued, were often no more mentally agile than healthy small children. Although hitting mentally *healthy* children was indeed an effective means for extracting obedience, he continued, it was useless in the case of people unable to grasp the meaning of punishment.[66]

The same kind of logic applied to all forms of mental illness; nurses were to bear in mind that the "laws" governing the mental apparatus of psychiatric patients differed from those of healthy people.[67] The use of force in psychiatric care was nothing more than a means for calming the patient down and therefore to be employed "in observance of the requisite humane consideration."[68] The only permissible justification for physical force of any kind was the threat of injury to the patient, to the nurse, or to others—and therefore such force was not allowed to exceed in degree the violence of the patient.[69] Most important, it was to be employed in a state of "iron self-discipline and self-control"; "[the nurse] must never allow himself to be worked up by the attacks and insults of patients; he must never lose patience and sympathy, must never repay evil with evil."[70]

Psychiatrists' goal, of course, was to maintain order while preventing patient abuse. When one thinks of the thankless character of nursing, the poor reputation of psychiatry, and the frequency of verbal and physical abuse by patients, it is not surprising that something more than procedural knowledge seemed necessary to achieve the desired results. Psychiatrists consequently aimed higher—specifically, they aimed for nurses' *internalization* of what psychiatry was and what their roles were within it. Success required that nurses perceive their work as something more than a series of "negative" tasks associated with restraint and supervision—that they embrace their crucial, "positive" role in Weimar psychiatry's attempt to replace punitive treatments of the past with the concept of *Erziehung*. To this end, psychiatrists had very specific ideas about what kind of person was suitable to become a psychiatric nurse, and about how he or she was to treat—and thus influence—the patient.

Let us begin on the level of appearances and general good character. Texts and articles of the Weimar Republic that instructed nurses in professional theory and practice routinely included, often at the very beginning, a brief section describing the necessary qualities of the model psychiatric nurse. Their point of departure was the maxim that psychiatric nursing demanded much *more* than general nursing. It was not enough to master the care of biological illnesses; the psychiatric nurse also had to possess the physical and emotional stamina to handle the varied and sometimes dangerous manifestations of mental illness. As such, it was not a suitable profession for just anyone, and certainly not for someone merely seeking a way to earn a living.[71]

This point required particular emphasis because psychiatric nursing was regarded by many as an occupation seized by those who were unsuited for anything else. In 1929, for instance, Senior Nurse Georg Sauer of the Waldheim institution described a conversation with a longtime acquaintance whose twenty-two-year-old son intended to become a psychiatric nurse "because he did not get on so well in his professional trade, his school grades were not good, he also did not have any real desire to work, he found learning difficult, and he therefore wanted to become a civil servant." This, the nurse told his colleagues, was one example (among many in his personal experience) of how misunderstood and undervalued their profession remained. In fact, he maintained, "precisely the best is good enough to become a nurse."[72]

Psychiatrists generally agreed that men and women were potentially equally suited—and equally necessary—for the profession of psychiatric nursing.[73] The suitable of both sexes were distinguished from the unsuitable primarily on the basis of performance and commitment.[74] A firm commitment to the charitable imperative was the essential prerequisite, since "in this profession one must often do more than is paid for with gold." This was not to say that nurses were to be left uncompensated: uncompensated work was "the most inhuman and humiliating thing there can be." Instead, emotional compensation (i.e., gratitude) was proffered as an appropriate complement to inadequate financial compensation.[75]

Psychiatric nursing presented a particular problem, however, because the mentally ill were often incapable of expressing even the most superficial thanks for the care they received. As a result, a good psychiatric nurse would be satisfied by the "professional activity in itself, the pleasure of success, of achievement." He or she took up nursing out of an "internal need" to help others that sustained a readiness to sacrifice leisure time and sleep.[76] Some of the rhetoric on good nurses' characteristics emphasized this inner compulsion to such a degree that psychiatric nursing took on the appearance of a religious calling. One psychiatrist, indeed, invoked this analogy explicitly when he described the male counterpart to the "motherly" female nurse. Women, he argued, derived their suitability for psychiatric nursing from their "motherliness," while men derived it from "priestliness." Both were inborn qualities of certain people that could be cultivated; they entailed enthusiasm for work, a willingness to sacrifice, and a desire to help "fellow human beings."[77]

Maintaining an appearance of respectability was, of course, crucial not only for earning patients' respect but also for enhancing the reputation of the institution in the eyes of the public. Nurses were not only to keep a neat appearance and speak politely to colleagues and patients; they were to emanate a calm, quiet propriety in all aspects of work: "Windows and doors must be closed softly; plates and utensils may not be clattered; keys may not be jingled. The walking of a nurse should be soft, not crashing about, not hasty. One should not whisper with other nurses or with a patient, particularly in order not to raise the suspicion in a patient that he is being talked about."[78] "Proper" conduct in one's private life was a subject that psychiatrists sometimes dismissed as obvious but nevertheless seldom failed to mention. It was particularly important to impress this on nursing trainees, who might at first fail to understand that the entire scope of their professional and private activities affected the reputation of their colleagues and of the institution—and thus fell under the purview of "professional" regulations. For example, "Relations with the opposite sex should be honorable and respectful. The pub should be avoided. The nursing trainee should seek recovery from the strenuous work and the air of the sickroom not in there but rather in sensible, not-over-done, gymnastics and other sports carried out in a similar way."[79] Physical exercise was the only genuine source of rejuvenation, he continued, but undoubtedly sports were preferred to the pub for image reasons as well.

Confidentiality was to be upheld at all times in matters medical and nonmedical. When speaking to patients' relatives, nurses were to respond politely to harmless, everyday questions and refer all questions about the patient's medical condition to the doctor.[80] Moreover, there was to be no gossiping. Nurses were required to refrain from casual discussions of their professional experiences in public even when specifically asked; "[the nurse] should avoid making himself 'interesting,' [but rather] should attempt to satisfy the curious inquirer with a few trivial words. The nurse is obligated to maintain silence about occurrences in the institution."[81] The temptation to speak informally or carelessly, and thus to "leak" information into the public sphere, seems to have been psychiatrists' main concern. They reminded nurses that the law called for a fine or a prison term of up to three months for anyone convicted of exposing private information about patients acquired in the line of duty.[82]

Nurses were also expected to *economize*. Whereas psychiatrists spoke among themselves about "economization" in terms of financial policy, in nursing parlance the word was basically equivalent to "not wasting things." The main objective was to use resources as sparingly as possible, and sometimes to make do with less. Nurse education on the topic was limited to marketing thrift as a virtue and as a practical necessity whose effects, contrary to what one might think, did indeed make a difference. Mixing organic and mechanical metaphors, one psychiatrist reminded nurses that "the working of the institution is an extraordinarily complicated and sensitive organism[;] just as with a watch, one little wheel takes hold of the other and any disturbance at any location must automatically affect the entire operation."[83] The same analogy continued to be used to stress the importance of even the most minor contribution.[84]

Patience and self-control were considered an "indispensable duty," especially in the many instances when nurses were provoked by verbal or physical abuse. It was, in the end, the most sensible way to handle such provocation, since "only through untiring patience and calmness will the nurse win influence over [the patients] and secure for himself the necessary predominance over them."[85] A nurse's impatience and loss of self-control could easily lead to coercion, and coercion ran counter to *Erziehung*. The proper way to secure patients' cooperation was to "give the patient the feeling that he is doing what he must do voluntarily and without force"—which sometimes required the passage of time.[86] For the sake of the institution's reputation, patience was also a "must" for personnel receiving and talking to relatives, even the unpleasant ones. One doctor remarked that nurses would come to find this easier by keeping in mind that many relatives displayed the same nervous or angry dispositions as the patients they came to visit, and the same restraint in judging them was therefore in order.[87]

Patience was also required in the face of administrative problems: nurses were encouraged to maintain their composure and cooperate with investigations of possible patient abuse. Administrators' potential public relations concerns in such cases are obvious, but nurses were advised that they too had a stake in these investigations: "Precisely where crazy ideas, pathological irritability, etc., play such a role, it is a duty to seek the truth twice as zealously, especially to protect personnel from false accusations and unsubstantiated mistrust."[88]

Obedience or Critical Judgment?

Nurses were expected to be objective, observant assistants of doctors, avoiding the temptation to compete with them in diagnosing a patient and reporting, instead, the "naked facts."[89] This medical responsibility was accompanied by a moral responsibility, namely, the preservation of the patient's trust in the doctor, which was regarded as "one of the most important healing powers at the disposal of the doctor."[90] Patients were never to overhear nurses complaining about a doctor, and nurses were instructed to avoid questioning doctors' orders in a patient's presence; both would undermine that trust.[91] The patient, according to one contributing nurse, should believe that "the doctor is absolutely right. . . . Then the doctor will be his best and truest friend."[92]

However, this brings us to an important qualification, namely, that nurses' mediational responsibilities did not entail constant reference back to a set of "rules" or the exclusion of independent thought: "The orientation toward one's duty may not, however, obscure the other qualities too much or destroy them; otherwise rigid, fossilized conceptions of duty arise, with which one can only harm oneself and others. A lot of well-organized people have been ruined by the rigid conceptions of duty in their environment."[93] The use of the mind in nursing had an unmistakably *active* dimension: doctors could make mistakes, Faltlhauser acknowledged, and this sometimes would result in an order that the nurse did not understand or had reservations about. In this case, it was "the legitimate right of the nurse . . . to express his doubts in the proper form or to ask for an explanation."[94] Thus affirming the ultimate authority of the doctor was in no way intended to shut off the critical capacity of the nurse.

This was so for two reasons. First, in addition to being susceptible to mistakes just like anyone else, doctors relied heavily on the observations of nurses and their competence in carrying out doctors' orders. Although nurses were supposed to include only the "naked facts" in their reports, they nevertheless required critical judgment to know which behaviors and symptoms were relevant. Since they saw patients for many hours at a time over the course of weeks and months, they were in the best position to note changes in a patient's condition. Even if they were discouraged from drawing their own diagnostic conclusions, they needed certain powers of insight to adequately fulfill the role of doctor's assistant.[95]

Doctors and administrators also had to rely on nurses' judgment with regard to the distribution of responsibilities. Overburdening a nurse could have serious consequences (such as patients' escaping, becoming disorderly, or committing suicide). Therefore, doctors and administrators realized, it was absolutely essential that a nurse be able to evaluate a situation in light of his or her ability and experience, and to inform a supervisor if he or she did not feel capable of handling a particular situation—if, for example, there were too many dangerous or agitated patients on a particular station.[96]

Third, and perhaps most important, nurses needed mental agility to function in daily life *in between* doctors' visits, even on the most basic level. They had to exercise foresight in heading off potential problems (keeping sharp objects out of patients' reach, keeping an eye out for unlocked doors or broken windows that could enable escape, and so forth). They had to base these preventive measures on a prior familiarity with individual patients' propensities. Above all, they had to be able to think on their feet when dealing with sudden problems or disturbances. The exercise of critical judgment was not simply a perk that psychiatrists offered nurses to make them feel involved. When practiced within the parameters of proper professional conduct, it was the cornerstone of institutional order and therapeutic success.

The Form and Content of Language

Psychiatrists clearly did not have a rigid or mechanical understanding of the responsibilities and requirements of the nursing profession. Nurses not only acted; they also served as examples and established a *presence* in the institution. What they did was no more important than the accompanying attitude and manner.

In this light, it is not at all surprising that rules governing speech figured prominently in psychiatrists' instructional texts. Speech was, in fact, one of the most important areas in which nurses' behavior was prescribed, because it was not only a means for extracting patient cooperation; it was also central to healing—to reconstituting the skills of sociability that mental illness destroyed.

The above discussion of work therapy has already suggested how potentially powerful a nurse's verbal influence on a patient could be: conversation during shared activity generated good-will, restored interest in the outside world, and encouraged the development of communicative skills. This "human" connection with the nurse was not only a result of organized activity, however; it was fundamental to the patient's daily institutional experience. Doctors and relatives appeared from time to time, but the nurse was in the end the "only person who connects the patient to humanity"; every word the nurse uttered in the patient's presence, and the tone of those utterances, were therefore of the utmost significance. "Just as the word of the mother supports and boosts the child, that of the teacher the schoolchild, that of the priest the *Volkskind*, that of the philosopher the chosen spiritual child, so does the word of the nurse support and boost the patient."[97]

Specific guidelines for nurses' speech included, most obviously, the imperative to speak *politely* to patients. This entailed the use of daily greetings, formal address (*Sie*), and the title the person carried in public life. It also entailed avoiding giving patients orders unless absolutely necessary. If a patient did not complete necessary tasks in an acceptable or timely manner, a good nurse attempted to awaken the patient's own initiative through calm, friendly, and determined suggestion and repetition. Constant commands would be perceived as burdensome by patients and would result in anxiety.[98] One contributing nurse advised his colleagues, "One should avoid under all circumstances everything that could cause the patient to see his nurse as a supervisor. Such patients will never feel good and will have no trust in their nurse. In psychiatric nursing everything depends on the patient's seeing the nurse as his friend who wants only the best for him."[99] *Deceit* was invariably to be avoided. Nurses were instructed never to lie to patients about, for example, the purpose of a transport. "It is under all circumstances impermissible to try to make patients obedient with trickery and lies. When necessary, force is ten thousand times better than deceit, trickery, and lies." There were two reasons for this: First, lying was in and of itself a "morally reprehensible means." Second, it was bound to backfire, because such patients acquired feelings of betrayal and mistrust that made their treatment all the more difficult. Force, experience showed, was easier for patients to forgive than deceit.[100]

This was not a call, interestingly, for the deliberate exposure of all truth. It was permissible—in fact preferable—to protect patients as much as possible from information that would upset their "emotional balance." In the event that relaying bad news was unavoidable, it was to be conveyed in proper form before the patient found out through some unfortunate coincidence.[101] Nurses were also instructed never to discuss medical matters with doctors or other personnel in front of a patient; voicing suspicions about a patient's intentions of suicide or escape, for example, would only encourage those entertaining such intentions and plant the idea in the minds of others.[102] Nurses should not underestimate patients' ability to understand what was going on around them.

They should not overestimate it, either: mental illness rendered patients impervious to the appeal of reason, nurses were told, and it was therefore useless to attempt to talk them out of their delusions or to mock them. It was also wrong, however, to *agree* with their crazy ideas or, for example, to humor such patients by agreeing to address them with titles that reinforced their fantasies ("Your Majesty," etc.).[103] Such agreement would constitute deceit. When patients pressured them for a response to their ideas, the proper course of action was to *listen, attempt diversion*, and *remain calm*. [104] Above all, nurses were to refrain from any display of agitation or excitement, if necessary turning unmanageable patients over to a doctor.[105]

Impartiality was an additional crucial requirement. Nurses were never, for example, to get involved in a dispute between patients and take the side of one or the other; this would presumably only deepen the problem at hand.[106] Even the appearance of favoritism was to be avoided—thus nurses were forbidden to accept even the smallest gifts of appreciation from relatives.[107]

The above guidelines, it will be noticed, focused on truthfulness, stability, and evenhandedness—the building blocks of trust. For without trust, the patient perceived the nurse as an (at least potential) adversary, was correspondingly uncooperative, and could be dealt with only through coercion. Weimar psychiatry, of course, sought to drive nurse-patient relationships of this description out of existence and to reconstitute them on the basis of psychological and emotional influence: "The modern, well-trained nurse . . . must influence the patient with his entire personality. [The patient] must come to trust him, [for then] he will more willingly obey. He must recognize in the nurse a friend, who means well toward him."[108]

This, however, brings us to a crucial point: friendship, trust, and the specific guidelines that fostered them were not only presented as reflections of human decency; they were part of a general strategy for extracting patient cooperation. In fact, a nurse charged with the supervision and care of a mentally ill person could *not* at the same time actually *be* a friend: "The psychiatric nurse must without exception be friendly to all patients. He may not, however, become friends with a single patient."[109] Psychiatrists insisted that a patient's trust was under no circumstances to be reciprocated—least of all toward patients who behaved themselves in order to put the nurse off guard. Even sincere, well-meaning patients would feel betrayed when an overly friendly nurse was forced under other circumstances to assert his or her authority.[110]

The behavior-as-symptom principle, then, affirmed the absence of guilt or "evil" among patients and gave rise to a professional ethic characterized by moderation, encouragement, and "humane" treatment. But at the same time, it affirmed the idea that nurse-patient relationships based on the reciprocity of goodwill were neither desirable nor possible. The patient was able—and in many cases predisposed—to return "real" friendship and trust with treachery. Thus paradoxically a certain "cold-bloodedness" was required of nurses in addition to "brotherly love."[111]

These imperatives were captured in the concept of "friendly resoluteness" (*freundliche Entschiedenheit*), whereby psychiatrists sought to steer nurses on a course between two extremes. They realized that encouraging too much friendliness toward patients would render those patients unmanageable and nurses ineffective in preserving order. They also knew that encouraging unfriendly, militant conduct would invite a problem equally destructive to the institution's stability (not to mention its reputation), namely, patient abuse. And in any case, psychiatrists' encouraging militancy among nurses would have been entirely inconsistent with their attempts to reconstitute psychiatric care according to the principles of *Erziehung*. Thus, to preserve *discipline* and therefore the very possibility of treatment, as well as the claim to be *humane*, they encouraged nurses to maintain a "friendly resoluteness and self-confident manner."[112]

Humanization and Utility

In light of this, the humanization of psychiatric practice during the Weimar Republic seems to have had something insincere about it: it remained on the level of propriety, guiding the form but not the content of nurse-patient relationships. The immediate goal, as we have seen, was to make the patient *think* or *feel* a certain way: she was to "see" the nurse not as a supervisor but rather as a friend and role model; he was to "say to himself" that the doctor was his best friend; if she "felt" that she was trusted, she would try not to disappoint that trust. Moral concepts—compassion, empathy, and truthfulness—were promoted for their ability to generate and manage specific *appearances*. Whatever humanitarian impulses were brought to bear on professional activity were channeled into an "ethics of utility" that kept them under strict control. Humane behavior thus found both its expression and its limits within the parameters of administrative and therapeutic utility.

This emphasis on the utility of moral concepts—and the discouragement of reciprocity—does not necessarily signify that psychiatrists were cynical about the humanity of their patients and were only paying lip service to increasing public concern for civil rights. Rather, this advice was an outgrowth of a moral and medical optimism that ultimately produced troubling conceptual obscurities. Dr. Wickel, for example, wrote an article for *Die Irrenpflege* in 1929 entitled "On the Dignity of the Human Being." As the title suggests, the author sought to remind nurses that they were charged with the care of human beings whose dignity as such was to be respected. "We must treat them in the same friendly, courteous way as other people, and as we ourselves wish to be treated."[113] For this reason, it was incumbent on nurses to honor the dignity of their patients by, for example, upholding standards of cleanliness and ensuring that patients were neatly dressed. Interestingly, however, this last remark led him to add that patients should not be permitted to forfeit (*einbüßen*) this dignity through uncleanliness or other violations of the rules of propriety and sink "below the level of an animal." In such circumstances, the nurse was to "make him into a human being again and give him back the dignity of a human being."[114]

This suggests that nurses' corrective influence was more than a contribution to a scientific-medical undertaking. It was part of a more general exercise in teaching patients to observe the dictates of *Sittlichkeit*, a conceptual catchall for traditional virtues such as orderliness, cleanliness, and respectability.[115] Since a lack of *Sittlichkeit* could be both the cause and the symptom of mental illness, it was to be battled on all fronts: "One of the most important tasks of nursing staff is combating unclean and unpleasant habits of some patients. Every disorderly behavior, lying around in dark places, on the floor, huddling in the corners, sitting for a long time on the toilet, spitting, carelessness in clothing, and so forth, are to be combated by personnel with strict consequences."[116] The powers of example and correction, it was hoped, would prevail: "Success can be expected only when ten and twenty times a day for months the same warning is repeated, the clothes are again and again straightened out and ordered, the patient is again and again picked up from the floor, and so on."[117]

Since illness and health could be "seen" only through behavior, therapy acquired the alteration of behavior as its focus. Conventional virtues were superimposed onto the discourse of sickness and health, the result being a *conceptual linkage of civilized behavior and mental health* in the theory and practice of *Erziehung*: animal-like behavior reflected the existence of an illness, and civilized, human-like behavior reflected its defeat.[118] Symptoms, in other words, were not morally neutral; they assumed a place on a value scale spanning the distance between animals and civilized humans. The most objective diagnostic language could thereby be deployed to reflect the moral status of the person as a whole.

We see this process at work in the use of the term *minderwertig* in Weimar psychiatric discourse. It is often pointed out that the use of the term has a long pre–National Socialist history, thus demonstrating that the Nazis were not the only ones who held psychiatric patients in contempt. The matter, as the current discussion suggests, is more complicated. Much of the time during the Weimar Republic, psychiatrists used the term to describe neurological capability—for example, certain patients had "psychopathic deficits" (*psychopathische Minderwertigkeiten*). Such characterizations presumed that there existed certain objectively verifiable standards for proper neurological function, and that the functioning of the mind of the patient in question was subpar. The term was not intended to reflect a judgment of the value of the person but rather to reflect their own image of themselves as good scientists.

The problem with the term *minderwertig* during the Weimar Republic is, rather, that it was used inconsistently. In one article the word could refer strictly to neurological phenomena, but elsewhere—sometimes in the same article—psychiatrists traveled down the slippery slope leading to the term's description of the entire person. At the end of an article on the treatment of "psychopathic deficits," for example, one psychiatrist wrote that "all psychopaths are by virtue of their inborn predisposition *inferior and therefore pitiable human beings* whom the healthy should protect and support."[119]

The patient's behavior made visible a mental condition that was understood as unhealthy, or not up to par; the very existence of that "condition," moreover, meant that the patient was forced to behave in an uncivilized or otherwise aberrant manner. Although innocent—indeed, pitiable—the patient was nevertheless incapable of functioning among the civilized, healthy population and was forced to reside on the other side of a psychological gulf that divided not only the healthy from the unhealthy but also the civilized from the uncivilized.

The patient's lack or limitation of reason thus eliminated one kind of moral "otherness" while reintroducing another: the patient was not responsible for acts of good and evil and therefore could not "be" a good or evil person; but that very inability to comprehend and uphold conventional virtues rendered patients somehow *beyond* good and evil—and therefore outsiders. There is even a sense that the mentally ill were in certain ways not fully human; but institutional psychiatrists do not seem to have entertained the Nazis' sinister notions about the implications of this. That is, they never, to this author's knowledge, referred to their patients as "lives unworthy of living" in the pages of *Die Irrenpflege*; rather, they spoke of *enabling patients to live "lives worth living."* As one psychiatrist put it, "Our purpose should be to support with particular love and enthusiasm those to whom nature has not been kind, so that the way to a life worthy of living is also opened to them!"[120]

This statement, of course, *implies* that the mentally ill person, before being cured, is living a "life not worthy of living," and this in turn has particularly grave implications for incurable patients. But these implications seem to have been a kind of "blind spot" for those invested in the art of psychological healing. As noted earlier, Weimar psychiatrists increasingly saw not a patient but rather a "possible case for discharge." Similarly, they saw not a useless or unworthy human being but rather a human being in need of being made fully human again. The patient was not, in short, thought about in isolation but rather perceived in connection with the task at hand, that of healing. Rather than speaking of Weimar psychiatrists' failure to recognize that all human life is worthwhile, therefore, we may find it more instructive to speak of their belief that a "life not worthy of living" existed only insofar as it was in the process of being cured.

Against the background of this therapeutic optimism, it becomes clearer why the creation of appearances was not perceived as psychological control or deception but rather as the simple magnification of what was true. Psychiatric staff, after all, understood themselves as protagonists in a great reformist adventure, a chief component of which was the abolition of coercion and the manifestation of moderation and goodwill in psychiatric theory and practice. Within this social and medical context, appearances—of the staff's good intentions, for example— more or less approximated the truth.

In positing the compatibility of utility and humane purpose, psychiatrists did away with the need to prioritize them—to think, for example, about the proper course of action when what was "useful" turned out not to be humane. Similarly, there was no need to think about the proper course of action when appearances no longer corresponded with the truth. It is tempting to ascribe a certain degree of significance to this observation in light of what was to come: that is, during the "euthanasia" program, nurses would encourage hesitant patients to drink all of the bitter "medicine" or else they would not "benefit" fully from it. These later developments point to the obvious dangers in stressing the importance of appearances—the danger that the integrity of the persons involved is compromised, that the truth becomes increasingly irrelevant, or, as would be the case ten years later, that appearances of goodwill serve as a smokescreen for a terrible truth.

THIS outlook left Weimar psychiatrists without theoretical precedents for confronting the economic crisis of the late 1920s, when the basis of their optimism evaporated once again. As the de-

cade came to a close, they confronted decreasing institutionalization rates and, even worse, increasing percentages of institutional populations that consisted of long-term cases with bad
prognoses. The hoped-for "filter function" of psychiatry did not
materialize, and the public and the state were becoming impa-
tient. Outpatient care was eliminated or drastically cut throughout the country; staff positions were eliminated; and in 1931
new legislation (*Polizeiverwaltungsgesetz*) placed the decision to
institutionalize completely in the hands of the law enforcement
bureaucracy.[121]

Psychiatrists responded to this state of affairs more or less as
they had in the immediate postwar years: if there was less to be
had, they would see to it that institutions simply required less.
To this end, they proposed various plans for rationalizing their
profession without compromising medical standards. The most
notorious suggestion came from Emil Bratz, director of the Wittenauer Heilstätten, who won a competition sponsored by the
German Psychiatric Association in 1931 with his essay "Can the
Care of the Mentally Ill Be Arranged More Cheaply, and How?"
Therein, he proposed that those patients with good prognoses
receive quality treatment, and those with bad prognoses be removed from regular institutional care and transferred to other
care arrangements that would cost only half as much.[122] Suddenly, psychiatrists were not simply arguing that patients' entitlements should be held in check by "availability," such that they
would have as much as, but no more than, the healthy population outside. They deduced moral inequality from an "objective"
medical diagnosis and proposed to reduce the entitlements of
certain patients accordingly.

It is therefore extremely interesting that in the midst of these
developments—that is, in 1930—Walter Morgenthaler published
a nursing textbook called *Die Pflege der Gemüts- und Geisteskranken*. Rather than limiting himself to the usual brief descriptions
of the qualities of the ideal psychiatric nurse, he devoted a chapter to describing in great detail a whole array of emotional and
psychological requirements—as well as rewards—in psychiatric
nursing. The chapter set out not only to convey information but

also to provide what we would today call assertiveness training. Most noteworthy in the present context are his comments to nurses on the question of entitlements. He wrote, "A temporary reduction even of that which is necessary for life can ... under certain circumstances be necessary and must be accepted by the individual. . . . Nothing is more deplorable than a person who, when he one time has to deviate from the usual way [of doing things], immediately complains about an infringement on his human rights."[123] This did not, however, imply that nurses must accept continuous deprivation: *It is not only the right, but also the duty of a person to defend himself against an ongoing reduction of the necessities of life.*"[124] Morgenthaler did not accept a facile elision of entitlements and prevailing conceptions of what was available. When deprivation became ongoing, or a matter of policy, prevailing notions of availability apparently no longer mattered. Individuals could and should manifest what they considered to be their own needs and entitlements; *it was not morally incumbent on them to accept what they were given.*

It is almost impossible to imagine that Morgenthaler's principle cut ice either among his colleagues or among nurses. After years of skepticism vis-à-vis eugenics, psychiatrists increasingly turned their attention to the *prevention* of psychiatric illnesses,[125] and in their zeal they became increasingly comfortable with denigrating "lives unworthy of living." In 1928, for example, one doctor warned psychiatric nurses in *Die Sanitätswarte* not to marry patients, citing in the process several anecdotes about disastrous consequences for those who had been foolish enough to do so in the past. Although the idea of sterilizing certain patients as a condition of their release was "enticing," for the moment it would perhaps suffice if popular enlightenment warned people against producing "lives unworthy of living."[126]

To be sure, this did not necessarily mean that such people should be killed; Dr. Baege wrote that "for eugenics, the occasionally occurring thought about the extermination of life unworthy of living is of course out of the question. This would undoubtedly be the surest method of hindering offspring; it is just irreconcilable with ethics."[127] For Dr. Kihn, however, it was not altogether a bad idea to kill such people, because then those who cared for them would be free for other purposes and the taxpayers would get a much-deserved break. Unfortunately, however, there were no legal prospects for such a move on the horizon because too many people were swayed by an exaggerated ethical concern.[128] Morality, in his view, was nothing more than a nuisance in these debates: "In the battle against inferiority, every measure that seems inexpensive and effective is permitted. Here there will never be definite norms for law and for humanity, according to which [we may] proceed. Experience shapes humanity and the law just as much as the other way around, law [shapes] experience."[129] Psychiatrists' task, Kihn continued, was doggedly to persevere in spite of hard times and apparent failure; perhaps a day would come when their efforts would bear fruit. He concluded on an eerily apposite note: "Here, it does not at all depend on us; we believe that we are swimming against the current and do not realize how we are carried along by it."[130]

4

The Evasiveness of the Ideal:
Private and Professional Obstacles

In THE WAKE of the previous discussion of the "ideal" psychiatric nurse, the following excerpts from the Berlin-Buch institution's administrative records seem to expose an unbridgeable gap between what was said and what was done:

In the case of Kr. and D., House 2, quiet and order were considerably disturbed, the female Nurse B. was abused by Kr. The nursing staff of House 2 felt disturbed by Kr.'s visit.

Nurse L., House 7, had a female visitor who was staying in his room, although he was on duty. In the room stood two made beds.

In the case of L.-Ku., House 7, several visitors were in the house the entire night. Disputes and an extended brawl erupted. The patients were disturbed in their sleep.

. . . . A patient complained that male Nurse K. lay in the bed of a female nurse during the day, changed his shirt there, and gave it to the nurse to wash.

Occasional complaints from female nurses have continued that, in cases where several female nurses occupy one room, visits from men are extraordinarily disruptive. The nurses felt embarrassed and also could not rest after night duty.

It has been discovered that in the women's cottages 4 and 6, men have remained visiting past 10:00 P.M.

In House 8 it was strongly suspected that a female nurse had had a night visit from a man. . . .

. . . . Female nurses cook for male nurses and are sought after by them for taking their midday meal.

. . . . Female nurse W. from House 2 once had sixteen people visiting who drank and made so much noise that the peace and quiet on the top floor of the house was disturbed and vigorous intervention was necessary.[1]

It is not in itself surprising or unusual that these "professionals," like most professionals, did not always behave as such. After all, fulfilling the professional ideal (namely, sacrificing leisure, sleep, privacy, freedom of movement and association) not only left little room for attention to private affairs but also demanded superhuman qualities and performance that were well-nigh unattainable. Unrealistic demands coupled with the "external" pressure of private concerns, however, provide only a partial explanation for the discrepancy between the ideal and the actual nurse. If we look more closely at institutional life during the 1920s, we see that even the most unencumbered nurse could also fall victim to disadvantageous administrative politics or succumb, in spite of prescribed rules, to the pressures of collective deviation.

PRIVATE LIFE AND PROFESSIONAL ORIENTATION: THE QUESTION OF COMMITMENT

The first question we need to address is, what kinds of people became psychiatric nurses and under what circumstances? For the most part, they came from working- or lower-middle-class backgrounds and had an elementary school education. Men often had worked for their parents, trained in a craft, or had a history of doing odd jobs; many women had trained and worked previously as domestic help. Some men and women were single parents; some had incurred debts. Their personnel files reveal a high degree of similarity in background but also a high degree of variability in individual life histories—variability that manifested itself in their everyday concerns, degrees of commitment, and professional conduct.

Some nurses had direct experience in the First World War and sought to make use of their skills after it was over. Managing station nurse T.P. of the Sachsenberg institution in Schwerin, for example, worked as a nurse for the Order of Saint John in a variety of war hospitals, volunteering at the end of 1917 to care for mentally ill soldiers "because these patients instilled in me a very special [kind of] pity." After the war, she pursued a career in psychiatric care.[2] Some male nurses had had similar experiences: Wittenau nurse Konrad Dauner, for example, worked in the medical corps during the war. Captured in France, he was later sent to Morocco and ended his service on the eastern front. After the war, and throughout the next ten years, he held a number of jobs in both general and psychiatric nursing in and around Berlin.[3]

Some nurses, particularly women, explicitly mentioned interest in the profession as the main reason they applied for a job. One Eichberg nurse wrote in an unsolicited application letter, "For a long time now I have had the intention to turn to this profession and also believe that I am suitable for it."[4] Her background was typical: her father was a railroad worker, she had attended elementary school for eight years, and she had performed office and household work before seeking employment at Eichberg.[5] She differed from most applicants insofar as her school performance was excellent and her written approach to Eichberg administrators was succinct, polite, linguistically above average, and professional in tone. Recognizing a stellar candidate, Eichberg employed her immediately.[6]

People also became nurses by requesting a "promotion" from some other form of institutional employment. Anja Reuter, for example, started off as a kitchen worker at the Dalldorf institution in late 1919 and asked to be made a nurse in early 1921. Her former supervisor, the institution's housekeeper, wrote, "In this respect there is nothing standing in the way of her wish. She is industrious and reliable."[7] This kind of in-house staff shuffling was useful for minimizing staff turnover: nurses with previous experience in institutional employment knew better than the uninitiated what was in store for them during daily life on the wards, and administrators had firsthand knowledge of their reliability.

Be this as it may, nurses often took up work with less than the
desired amount of education and commitment. The director of
the Winnetal institution in Württemberg, for example, lamented
in 1930 that nurses for the most part had only an elementary
school education, and not a terribly impressive one at that.
Moreover, they usually had no intention of making psychiatric
nursing a lifelong occupation; they came mainly from rural areas
and took up nursing because they currently couldn't find a job,
a relative had worked at the institution, or for a variety of other
reasons. To be sure, men generally tended to stay on after they
realized that nursing was physically easier than other potential
jobs and afforded lifelong financial security for them and their
families. Female staff turnover, however, remained at 25 percent
per year owing to marriage, caring for elderly parents, and the
"greater availability of jobs" for women.[8]

Although high staff turnover among women was a common
subject of complaint among administrators, it by no means came
as a surprise. Women continued to leave nursing once they married throughout the Weimar and National Socialist years; and
even if administrators complained about staff turnover, they
prepared the paperwork for these departures as a matter of routine.[9] Women also sometimes left to care for sick relatives or otherwise attend to family crises and later returned to work. Entering and leaving the workforce according to the evolution of their
private lives, they constituted the "movable parts" of the social
machine.

For female nurses themselves, this meant that they were subject to competing imperatives: their professional "code" demanded unflagging professional commitment, while social
mores called on them to keep an eye out for the potential husband—to *divide* their attention and energy between work and
preparation for life-after-work. They were expected to devote
themselves to their highly challenging and fulfilling duties
while at the same time plotting their "escape."

Did women perceive this contradiction, and if so were they
troubled by it? An interesting poemlike text from a 1919 issue of
Die Irrenpflege, "Conversation between a Nurse and a Farmer's

Wife," suggests that women themselves did not entertain the possibility that professional and domestic life were compatible, nor did they have their hearts set on living the life of the "modern woman," even if they found it tantalizing. In the first stanza of this text, Nurse Bertha, who has worked a long time in the city, returns to her hometown and strikes up a conversation with her friend Lenerl, a farmer's wife. "You know, I'm a modern [girl], and I've got what's 'in' today, a profession," she exclaims, and tells of the forty patients whom she feeds, dresses, and washes. In an assertion of her independence, she adds, "We modern girls don't gaze after men anymore."

Lenerl is skeptical but adds that in any case she has no cause for envy. Look at my husband and my house, she says, and at my cow, chickens, and other animals: "You have to slave away for strangers, I just look after my own." While Bertha is being ordered around by doctors, Lenerl presides over her domestic world, where the logic of work and reward is clear, and where those rewards appear tangibly before her. Bertha replies that Lenerl is bossed around as well, namely, by her husband, whereas she is guided solely by *intelligence*. "Intelligence," Lenerl scoffs, "What's that? Is that a modern thing?"

Bertha does not say; rather, she proceeds to add that nursing does not entail only the fulfillment of duty; there are also many pleasures. In her institution she enjoys theater, dancing, coffee hours, and music. But don't be angry, she coaxes her friend; let's end this dispute. In an attempt to close the gulf between them that the exchange has created, she says, "Secretly I'll confess to you, Hansel is making my heart ache, and if he should propose sometime soon, I'll have to think about it once again." She is well versed in the appealing aspects of professional life but admits that she, too, ultimately prefers husband and home.[10] The apparent contradiction between professional and social expectations seems to have been reconciled by tacit agreement among all concerned on the priority of marriage.

This is not to say that women's experience was always reducible to a rigid and, in certain respects, romanticized career-then-marriage progression. Nurse Elsa Gartner, for example, informed the Wittenau administration in April 1931 that she would be leaving her job in September on account of marriage—but withdrew the notice one month later because the engagement had been broken off.[11] Since the broken engagement involved a Wittenau senior nurse, she simultaneously requested a transfer to another institution. In the meantime, she was absent from work on account of "nervous exhaustion."[12]

Nurse Gartner was generally liked by Wittenau administrators, despite the fact that she suffered from psychological problems of her own and had spent four weeks in a sanatorium the previous year.[13] More than willing to oblige in the current crisis, they turned to the city administration. "In the interest of the nurse and of [her] duties, we request [you] to expedite the transfer."[14] Finding a suitable nurse for an exchange proved easier said than done. Fortunately, however, Nurse Gartner eventually recovered from her emotional problems and decided that she would prefer to stay at Wittenau after all, thus bringing the administration's involvement in the affair mercifully to an end.[15] She married a salesman in 1935, after which her career at Wittenau, as per routine, came to an end.

Administrators' involvement in nurses' personal affairs was not, then, always reducible to bureaucratic procedure in which they were, like it or not, entangled. Rather, it was a matter of good management: heeding developments in employees' private lives was in the interest of administrative efficiency and staff morale. Many administrators were no doubt sensitive and well intentioned in such situations. The fact remains, however, that female nurses did not, as a result, have the option of keeping their private affairs private. In the case of a broken engagement, their pain and humiliation was exposed and eventually became part of their professional record.

Other nurses were single mothers subject to the pressures of both parenthood and professional responsibility. Wittenau nurse Reuter was one such single parent whose son lived in the "Home for the Homeless." She was supposed to provide financial support for him, but the local social welfare association reported to Wittenau in December 1929 that she was behind in her payments.[16] Almost one year later, she was pressured to take the son into her own care and to find a training post for him. This was impossible, she claimed, because she did not have a permanent living arrangement for herself, worked around the clock (morning, afternoon, and night shifts), and thus could not look after him properly. Moreover, she believed herself to be "too good-natured . . . and precisely here in the big city, he could fall too easily into the wrong hands."[17] She managed to keep the social welfare bureaucracy at bay until 1933, when she was sued for missing payments. The son eventually took up residence with her parents and trained to become a barber, entering the military in 1936.[18] But in the meantime, ongoing personal problems took their toll; she was absent from work for most of April, September, and October 1931 on account of a nervous ailment.[19]

This brings us to an issue that nursing texts generally avoided, namely, the fact that many nurses were driven to nursing by financial need and fought bitterly for their positions on precisely those grounds. Nurse Peter Zewen of Berlin was a particularly desperate case, holding fourteen short-term jobs during the Weimar Republic, eight of which were temporary nursing positions. He was unemployed approximately eighteen months of the time. His work was consistently good and the dismissals followed without exception from forces beyond his control, such as the end of a temporary position, dissolution of an enterprise, or, more often, lack of business. Against this background, it is not at all surprising that, shortly before the end of his one-month stint at the Herzberge institution in 1930, he wrote to the administration begging for an extension. He had a wife to support, he reminded them, and before this job, he had been unemployed six months and had incurred debts. "There are after all younger, single colleagues who have been there longer and do not have to leave until the beginning of October. I have done nothing wrong and am in the profession with body and soul."[20]

He was allowed to continue for an additional two weeks, but before this time had elapsed he had sent another missive to the administration. "Please do not regard me as an unthankful person if I once again trouble you, dear Herr Director, with this letter. But think about what a person will do out of desperation to free himself from economic need, if the opportunity permits. . . ."[21] The letter contained a variety of appeals to sympathy, from a brief mention of an on-the-job accident the previous month (he was bitten by a patient)[22] to expressions of regret that he had been unable to pay the fees for nursing courses which would have enhanced his professional performance. In spite of this, he reminded the director, he invested body and soul in his profession—a fact that his supervisor could confirm—and would be "eternally grateful" if the director could continue to employ him.[23] This time his appeal was unsuccessful, and he would have to wait four months until his next temporary position at Berlin's Wuhlgarten institution.

Other nurses took to moonlighting even though such activity was forbidden by their work contracts and created problems with the institution's surrounding community. Eichberg nurse Paul Scharf, who routinely performed barber services at the institution, outraged local barbers in late 1922 by selling his services privately after his shifts. The barbers' guild of Biebrich (today part of Wiesbaden) complained to Eichberg's administration, which in turn warned Scharf that performing work on the side was forbidden. Scharf, however, had denied the charges and continued his trade, according to three local barbers who pursued the matter with the local government in Wiesbaden. Work materials were expensive, they explained; local barbers could thus lower their prices only a certain amount if they were to stay afloat, and certainly not low enough to compete with Scharf. Scharf was ruining a local trade as well as, they reminded the administrator, violating a ban imposed by his employer. It was a sound case: Scharf was subsequently warned a second time and threatened with dismissal if he continued. This second warning worked.[24]

Nurses who performed work on the side, however, were not necessarily scheming profiteers. Many who lived in rural areas performed such work within a communal system of nonmonetary exchange that administrators, in fact, respected. For example, in spring 1927 the local shoemakers' guild somehow found out that two Eichberg nurses had done odd shoe repairs for people in their neighborhood over the past year, and lodged an official complaint with the head of the regional government (the *Landeshauptmann*), who was officially their employer. Government administrators' investigation of the matter revealed that Nurse Dunkel had done this work as compensation for work performed on his house by a former tenant—not for money. Nurse Kohl had done the same for two widows (one of whom had been married to an Eichberg nurse), and for a man who had formerly done some metalworking for him. "According to this account, it concerns nurses' labor that is performed as compensation for other services, which is usual in rural areas." For formality's sake, however, he reminded the nurses that private employment on the side was forbidden.[25]

Thus, having begun with the observation that motivation and professional conduct at times did not even approximate the ideal, we can now begin to understand why such lofty professional standards were well-nigh impossible to maintain: nurses experienced a variety of extrainstitutional pressures and temptations that could and did distract them from devoting their undivided attention to their work. The realities of life off-duty, however, were not the only operative factors underlying deviations from professional norms. Contradictions between the ideal and the actual within institutional life, as we shall now see, exerted their own specific pressures on nurses.

PROFESSIONAL AND PRIVATE LIFE UNDER ONE ROOF

The guiding principles of interstaff relations were ideally camaraderie and cooperation. On the basis of personnel records, it is difficult to say with certainty to what extent this ideal was generally upheld; it is certain, however, that those relations were extremely fragile. One reason for this was the rather mundane fact that nurses living in-house were confronted with the same faces both on duty and off, in a highly stressful environment, with no private space to which to withdraw, twenty-four hours a day. Polite relations, not to mention a sense of humor, were not always easy to maintain.

To the contrary, tempers could flare at the slightest, most harmless provocation. In February 1919, for example, at Eichberg, Nurse Knoll complained of harassment by his roommate, Nurse Mettler, in the wake of a practical joke. Mettler had allegedly returned to their room after his evening off, said, "Get up," and convinced Knoll that it was 6 A.M. and time to rise. Knoll had jumped out of bed and gotten dressed before being informed by another roommate that it was actually only 2:30 A.M. Nurse Knoll, not at all pleased, reproached Mettler, whereupon Mettler allegedly attacked Knoll, choked him, insulted him, and tore his jacket. Knoll added in conclusion that he believed Mettler to have been drunk.[26]

The investigation of the matter turned up several qualifiers to the story, namely, that the practical joke and the brawl had taken place on separate, consecutive evenings. Mettler claimed to have just returned to the room after his evening off when Knoll asked him whether it was time to get up. "Completely harmlessly," Mettler replied, "I said yes."[27] Knoll had not found the joke funny and had become angry; nothing more, however, had occurred on that evening. The following night, Knoll, whom Mettler believed to be drunk, had verbally harassed Mettler until the latter lost control and grabbed Knoll by the jacket. Knoll tore himself free, ripping his jacket in the process.[28]

Four other nurses who had witnessed the episode testified that Knoll was drunk, not Mettler, and that Knoll had certainly taunted Mettler relentlessly prior to Mettler's assault—in short, had asked for it.[29] This was apparently of no interest to the administration, however, which simply wanted to put an end to the matter. Disregarding most details in several pages of "testimony"—the counteraccusations, hearsay, and suppositions of both parties involved and their witnesses—it limited its concern to indisputable violations. In the end, the director reported, "K[noll] and M[ettler] are summoned. M[ettler] agrees to pay K[noll] for damages [to the jacket] and asks to be excused. Knoll is satisfied by this. Thus the matter is considered closed."[30]

The Politics of Authority and Betrayal in Everyday Life

Interstaff disputes involving patients were, as one might expect, a more serious matter for nurses on account of their disciplinary implications. Forbidden to physically coerce patients, and in any case outnumbered by them, nurses relied on their appearance as moral authorities to hold dozens of unpredictable and potentially unruly people in check. Patients who witnessed disputes among staff members discovered that their nurse was, in fact, *not* a model of decorum who was always under control but rather a being subject to the same human "vices" as they were. Moreover, a nurse who was not respected by his or her colleagues, or, worse, was reprimanded by a superior, gave patients no reason to heed his or her orders thenceforth. Once their vulnerability had been exposed during the course of some kind of interstaff row, nurses often found that, in the process, their authority had evaporated.

We see how sensitive nurses were to this possibility if we consider an incident at Berlin-Buch in September 1928, when Nurse Blau was reported by Senior Nurse Bersch for insubordination. The dispute arose after Nurses Blau and Knippel were caught in the garden in the forbidden act of taking a photograph on institutional grounds. Senior Nurse Bersch had intervened, asking them what was going on and reminding them that taking photographs was forbidden. Later, Nurse Blau stormed into his office, furious over having been reprimanded in front of patients.[31] Nurse Knippel had, for the purposes of assisting Nurse Blau, left his keys unattended on a table inside the building. He was, he later explained, convinced by the proximity of other nurses that the keys could not be stolen, but he was in any case reported along with Nurse Blau.[32]

During the investigation, Nurse Blau explained that he had recently bought himself a camera and, since he was not familiar with the instrument, had asked Nurse Knippel (an experienced photographer) to show him how to handle it. He knew, of course, that it was forbidden to take photographs, but he had only intended to make a private photo.[33] (After Nurse Knippel reported that he was only demonstrating how to *position* the camera, Nurse Blau changed his story accordingly, adding that he had no plates and couldn't actually have taken a photo even if he had wanted to.)[34] Senior Nurse Bersch had "screamed" at them in the presence of patients. Nurse Blau had merely gone to his office later to explain to him "in a calm way" that the camera was his own private property, and that *he* wasn't in the habit of making reproaches against Senior Nurse Bersch—when, for example, the latter shaved himself while on duty with soap that belonged to the city of Berlin.[35]

Senior Nurse Bersch refused, for his part, to agree that he had behaved offensively toward the nurses in any way and added on the side that he shaved with his *own* soap. He admitted, however, that perhaps he had spoken a bit loudly in the garden because they were outside, not in a closed room.[36] His tone, which of course is impossible to reproduce in a written file, seems indeed to be the crux of the matter, because even Nurse Blau admitted that, as far as content was concerned, Bersch had merely asked what was going on and reminded them that taking photographs in the institute was forbidden. Even so, however, he felt that Bersch had behaved "improperly. . . . so that I felt that I had been shown up in front of the patients. I couldn't possibly put up with this behavior."[37] Nurse Knippel also reported during his interrogation that "B[ersch] has recently and sometimes in the presence of patients behaved very inconsiderately toward me."[38]

There is no evidence in Nurse Blau's file that the administration formally acknowledged any wrongdoing on Senior Nurse Bersch's part, although it is certainly possible that he was informally requested, in the interests of staff morale, to observe the "rules of language" more closely. The central concern was what could be *unequivocally* recognized as wrongdoing on the basis of everyone's accounts. In that regard, it was clear that (1) Nurse Blau had made preparations to take private photos in a garden full of patients; and (2) Nurse Knippel had negligently left his keys unattended. The latter was, in the end, dealt with more severely on the basis of the security risk involved: he received a warning because of the danger that his keys could have been taken, while Nurse Blau received only a formal reprimand.[39] Be this as it may, the case indicates that nurses took their appearance of authority vis-à-vis patients very seriously indeed.

We can better understand *why* nurses were especially fearful of shattered authority if we turn to an incident at Berlin-Buch in 1926. Around 10 P.M. one evening in late November of that year, Nurse Siebert had difficulties controlling a violent patient and learned, after sending a colleague in search of the senior nurse, that neither the senior nurse nor her representative was to be found anywhere in the house. In the meantime, Siebert attempted to control the other forty patients under her supervision, but with less and less success. The unruly Patient W. had a bloody nose, was crying, and kept getting out of bed; another patient requested water, and other patients were becoming excited and unmanageable in the midst of all the commotion. Nurse Siebert sent her colleague in search of the senior nurse once again, this time with success.[40]

Senior Nurse Hamm entered the room cursing and uttering complaints about how the nurses didn't know how to handle patients. A short while later, as she stood among the patients combing Patient W.'s hair, she said, "The patients are treated like beasts" and "The nurses sit around and do handicrafts and do not look after the patients."[41]

Besides being untrue, Nurse Siebert later told the salaried employees committee (*Angestelltenrat*), these statements had had disastrous disciplinary consequences: the patients had become excited and unmanageable and complained about all the nurses. Patient W. had gotten out of bed frequently during the night and sat on the floor. Moreover, this kind of talk was not an isolated incident; she and other nurses had repeatedly been chastised in front of patients by the senior nurse. The result was that "the nurses thus lose all authority over the patients; the patients will not listen to the nurses anymore but rather become unmanageable and refer instead to the senior nurse. Thus the work of the nurses is unnecessarily made considerably more difficult."[42] The committee agreed with her and ruled that Senior Nurse

Hamm must apologize.[43] Nurse Siebert, personally insulted and professionally undermined by a superior, seemed to have "won" the dispute.

Two other factors, however, are of interest: first of all, buried in this anecdote is the absence of the senior nurse during her shift—a serious violation, if true. Indeed, the chairman remarked that Senior Nurse Hamm had been seen in the vicinity of the Berlin-Buch station around the time of the incident. In the end, however, no disciplinary measures were taken against her for leaving her post. She denied having been out of the house, and there was no other proof of a violation, but the heart of the matter seems to be her "place" among all the participants in the dispute. That is, she was opposed to Nurse Siebert and allied with the administration.

This alliance had grave implications for Siebert, because the bloody nose and general disorder during the night in question prompted the administration to lodge countercharges of "unsuitability" against her and the colleague who had assisted her. Several patients were questioned in connection with this charge and reported having been mishandled (although they didn't say by whom).[44] Siebert reported two weeks later, however, that one of the patients had approached her, crying bitterly, and said that "she [Siebert] shouldn't be angry at her any more; she had been constantly ordered by Senior Nurse H[amm] simply to say that she had seen Nurse S[iebert] striking Patient W."[45] The administration responded to this news by questioning the credibility of a mentally ill patient and concluding that there did not seem to be grounds for any particular action against the senior nurse.[46] In the end, thanks to its unflagging support, no disciplinary action was taken against her.[47]

We see, then, that nurses were expected to control dozens of patients with the only viable tool at their disposal, namely, their appearance as an authority. They were instructed to "fall back," so to speak, on the authority of their superiors in the event of disciplinary problems. Yet when a senior nurse undercut their authority in the presence of patients, thus betraying them in the most damaging way possible, the administration supported senior staff in the face of the most incriminating evidence. Even worse, it betrayed the nurses as well by blaming them for the chaos caused by the senior nurse's behavior.

This was not a unique incident at the Berlin-Buch institution. One spring evening four years later, Nurses Degen and Kratz had difficulties calming down a patient who refused to stay in bed. Nurse Degen sent Nurse Kratz in search of Deputy Senior Nurse Gimbel to request permission to transfer the patient to another station. Gimbel, however, neither responded verbally nor opened her door in response to the knock, despite the fact that she had been seen fifteen minutes earlier and was therefore certainly still awake. The next day, Nurse Degen explained to Nurse Gimbel that the patient had assaulted her. Gimbel was unsympathetic, to say the least, chastising Nurse Degen for sending someone for assistance and remarking that if she was afraid of the patients, she was not a suitable nurse. This response brought Nurse Degen to tears, to which Gimbel responded, "She is more excited than a mentally ill person."[48]

In her own defense, Gimbel claimed not to have heard the knock; moreover, she had said that Nurse Degen was crying like a "sick person" (*Kranke*), not a "mentally ill person" (*Geisteskranke*). Since there was no way of proving that she had indeed heard the knock, the Berlin-Buch administration did not see any reason to discipline her on the basis of these claims. It simply suggested that the problem could be avoided in the future through the installation of electric bells on the doors.[49]

This was a far from satisfactory solution to the problem from the salaried employees committee's point of view. The following month, it lodged a complaint with the staff council charging the administration with an "inadequate investigation" of the case and taking unsatisfactory measures against Gimbel. In particular, it called the administration's attention to the potential problems that could arise from its superficial treatment of the complaints: "When the deputy director in charge does not address the established grievances of nursing personnel as requested, then it is demonstrated that a completely unsuitable and unusable deputy senior nurse is being protected in an irresponsible way. Thus the staff's faith in justice could possibly be shaken. The nursing personnel are thereby depressed; pleasure in work and in the profession is diminished. Also, the patients could thereby possibly be endangered."[50]

The investigation thus continued, with Gimbel adding an interesting further defense: even if she *had* heard the door, it was not her job, as deputy senior nurse, to respond at that hour of the night when the "real" senior nurse, Holz, was in-house. The senior nurse, she reminded the committee, was a civil servant and thus obligated to be available around the clock, whereas she was "subject the same contract as the other nurses and had already worked [her] eight-hour shift (2–10 P.M.)."[51]

This in itself says a great deal about her degree of professional dedication, but the committee's review of other complaints over the course of the following months revealed her to be extremely unpopular among her colleagues as well. Her alleged offenses, however, were considered minor and in any case unprovable. The Berlin-Buch administration defended her to the end, adding in this second round of investigation that it had warned her about derogatory language like "crying like a mentally ill person"—regardless of whether "sick person" or "mentally ill person" was the offending term.[52] After six months of discussion of the case, the city administration (which, as her "official" employer, was of necessity entangled in the proceedings) was beginning to lose patience, chiding the staff council for spending far too much time on the case and exaggerating its seriousness through the use of juridical language.[53] In March of the following year, it put a formal end to the matter by conceding that Deputy Senior Nurse Gimbel could have been more circumspect on certain points but flatly rejecting the employees committee's demand for her removal.[54]

Lower-level nurses were thus victims of a double standard: they were expected to control patients through the manifestation of authority even after that authority had been deliberately shattered by precisely those who were supposed to support them. The salaried employees committee, we have learned, was quite aware of the psychological gravity of this betrayal in the eyes of the nurses and its implications for their morale. It also, not at all incidentally, exercised enough leverage in these cases to save their jobs. But it did not have enough leverage to break the bond of solidarity between higher-level nursing staff and an administration that did not take nurses' complaints nearly as seriously. The Berlin-Buch nurses sought impartial mediation of these disputes but found themselves sent back to their wards for business as usual.

THUS we see how interstaff politics and administrative favoritism of senior staff could derail nurses' efforts to live up to the professional ideal. With this last example, however, we have touched upon yet a further dimension of the problem that could spoil even the most concerted attempts among nurses to conform to the norms of professional conduct, namely, the fact that they were responsible not only for their own conduct but also for any trouble their *patients* got into while under their supervision.

Just how serious even a minor oversight could become is revealed by an incident at Wittenau one morning in July 1932, when Nurse Weber was supposed to accompany a patient from her sleeping quarters downstairs into the main rooms of the institution. As the senior doctor later reported, she had instead simply let the patient go on her own. This, of course, constituted a violation of the "no trust" rule—that is, nurses were never to place their trust in patients on the basis of their own assessment of a patient's reliability or goodwill. Some patients, psychiatrists warned, would betray that trust and use their freedom to escape.

This, in fact, is precisely what had happened. The patient had not gone downstairs but rather had gone to the unlocked nurses' dressing room on the top floor, dressed herself in a nurse's clothing, proceeded to an unlocked room in which two nurses were sleeping, taken a bunch of keys from there, and escaped. Luckily, the patient had been apprehended at the rear exit, but Nurse Weber was issued a warning.[55] This was the end of the affair; the rest of her career passed relatively uneventfully, and she remained at Wittenau beyond her twenty-fifth year of service until her death in 1943.[56]

The patient's escape produced a blemish on Weber's record because it was a clear act of negligence. Weber was aware of the procedural requirement to watch patients at all times and of the more abstract, but no less clear, requirement never to place one's trust in a patient. From an administrative standpoint, Weber's violations were obvious and had been easily avoidable. From the perspective of nurses, however, such mishaps were not always completely avoidable for the simple reason that, as in any professional environment, rules were occasionally ignored—sometimes out of laziness, but sometimes in recognition of the fact that cutting corners was far more sensible in certain circumstances than blindly following cumbersome rules; indeed, to the overburdened and exhausted nurse, such abberations could even have appeared to be justified. Everyone in the work environment participated in a kind of solidarity of silence that kept minor and inconsequential violations out of administrative view. The stakes for psychiatric nurses in this game of chance were high, however, because an act of negligence that on one day was without consequence and quickly forgotten could, on another day, land a nurse in court.

Precisely this came to pass at Eichberg in early April 1931, when Patient S. killed herself by jumping off the roof of a building. She had done so with the help of Patient M., who was in possession of a key to virtually all the doors in the house except the main door, including that leading to the roof. On the fateful evening, the suicidal woman had apparently arranged to meet Patient M. at this door, tricked the latter into opening the door for her, and jumped to her death. Nurse Greta Becker, who had night duty at the time and had given Patient M. the key, was tried by the district court for negligence later that month.[57]

Nurse Becker defended herself with the argument that Patient M. was a long-term patient who was "absolutely reliable" and "enlisted in the most varied types of work." For this purpose, she was routinely given the station key when necessary by all nurses on the station with the knowledge of the senior nurse. (To be sure, Nurse Becker could not say whether the house's doctor or the director was aware of the procedure.)[58] This was apparently a suitable enough defense to cause the district attorney to suspend the trial one month later.[59] The head of the local government (*Landeshauptmann*) ordered that a new lock be put on the door to the roof taking its own key and no others.[60] Although it is unclear whether the case was pursued in other directions (against, for example, the senior nurse who knew that the key was routinely given to the patient), Nurse Becker did not suffer lasting administrative consequences; she remained in service at Eichberg until 1947.[61]

The formal acknowledgment of a violation and the initiation of disciplinary procedures depended, then, on its consequences. Becker, after all, wound up in court not because a patient under her supervision had a key without formal permission, but rather because this state of affairs had enabled a patient to commit suicide. Had nothing extraordinary happened on that night, we can be fairly certain that the key would have been given to Patient M. as usual the next day: that is, she would have remained the object of a tacit, *collective* trust which saved nurses the trouble of being constantly pestered to lock and unlock doors for patients. Questions of accountability for this state of affairs could be indefinitely postponed in the minds of the nurses involved because it was deemed highly unlikely that they would ever crop up, and because they could take refuge in the "gap" of accountability created by the collective, silent nature of sanction: no one had explicitly permitted Becker to give the patient the key; but no one forbade it either, and everyone knew. This case suggests that everyday institutional life contained mechanisms for accommodating, both psychologically and legally, certain violations of professional duty. Central to the process was *keeping such violations in the realm of collective silence* and hoping for the best.

The case begs the question of how nurses responded when questions of accountability could no longer be postponed— when injury, escape, or death shattered the solidarity of silence and demanded the location and articulation of accountability.

Nurse Becker, as we have seen, defended herself by reminding the court that, although she was guilty of giving the key to the patient, the collective, silent, ongoing character of the procedure somehow rendered her *less* responsible for its tragic result. This feeling that violations were somehow beyond reproach if they were common or routine was not unique—in fact, it manifested itself in the most common, unspectacular violations of staff discipline. For example, when caught sleeping on duty one night in 1921 and subsequently lectured by the senior nurse, Eichberg nurse Mettler allegedly retorted, "Go ahead and report me, you only check up on me, the others—never." (Mettler himself only admitted to saying, "If I've made a mistake, then report me," but was fined five marks for "impertinent behavior" toward the senior nurse.)[62] In his eyes, being disciplined for a violation of regulations per se was not as traumatic as being singled out while others went unchecked and, thus, unpunished. This episode reflects a more general phenomenon: discipline from a senior nurse was perceived as a breach of a tacit understanding whereby everyone looked the other way when minor rules were broken. (Hence the almost invariable response of pointing fingers at the unchecked violations of other nurses.) A nurse who happened to be the one "selected" for punishment thus felt unjustly treated.

By making explicit reference to the existence of such an understanding and to the fact that the senior nurse had betrayed it, Mettler (and, even more vividly, Blau) introduced psychological weapons into the dispute. Although their position at the bottom of the medical hierarchy rendered them helpless in the face of disciplinary procedures, they attempted to exploit what little manipulative power they had: the power to accuse superiors of violating the informal, but abundantly clear, norms of the nursing "community" within the institution, and to recharacterize discipline as the arbitrary abuse of power. This phenomenon poses the possibility that lower-level nurses verbally pressured *each other* to respect the informal rules and "secret" violations of the staff community as well.

The Limits of Mitigating Circumstances: A Case of Abuse

Up to this point, we have encountered a variety of institutional circumstances that contributed to nurses' deviations from the ideal: the stresses of collective life under one roof, the betrayal of colleagues and administrators, the unpredictability of patients, and the tension between rules and collectively sanctioned (or at least collectively tolerated) deviance. But if this last item was part of the nurse's problem, we have seen that it was also part of the solution: having had the misfortune to be singled out and accused of "bending" the rules in a way that was general and routine, nurses could invoke that very collective nature of the practice as a moral alibi—with the resulting claim that perhaps they had done something wrong, but they should not be held responsible for it. In other words, the more general discrepancy between the ideal and the actual in daily institutional practice not only tempted nurses to stray from prescribed rules; it was *appropriated* by them and used in self-defense when their errors became visible and subject to discipline.

We have seen above how this process worked among generally well-meaning nurses; but in addition, the case of Wittenau's Nurse Herta Meyer demonstrates that mitigating circumstances were marshaled by nurses who had not simply strayed from the rules but were guilty of patient abuse. The daughter of a shoemaker with an elementary education and household training, Meyer was typical of women who took up psychiatric nursing during the Weimar Republic. She was hired at Wittenau in 1920 and proved to be somewhat of an administrative problem from the beginning: she was frequently late for work, sick, and suspected of faking illness.[63] She was also disciplined in 1925 for treating a patient "not according to regulations" after the suspicion of abuse could not be confirmed.[64]

An episode in April 1931 would prove her undoing. Patient C. wrote to her parents,

Dear Mother and Father,

Take me out of here, I've been beaten by a Nurse M. Arm twisted, towel bound around [my] mouth, towel then wrapped around [my] throat, then she hit me on the head, then she tore my jacket off my body. All the patients [who now admit that they saw] it can describe it to you. I would like to ask [you] to come from the 25th to the 29th [of April]. Write to Senior Doctor P. that I would like to get out of here.[65]

This was in itself clearly a serious matter, if true; but in addition, Doctor P. reported that one week earlier he had issued a severe warning to Nurse Meyer because she had tied the hand of an unruly patient to a bedpost, causing swelling and temporary neuroparalysis. At the time, he had refrained from making a formal report of the incident, but the present situation called for a thorough investigation of Nurse Meyer's recent conduct.[66]

Dr. R. and his colleague Dr. P. confronted a terribly vexing problem: the possibility that a patient's psychosis could produce a false accusation. The problem was particularly acute in this case because the accused party was an eleven-year veteran. Patients could lie; but they also could tell the truth. Moreover, nurses could lie as well, especially when their jobs were at stake. The doctors could not simply mediate the dispute "from the outside" by hearing testimony; they had to bring their professional expertise to bear and evaluate the credibility of those involved.

Thus they began their investigation by identifying six patients and seven female nurses who had something to say about the course of both events, and each doctor proceeded to take separate detailed statements from all of them. Patients' mental condition and the coherence of their separate accounts were then assessed and a general evaluation made of their credibility. Proceeding in this fashion, Drs. R. and P. soon learned that the incident had occurred during lunch one day after the patients had returned from their morning's work. Patient C. had asked for more sauce from Nurse Roos, who was about to oblige when Nurse Meyer intervened and said no, she should not be given any more. Patient C. then refused to finish what was left on her plate.

From that point, the picture of what had happened was not entirely clear. The seven patient witnesses interrogated the following week were virtually unanimous in stating that Nurse Meyer had twisted the patient's arm, wrapped a towel around her mouth and/or her neck, and dragged her from the table with it. Some also noted that Patient C. screamed, "Help," "I'm suffocating," and threatened to bite in self-defense; that Nurse Meyer hit her head against the wall, slapped her, and tore her jacket off.[67] The only patient who disputed the accusation was put forward for questioning by Nurse Meyer herself and was, as the doctors noted, an "outspoken liar of a pathological type."[68] No other nurses witnessed the incident itself, but Nurse Roos, who had left the room beforehand to throw the remaining sauce away, deemed Nurse Meyer's denial of a second portion unwarranted. Moreover, several senior nurses reported patient complaints about Nurse Meyer's "rough treatment."[69]

Nurse Meyer gave a radically different account of the proceedings: Patient C. had become disruptive after being denied more sauce, pushed her food onto the floor, tipped over a chair, and tried to bite her. Nurse Meyer had tried to calm her down by talking to her and *holding* her arm. Patient C. had violently twisted herself around, thus injuring the arm. Nurse Meyer had only grasped a towel to wipe off Patient C.'s mouth. As for the case of the patient tied to the bed, she maintained that she had *found* the patient in this condition.[70]

Here, Meyer presented a classic (if unconvincing) self-defense argument and, in so doing, attempted to exploit one of the chief dilemmas in psychiatric administration. On the one hand, as we have seen earlier, nurses were absolutely forbidden to strike or otherwise abuse patients, despite being provoked on a daily basis by behavior that was, by all appearances, deliberately perverse and aggressive. On the other hand, they *were* permitted to defend themselves with certain prescribed techniques and had ample occasion to do so; nurses were often injured and in rare cases even killed by patients. The problem of distinguishing abuse from self-defense in individual cases and on the basis of conflicting testimony, in other words, was a very real one, and it presented Meyer with the opportunity to cast the alleged abuse in an entirely different and, from her perspective, more favorable light: she had not twisted the patient's arm; she had held the arm and the patient twisted her body(!). Although splitting hairs, Meyer knew that this portrayal—if accepted—was the difference between accidental injury and abuse, between saving her job and landing on the street.

Alas for her, it was not accepted. Interrogation of other nurses did not produce any clarification of her guilt or innocence in tying the patient to the bed; but Dr. R. concluded that regardless of this, and even by the mildest interpretation, the lunchtime incident was a "gross violation of regulations and strong suspicion of direct abuse." He proposed that she be dismissed.[71]

Over the course of the following year, Nurse Meyer made a number of attempts to save her eleven-year-old career; she was allowed to continue working on a different station for the first five months of that time. First she took her case to the employees committee, which supported her against Wittenau and the city of Berlin during her trial before the labor court (*Arbeitsgericht*). The committee argued that Nurse Meyer's behavior constituted not abuse but rather "inappropriate" (*unzweckmäßig*) treatment; a simple warning would have been commensurate with the seriousness of the violation. It deemed dismissal an "undue hardship." Wittenau argued, to the contrary, that the testimonies of patients were coherent and consistent on the main points and adequately sustained the charges at hand. Moreover, this was not an isolated incident; Nurse Meyer had already been the subject of abuse allegations and had received a warning.[72]

In the first round of court proceedings in September 1931, the court claimed not to be able to determine with certainty that the incident was a case of abuse and not self-defense, and sought instead to introduce a compromise: a transfer to the Herzberge institution would allow her to continue work and would satisfy Wittenau's desire to be rid of her. The city of Berlin, however (which, together with Wittenau, was the defendant) refused to retain her in any of its institutions. She was not to be allowed to return to work.[73]

The compromise having been rejected, the trial was to proceed. In the meantime, Meyer tried another tactic. She presented her case to the mayor of Berlin in a long, sentimental letter that she began by congratulating him on his silver wedding anniversary before proceeding to the matter at hand: she had been the victim of grave injustice, and she was turning to him, as her "highest superior, in whom I trust," to defend her.

The first strategy she deployed was to attack the credibility of the witnesses. She had been accused of forcibly feeding a patient, and "even though these patients are longtime mentally ill [persons], this accusation against me was strangely enough believed by the doctor!" Second, she appealed to his sense of justice. The Wittenau administration had rewarded her cooperation in the investigation with dishonesty and betrayal: she had agreed to a transfer to another station at Wittenau with the prospect of a later transfer to Herzberge; moreover, during an informal conversation in the institution's garden several days previously, the director had reassured her that she would soon receive word of a decision in her favor—but she was still dismissed!

Third, and finally, she sought to awaken his sense of sympathy. Holding nothing back, she detailed her history as a respectable, industrious person and a devoted daughter and sister: since her father's death in 1926, she had cared for her mother and prevented her from becoming a burden to the community. One brother had been killed in the war; the other had been blinded and lived with their mother. She had supported five of her siblings, providing some of the money for their professional training. With no job, she could not possibly continue to fulfill her familial responsibilities.[74]

There is no evidence in Nurse Meyer's personnel file as to whether this letter was answered, but it did not ultimately alter the final outcome: in November 1931 the court ruled that the dismissal should be upheld. The question of whether it constituted an "undue hardship," it explained, could be evaluated only in conjunction with the rights and responsibilities of the defendant. In this case, Wittenau administrators had an obligation to the public to ensure that those entrusted to their care were nursed and not abused. The interests of the patients took priority, and the existence of a reasonable doubt about the reliability of their caretakers was sufficient cause for dismissal. The available testimony, in its view, sustained that doubt.[75]

Nurse Meyer refused to accept this, but the employees committee declined to pursue the matter, deeming an appeal "pointless." She next took her case to a lawyer, who apparently intended to pit the testimony of unreliable, manipulable psychiatric patients against that of a mentally healthy veteran nurse, and to "reveal" a bit of intrigue on Nurse Meyer's station whereby Patient C. had been encouraged by another rival nurse to stir up trouble.[76] This case went before the district labor court (*Landesarbeitsgericht*) but was immediately dismissed as "pointless" as well; the lawyer withdrew the appeal, and the city of Berlin considered the matter closed.[77]

The suicide of Dr. R. in May 1932 presented Meyer—or so she thought—with another opportunity to open her case. In a letter to the Wittenau Directorate, she noted that according to the *Berliner Volkszeitung*, Dr. R. had increasingly distanced himself from his family and colleagues during his last months of life and devoted his entire interest to the "pitiable patients." This fact, she believed, cast the administrative investigation of her case in a different light: the interrogations carried out by Drs. P. and R. were, owing to Dr. R's condition, naturally predestined to support Patient C. She was not guilty of abuse but, rather, a victim of untimely circumstances.[78] Although she combined this reasoning with reminders about her personal woes and disciplinary injustice at Wittenau, the administration remained unmoved: Dr. P. wrote a memo in which he reiterated the validity of the investigation, adding that the incident in question had taken place several months before the onset of Dr. R.'s depression. The administration sent her a brief note formally rejecting her request several days later.[79]

This response was in no way satisfactory to Meyer. In another long missive to the director, she reiterated her claim that the proceedings were biased and arbitrary, that psychiatric patients are

not reliable witnesses, and that she had been duped by a hypo-
critical employees committee that made a token defense but in
the end did not want to bite the hand that fed it. Moreover, she
added, "You, Herr Director, told me yourself during a meeting
in the institution's garden that I should just wait, the affair
would come out to my advantage and was not yet over, and so
forth. I hung on your words because you know me so well and
treasure my work capability, which is certainly just as valuable
as any other in the operation of the institution."[80] Meyer's attempt to stir the director's sense of guilt in this fashion was unsuccessful; three days later, he curtly responded, "The decision
given to you on June 8, 1932, must remain."[81]

INVESTIGATING patient abuse was, regardless of the incident in
question, an exceedingly ugly affair for all involved. Patients
themselves, who were utterly helpless vis-à-vis their caretakers,
could never be certain that their accusations would be taken seriously. Administrators were legally responsible for mediating
the claims of nurses who, although sane and often experienced,
had good reasons to cover up abuse, and of patients, whose
medical condition *could* produce false accusations. Nurses, finally, lived with the possibility that they could be falsely accused
and unfairly dismissed, and the demand to cooperate in investigations of false accusations must have been difficult to swallow:
they were, after all, asked to accept gracefully the suspicion that
they had not simply broken a rule but assaulted an innocent and
defenseless person. As the official bearers of that suspicion, administrators were put in a terribly awkward position.

Precisely this awkwardness, however, could work to the advantage of those guilty of abuse; such nurses could attempt to
save their jobs and their honor by incredulously denying the
charges (thus possibly exerting psychological pressure on the arbitrators), exploiting the false-accusation issue, splitting hairs
over who held and who twisted an arm, pointing to other violations that went unpunished, and invoking a variety of other
potentially mitigating circumstances. For them, too, a "gap" presented itself whereby they could attempt to escape accountabil-

ity. They simply had to *create the appearance* that things had not happened as the accuser reported them, and that the accused was in fact the victim.

As we have seen earlier, this was attempted even if—and perhaps especially if—one could not entirely free oneself of guilt. Nurse Meyer maintained that even if she were guilty of a violation of official regulations, the penalty was too severe. Realizing that she faced damaging testimony, she was apparently ready to concede wrongdoing and accept punishment up to the point where it cost her that job. Most important, in her view, was that she portray herself convincingly as a victim; consequently, her arguments appealed to administrators' sense of sympathy and justice. Avoiding discussion of the incident itself, she attempted to place her own person and her own miserable fate at the center of the administration's deliberations and, perhaps, awaken a sense that, as her *employer*, it had a certain responsibility to protect her, as an *employee*, against damaging allegations.

If it is indeed true that the director spoke privately to Meyer in the institution's garden and assured her that she would be retained, she may in fact have had some measure of success. That is, administrators may very well have been divided among themselves over whether to retain Meyer or dismiss her in the interests of the institution's reputation. The incident's resolution would thus have been a far less straightforward matter than the verdict would lead us to believe.

Be this as it may, it is nevertheless the case that, when it came time for a decision, strong suspicion of abuse could not be brushed aside. What Meyer failed to understand (or perhaps understood but could not overcome) is that Wittenau and the city of Berlin in no way felt bound to a principle of "innocent until proven guilty" or obligated to heed nurses' personal problems. They were not only her employer; they were also, and in the first instance, keepers of the public trust. When disputes of this nature arose, the institution's primary responsibility was to the public that entrusted its family members to their care. Upholding that responsibility meant that the "rules" of democratic jurisprudence, which gave the individual the benefit of the doubt, did not apply. Rather, the existence of a reasonable doubt about the employee's reliability was sufficient cause for dismissal. Nurse Meyer could deploy arguments that called the validity of the investigation into question and pointed to her impending financial ruin, but she was unable in the end to dispel that doubt. The ability of appearances and mitigating circumstances to salvage the career of a less-than-"ideal" nurse thus found its limit in a violation that was not only severe but also, and more important, known beyond the institution's walls.

5

Cleaning House in Wittenau:
1933 and the Law for the Restoration
of the Professional Civil Service

THE YEAR 1933 brought the end of employees committees and due process in institutional management. Trade
unions were abolished, the compulsory German Labor Front
took their place, and the National Socialist Cell Organizations
(NSBO) saw to it that the Party remained intimately involved in
hiring and firing decisions.[1] In psychiatric institutions, as in the
population at large, this first year of National Socialist rule
would bring with it a bureaucratic restructuring whereby not
only rules and precedents but also people would simply be done
away with—albeit under the *guise* of legal sanction—in accordance with Party mandates.

A cornerstone of this process was the "Law for the Restoration
of the Professional Civil Service" of April 7—a misnomer that
could not disguise for long the Party's intention to effect personnel changes neither legally nor in a spirit of restoration but
rather to purge politically unreliable or otherwise undesirable
elements and demand *Kadavergehorsam*, or corpselike obedience, from the rest.[2] When one considers that the decree encom-
passed not only Germany's 1.5 million civil servants (*Beamte*)
but also thousands of workers (*Arbeiter*) and salaried employees
(*Angestellte*) in public service,[3] it becomes clear why it had great
potential for disrupting essential public services and of alien-
ating a politically and economically significant sector of the
population.[4]

It was thus much to Hitler's detriment that he and his party, although deeply suspicious of the Weimar civil service, had no clear ideas about the future function of this institution when they took power in early 1933 and produced half-baked "legislation" as a result; the decree can be considered a seriously thought-out policy statement only insofar as it manifested the intention to eliminate Jews and Communists. Although the decree's architects recognized the need to sustain some semblance of fair treatment, they did not initially foresee that doing so, and doing the job thoroughly, would require that virtually *everyone* eligible be subjected to the time-consuming, paper-pushing review process which was originally foreseen only for people who could already be "assumed" to fall under specific paragraphs. The decree was intended to be fully implemented by September 30, 1933, but this administrative snowball effect required that the date be pushed forward to the end of March 1934. It would not be long before the decree's effects would begin to be rolled back; by the end of 1935, some people dismissed under the law were being considered for rehiring. After the war broke out, many more would find that the force of circumstance had created a new place for them, too, in public service.[5]

Implementational difficulties were accompanied by precisely the kind of alienation the decree's architects had hoped to avoid. Karl-Dietrich Bracher writes, "In fact, during the application time of the civil servant law there existed no more reliable guarantee of civil servant rights. . . . uncertainty spread swiftly and widely until it was all-encompassing, so that the fear of being affected was no less devastating than actually being affected."[6] The decree (hereafter referred to as *Berufsbeamtengesetz*, or BBG) thus not only reconstituted the racial and political profile of civil and public service; it also reconstituted the criteria of professional survival in such a way that an individual could no longer predict, and thus control, his or her fate. There is, thus, a great deal to be learned about the BBG—and a great deal to be learned *from* it—if we consider not only the numbers of people dismissed but also the discourse surrounding its implementation and other psychological "indicators" that escape interpretation through quantification.

Statistical information on the number of firings among psychiatric nurses is in any case currently inconclusive. Particularly unfortunate for the current study is the absence of documentation of the number of Wittenau personnel dismissed under the BBG—although witnesses estimate that 30–40 people (an unspecified percentage thereof being nurses) were dismissed out of an approximate total of 400–500 nurses.[7] Available figures for the Berlin-Buch institution suggest that approximately one nurse in nine was dismissed.[8] But sample statistics from other institutions leave the impression that, generally speaking, the decree was at best an incidental event for psychiatric nurses in 1933—or at least one whose effects were limited to a small number of them: at the psychiatric institution near Konstanz, only two male nurses (former members of the German Communist Party, or KPD) were dismissed out of at least 60 nurses; former members of the German Social Democratic Party, or SPD, were permitted to remain.[9] At the Waldheim institution in Saxony, there appears to have been only one dismissal out of approximately 60 nurses, and no other sign of administrative turbulence.[10]

While this may have indeed been the case at some institutions, several richly documented cases of BBG dismissals from the Wittenauer Heilstätten demonstrate that administrative business-as-usual cannot have prevailed everywhere.[11] While one must be careful not to exaggerate the results of a case-study analysis, the story of the BBG's implementation at Wittenau offers a glimpse into the psychological ramifications of the BBG. It suggests that for administrators, for dismissed nurses, and for their colleagues who remained, the decree was by no means incidental but rather a point around which survival instincts, opportunism, and political and apolitical emotions crystallized, and whose precedents would shape future administrative practice.

By way of orientation, let us briefly examine the formalities of the review procedure at Wittenau, over which administrative director Karl Braasch (who called himself the "King of Wittenau") presided.[12] The first observation to be made is that, consistent with the general observations above, implementation of the BBG at Wittenau was characterized in its early months by confusion and lack of formality. Although the decree was issued on April 7, some nurses who would be later dismissed under the anti-Communist paragraph of the law received memos as early as March 25th informing them of their impending dismissal: "At the instigation of the Prussian state commissioner for the Health Service of the city of Berlin, you are hereby provisionally dismissed from public service effective September 30, 1933."[13] Another memo issued on April 25th ventured closer to the matters at hand: "On the orders of the state commissioner in observance of the duties of the city medical adviser, the termination of your employment as nurse effective September 30, 1933, announced on March 25, 1933, will go into effect at the given point in time on suspicion of views hostile to the state."[14] Ideological zeal notwithstanding, however, Party bureaucrats apparently realized that dismissal based on "suspicion" alone would never do. After all, it might miss those lucky enough not to have been denounced; but in addition, its glaring lack of due process would undoubtedly cause widespread alarm among those potentially subject to dismissal. Thus their next move in a long series of implementational clarifications and revisions was to introduce questionnaires that asked for personal information, family history, and the details of all former political activity. (As noted above, these were originally intended to be required only from candidates who could already be "assumed" to fall under one of the law's provisions.) Indeed, Wittenau nurses, including those whose only known liability, if any, was absenteeism, dutifully filled out the *Fragebogen zur Durchführung des Gesetzes zur Wiederherstellung des Berufsbeamtentums vom 7. April 1933 bei Angestellten und Arbeitern* (hereafter referred to as *Berufsbeamtengesetz*, or BBG, questionnaire).[15] If nothing damaging was reported, and suspicion of political unreliability did not already exist, the Wittenau administration decided whether to try to dismiss the nurse for other, nonpolitical reasons—which, as we shall see, was absolutely permissible under the sixth "unpolitical" paragraph of the decree, enabling dismissal "for the simplification of administration."

Those who reported membership in a "Marxist" party or were suspected of harboring left-wing sympathies were instructed to fill out an additional *Fragebogen gemäß Anordnung des Staatskommissars in der Hauptstadt Berlin vom 8. August 1933* (hereafter referred to as supplemental questionnaire). The questions to be answered were as follows:

1. Have you declared your withdrawal from the (Marxist) party? Simply ceasing dues payments can by no means count as a withdrawal.
2. When and to whom did you properly declare your withdrawal? What proof can you provide for it?
3. Was a declaration of withdrawal somehow impossible because the party was dissolved in the meantime?
4. Are there witnesses who are recognized as nationally trustworthy, who can testify that you [had] already expressed your support for the National Socialist government in terms of participation before March 5, 1933?[16]

Next, the representative of Wittenau's NSBO reviewed the information given and, on the reverse side of the supplemental questionnaire, filled in a form asserting or denying that the nurse had "proven through his/her personal behavior that he/she wants to participate in constructing the state in the spirit of National Socialism and is also suitable for it."[17] At that point, as we shall see in more detail shortly, the Wittenau administration decided whether to make a recommendation for dismissal and sent its paperwork to the Office of the Mayor for approval. The next stage was formal dismissal issued by Brandenburg's governor (*Oberpräsident*) effective September 30, 1933, at the latest, which could be appealed by the nurse within two weeks. (As noted earlier, the period of implementation was later extended to the end of March 1934.)[18]

At this point, it is already clear that nurses with former left-wing affiliation were going to have a difficult time saving themselves from dismissal if they had not *explicitly* renounced that affiliation and then *actively* demonstrated support for National Socialism. The supplemental questionnaire reveals that simply ceasing dues payments did not count; lapsing into political inactivity was not enough. In addition, we have a "preview" of another important element in the review process, namely, the testimony of third parties. The fourth question suggests that it was not enough for nurses of questionable political reliability to affirm their commitment to the National Socialist State themselves; they had to *demonstrate* through the testimony of others that they meant what they said—or at least had convinced others accordingly. Already, we see a pattern emerging where nurses were guilty until proven innocent.

Due Process and the Art of Convincing: The Dismissal of Ex-Communists and Socialists

The second paragraph of the BBG read in part as follows:

> §2
>
> (1)
> Civil servants, who became civil servants after November 9, 1918, without the required or usual educational background or other suitability for their career, are to be dismissed from service. . . .[19]

This paragraph aimed to oust civil servants whose appointments during the Weimar Republic had been strictly acts of political patronage—the so-called *Parteibuchbeamte*.[20] Predictably, it simply substituted one form of political patronage for another, since the clause "or other suitability" provided a basis for exempting National Socialist sympathizers from §2 dismissals and ensured that Communist civil servants would go—as an addendum of April 11 made clear:

> to §2
>
> (1)
> Unsuitable are all civil servants who belong to the Communist Party or to Communist aid or reserve organizations. They are therefore to be dismissed.[21]

The second implementation ordinance of May 4, 1933, extended these measures to salaried employees and workers in public service.[22]

Theoretically, Wittenau's salaried nurses with a history of Communist involvement could be excepted from dismissal if they had belonged to a party or association that supported the National Socialists for "a rather long time"—or at least since January 1931.[23] Thus administrators were not simply to dismiss nurses with former left-wing affiliation; they were, rather, to identify this blemish on the nurse's record *and* consider it alongside potentially redeeming variables such as time and duration of membership, subsequent attempts to "atone" for this political "error," and Party representatives' estimation of the nurse's overall political reliability. Research for the current study turned up several mixtures of these factors which suggest that, contrary to the possibilities of redemption embedded in this procedural formula, the outlook for nurses with a history of Communist association, no matter how minor, was very bleak indeed.

Friedrich Blau, whom we encountered in the previous chapter, entered psychiatric nursing in 1926 and, after several transfers, landed at Wittenau in January 1931. He had been a member of the Communist Party relatively recently (1929–1932) when he filled out his BBG questionnaire, and had no serious political involvement since that time. He was, on that basis alone, a clear case for dismissal, and dismissed he was; it is instructive, however, to take note of the arguments on his own behalf that the administration chose to ignore, which he appended to his BBG questionnaire.

He had, he admitted, belonged to the KPD from 1929 to the end of 1932; his membership, however, had nothing to do with political inclination. He was a disabled war veteran with a wife and five children to feed. A foot injury prevented him from finding work, and his multiple applications for orthopedic shoes had been repeatedly rejected during the early Weimar years. His attempts to survive within the parameters of the existing health and labor bureaucracies, in short, went nowhere—and only with the help of the Communist Party had he finally been able to acquire both the necessary shoes and suitable employment. "After this time," he wrote, "I was constantly encouraged to become a member of the party and reminded each time of the advantages I'd had . . . and in 1929 I was talked into it and became a member. What I . . . have to recognize is that I was fundamentally misled."[24] He added that he had not taken part in the KPD's activities, such as collecting signatures or membership drives; he had not participated in demonstrations because of his foot ailment. In 1932 "irregularities" were discovered in the conduct of his local branch of the party in Berlin's Wedding district, which as a consequence withdrew from the International. He had taken the opportunity at that point to withdraw from the party itself.[25]

Blau had, quite harmlessly, supported a party that had done something for him—not, in itself, such a heinous act by most accounts. But, apparently quite aware of the magnitude and nature of recent political developments, Blau knew better than to present this kind of defense. Rather, he attempted to offset the damaging implications of KPD membership by claiming he had joined under duress. To be sure, he acknowledged, membership itself *suggested* hostility to the National Socialist State. To assume this in his case, however, would be a grave error, since his membership was nothing more than the innocent mistake of a well-intentioned family man and war veteran whose needs had been cruelly ignored by decadent and thankless Weimar bureaucrats.

It is instructive that administrators remained unmoved by his defense, dismissing him on the basis of §2 at the end of July 1933. As he rejected Blau's appeal in October, Braasch revealed the fatal weakness in his argument: "B. belonged to the KPD from September 1929 until December 1932. His claim that he only let himself be talked into joining the KPD seems hard to believe, since he belonged to the party over three years. . . ."[26] Braasch also enlisted the NSBO in documenting Blau's failure to demonstrate support for the National Socialist State. Blau not only failed to convince administrators of his political gullibility (and thus innocence) in 1929; he also failed to convince them that he had in the meantime learned his lesson.

This case begs the question of whether Blau might have "survived" professionally if his KPD membership had been a thing of the distant past. A possible answer can be found if we turn to the case of Robert Wendel, who began at Wittenau in 1928 as a garden worker and was made a nurse three months later. Wendel admitted in his BBG questionnaires that he had belonged to the KPD for ten months between 1920 and 1921. However, he explained, "the undersigned regarded it as beneath his dignity to confront the party, to which he had belonged ca. one year, in writing, since [its] goals and endeavors were no longer compatible with my [*sic*] political outlook."[27] In a further attempt at self-defense later that year, he wrote, "When I saw the rise of the National Socialist German Workers' Party [NSDAP] in the elections of autumn 1930, I considered myself from then on to be a sympathizer of the . . . Party. . . ."[28] At the request of the Wittenau administration, Wendel also presented statements from other people testifying that he had voiced support for the nationalist movement.[29]

In light of these concerted attempts to demonstrate his political atonement (not to mention the fact that his membership lay a dozen years in the past and had lasted all of one year), it may come as a surprise that Wendel was also dismissed without much ado on the basis of §2. The problem, as Wittenau's NSBO representative delicately put it, was that Wendel had not yet (adequately) demonstrated a readiness to participate in the construction of the National Socialist State.[30] The NSBO's assessment (whatever its basis), plus the blemish of Communist Party membership, were sufficient to override any third-party testimony regarding Wendel's political metamorphosis (even, apparently, if the administration had invited Wendel to defend himself in this manner).[31] Wendel appealed the decision but was flatly rejected on the same grounds in April 1934.[32] His case suggests that professional survival for former KPD members rested neither on what a nurse claimed to believe, nor, necessarily, on what others reported about him or her. It rested on whether those in charge could be *convinced* of the nurse's support of the National Socialist State.

But how to convince? If mere words could not turn the odds in a nurse's favor, could formal pro–National Socialist affiliation help? If we consider the case of Nurse Peter Winkler, we receive a tentative "no" for an answer. Winkler was a veteran at Wittenau in 1933; he had worked there without significant incident since August 1914. In his BBG questionnaire, he admitted to having belonged to the KPD from January 1 to February 15, 1933. This information was underlined several times by administrative reviewers and sealed his fate, despite his additional claims that he had joined the NSBO in March 1933 and the NSDAP one month later.[33] The NSBO representative deemed him politically unreliable, and the Wittenau administration drew up a §2 dismissal effective September 30, 1933. The Office of the Mayor and State Commissioner Dr. Lippert were in full agreement.

Winkler issued an appeal that was immediately and unequivocally rejected by Wittenau: "The appellant was dismissed without notice on September 30, 1933, because he belonged to the KPD from January 1, 1933, until February 15, 1933. By joining the KPD in January 1933, W[inkler] consciously placed himself on the battlefront against the National Socialist movement. His further employment in public service can therefore not be supported. . . ."[34] Once again, the Office of the Mayor agreed; his appeal was flatly rejected.

Winkler's fate was sealed not only by KPD membership itself but, more specifically, by the timing of that membership. This was clearly not the case of a person who was compelled to join during less turbulent times or was unable to grasp the political implications of his activities. It also was not the case of someone who merely failed to demonstrate a willingness to participate in the construction of the new state; Winkler had deliberately placed himself in opposition to the National Socialist movement precisely when it needed his support most. Joining the KPD at that particular time was, in the eyes of those reviewing his case, politically perverse—an act certainly not to be undone by his joining the NSDAP two months later. Indeed, it is probable that this U-turn only worsened the case against him; after all, joining two mutually hostile parties in the course of four months does not by most accounts represent a credible evolution of political consciousness. Winkler exposed himself as a political chameleon whose actual allegiances remained a mystery; he may have been even more dangerous in the eyes of National Socialists than an outspoken Communist would be.

Winkler was, then, a nurse who was about as politically unreliable as one could imagine; the same treatment, however, was accorded to others for left-wing affiliation of a far more innocuous nature. Agnes Jost, for example, came to Wittenau in 1921 as a war widow with one child to support.[35] She had worked there over ten years without incident when the National Socialists came to power, but in April she was issued a dismissal effective September 30, 1933, on account of "suspicion of views hostile to the state."[36] Wittenau's NSBO elaborated the following month: "Nurse A[gnes] J[ost] said off duty that she is indeed in the NSBO, but Communism couldn't be gotten out of her heart."[37] A certain Herr S. was named as the source of this information; but when interrogated by the Wittenau administration several months later, he denied having said this and, for that matter, knowing Nurse Jost in the first place. A Communist Party member had simply told him that Jost was sympathetic to Communism, and he had passed this information on to the chairman of the salaried employees committee, thereby cautioning him about accepting Jost as an NSBO member.[38]

Nurse Jost filled out both the BBG questionnaire and its supplement and claimed never to have belonged to any political parties or unions. She had merely been a member of the Revolutionary Trade Union Opposition (*Revolutionäre Gewerkschafts-Opposition*, or RGO) for three months in 1931, unaware at the time of its Communist orientation. Her membership sufficed to prompt a §2 dismissal, despite the fact that Wittenau's NSBO representative asserted that she had indeed shown that she was willing to participate in the construction of the National Socialist State, and despite the fact that no one else could be found to confirm the suspicion of "views hostile to the state" which Herr S.'s (mis)reported information had created. Nurse Jost appealed the decision but received little sympathy from the Wittenau administration. After all, as Braasch noted in a memo to the Main Health Office (*Hauptgesundheitsamt*, or HGA) in November, she had not joined any pro–National Socialist parties or associations after her RGO membership in 1931.

We see, then, that even in a case where the "evidence" provided by a denunciation turned out to be rather flimsy, not much damaging evidence could be assembled to replace it, and the NSBO supported an employee, Wittenau administrators heeded and disregarded evidence as they saw fit. There was no way to guarantee one's success in this art of convincing, no predetermined, reliable course of action. Although Wittenau administrators subjected all former KPD members to the same review process, it is difficult indeed to discern the logic behind their deliberations. Although they tried to sustain the appearance of due process, they reserved final judgement for themselves—behind closed doors, on whatever grounds they saw fit. Evidence on nurses' behalf was allowed—even requested—but administrators reserved the right to disregard it. They could always introduce a hard-line interpretation of the law to justify their decision.

POLITICAL UNRELIABILITY AND THE POWER OF DENUNCIATION: BBG §4

We have, up to this point, suggested that self-reported membership in the KPD or a Communist-oriented organization constituted the formal basis on which nurses were dismissed, and that the professional consequences of Communist affiliation in 1933—namely, dismissal under the BBG—were virtually impossible to avoid. In addition, however, Nurse Jost's case demonstrates that a simple denunciation was quite sufficient to start the gears of the BBG machinery rolling, and with similar consequences. Indeed, although the questionnaires were no doubt useful in buttressing the apparent legitimacy of dismissals (employees condemned themselves, so to speak, by reporting left-wing affiliation and rendering their dismissal a matter beyond administrators' control), the March and April memos suggest that Wittenau's administrative "housecleaning" got off the ground in precisely this manner: through the migration of informally exchanged information through the staff hierarchy until it reached the ears of those in charge.

The BBG's §4 aimed precisely at this non-Communist, yet allegedly politically unreliable, group. It applied to salaried and unsalaried workers, as stated in the second implementation ordinance:

> §4
>
> Persons signed up for public service (*Dienstverpflichtete*), who on the basis of their prior political activity cannot offer a guarantee that they stand up for the national state without reservation, can be dismissed without notice through a unilateral declaration of the employer [*Dienstberechtigte*]. . . .[39]

We should not, then, be misled into thinking that the point of the review process was to pursue the details of formal membership; it was, rather, to evaluate whether an employee had demonstrated support for the National Socialist State. While formal left-wing affiliation was certainly a handy and, in most cases, invincible weapon for "proving" an employee's political unreliability, the case of Erika Macher demonstrates that it was by no means necessary.

Erika Macher was a single mother who worked throughout the Weimar years as a substitute nurse at various Berlin psychiatric and general hospitals.[40] She nursed at Wittenau from early 1929 until March 1932, when the administration cut back on personnel and dismissed her for below-average performance.[41] She requested to be retained in the institution as a cleaning woman, however, noting that she was a single parent with a twelve-year-old son to support. The administration obliged.[42]

It was, then, as a cleaning woman that Macher received notice of her dismissal "on suspicion of views hostile to the state" in spring 1933.[43] For reasons that are unclear but possibly suggest administrative confusion over the implementation of the BBG, the date of dismissal was changed several times and the dismissal itself was lifted in May.[44] During the summer, when the BBG review process was in full swing, she reported in her supplemental questionnaire that she had never belonged to a (political) party.[45]

In early September, however, the administration received the ammunition it needed to dismiss her; Macher's colleague S. reported:

> On Friday, September 1, a conversation took place in the kitchen of the reformatory between the assistant L., the maid M[acher], and myself. Assistant L. was very excited and declared that there would soon be war again. Trouble, [she said,] was produced by the fact that only SA and SS [members] were integrated into the work process, while all the others got no work. The police were, of course, on the side of the SA and SS. Misery was increasing daily, and she had never experienced such a state of affairs. She maintains that she was raised completely patriotically. In addition [she said] that an acquaintance of hers had been stopped by an SA man without reason while on a walk, and that this SA man had placed a revolver on his chest. She cursed the SA and SS and *was supported in this by M[acher].* . . .[46]

Macher, much to her detriment, admitted that she had indeed conversed with L. in this spirit. She undoubtedly incriminated herself further by elaborating on her own contributions to the conversation—namely, that "my brother has already been unemployed three years, and when he went to the employment exchange to request a job, he was told that the SA and SS had to be taken care of first. . . ." When her brother had been asked why he himself had not joined the SA, Macher continued, he had retorted that the few "peeps" of unemployment assistance weren't enough to cover the cost of the uniform. "I must admit," she concluded, "that I'm somewhat annoyed because around four weeks ago my house was searched to determine whether I have Communist rabble-rousing material[;] . . . nothing was found, however."[47]

In all likelihood, this was enough to seal Macher's fate; but the administration proceeded to take a statement from L., Macher's conversation partner, who accepted some parts of S.'s account while denying others, and again from S., who reiterated her account and reminded her audience of her National Socialist views.[48] It deemed Macher and L. eligible for dismissal under BBG §4, and by mid-September the HGA had drawn up the paperwork. Macher, it reported in its official explanation, "has . . . not as yet demonstrated through her personal behavior that she wants to participate in building the state in the spirit of National Socialism. We also consider her unsuitable for it, since according to the accompanying file she is a killjoy [*Miesmacherin*]."[49] Macher appealed the decision, but the central personnel administration of the HGA defended its decision by noting that Macher had cursed recent developments, "in particular the behavior of the SS and SA." The NSBO representative had expressed doubts about her political reliability, making her unsuitable as an employee in a home for "problem" (*schwer erziehbare*) children.[50]

WE SEE, then, that for administrators, the presence or absence of formal left-wing affiliation was only one of several factors figuring into an employee's political profile. When such affiliation existed, these previous cases demonstrate, it was the primary basis of dismissal; when it did not, suspicion of political unreliability generated by a denunciation was an adequate substitute. Nurses could be cast into an administrative spotlight through no initiative of their own and, once ensnared in a thorough "investigation" of their prior political activities, could be out of a job within six months if they could not prove the charges against them to be trumped up. The impression gained from these cases is one of complete helplessness on the part of individual nurses because of the lack of procedural integrity. Taken as a group, their cases present political blemishes of varying degrees and different attempts to overcome them. The review process itself, guided as it was by the completely subjective question of whether a person had demonstrated willingness to work on behalf of the new state, wore the guise of due process to mask what the case of Heide Turner begins to demonstrate: that the Wittenau administration used its enforcement of the BBG as a means for pursuing its own agenda in the nonpolitical sphere of staff management.

Heide Turner began work at Wittenau in April 1920. She was apparently a competent nurse so long as she was there; her file consists mostly of sick reports. She, too, was the recipient of the March and April memos, which informed her of her pending dismissal "on suspicion of views hostile to the state."[51] Her first brief response, in the form of a note to the state commissioner, was "I'm aware of no conduct hostile to the state." A few days later, she sent a long letter to a city official and the state commissioner detailing her personal history, in which we learn the source of this "suspicion":

I take the liberty of responding as follows to the termination of my employment as a nurse, which was pronounced on April 18, 1933, on suspicion of views hostile to the state.

I am [not] and was never hostile to the state. I was raised ... German and nationalist. From age seven onward I was raised in the orphanage of Driesen/Neumark, since I was an orphan. Later I had jobs. . . . [and] my certificates are available as references. My only brother took part in the war . . . and fell on November 10, 1914. That I am suspected of views hostile to the state is something I must reject on the basis of my entire outlook and socialization.

If an accusation is made because of my former membership in the SPD, I must point out that I indeed had a formal membership in this party, since there was . . . a certain obligation there to join, especially since the leading civil servants and . . . doctors, as well as the great majority of personnel, were members of this party[;] but [I] never had an inner attachment to this party. I have been working at the Wittenauer Heilstätten thirteen years and have always carried out my work to the fullest satisfaction of my superiors. I would kindly ask you to review my termination again, since in my opinion personal factors may be involved.

I emphasize once again that I am not conscious of any views hostile to the state and stand firmly behind a nationalist Germany as I always have. In hopes that my request will be honored, yours faithfully, H[eide] T[urner][52]

Her argumentative strategy is similar to that of Friedrich Blau, who also declared his support for the new state, invoked war experiences as proof of nationalist orientation, explained his leftward swing as a result of pressure, and characterized his involvement as devoid of emotional commitment. In addition, Turner attempted to defend herself in her supplemental questionnaire by providing the names of three people who could attest to her political reliability.[53]

Again, as with Nurse Blau, Braasch remained unconvinced; besides, he had reasons of his own for favoring her dismissal. In addition to having belonged to the SPD, he wrote in a letter to the HGA, Turner had been sick frequently (four hundred days since 1927). "Because of frequent illness of nursing personnel," he explained, "difficulties in allocating and maintaining work have repeatedly occurred. Thereby the proper care and supervision of patients suffer, so that we are forced to remove personnel apparently not physically suited for psychiatric care." As if this were not enough, Nurse Turner gave administrators reason to doubt her suitability for service to the public in "moral respects": "As we have learned, since March of this year T[urner] has been living in sin with the servant R.B., [who] was dismissed without notice from here on account of theft of food from the institution's stock. B. is married and the father of two children. He left his family unprovided for and moved in with T[urner], with whom he lives together. In the interests of the reputation of the institution and of the nursing staff, we therefore consider it appropriate to remove Nurse T[urner] from public service. . . ."[54] Nurse Turner, then, had not only failed to demonstrate political reliability; she also was a morally degenerate, administrative burden.

These latter considerations remained in the background of the review process, however, most likely because the evidence of political unreliability—indeed, political hostility—was so compelling. Although it is obvious that someone had denounced Turner many months earlier, administrators drew up protocols in which Turner's political unsuitability was "documented" by colleagues. One week before Turner was to be dismissed, they took the following statement from Nurse L.F.:

> I can only confirm that Miss T[urner] recruited for the SPD after January 30, 1933, and paid dues for the trade union. She behaved particularly spitefully toward me and Miss M. because she knew that we were "Nazis." According to her, all "Nazis," including doctors, should be mentioned by name in the journal *Sanitätswarte*, which belonged to the Association of Free Trade Unions, and "thrown out." In the affair concerning Stormtrooper Maikowski, who fell on January 30, 1933, Miss T[urner] said that she would never go into the Dome again because the murderer Maikowski had lain in state there.[55]

Another nurse signed an almost identical statement. Not surprisingly, Nurse Turner was dismissed as planned. Wittenau's administration sent her a certificate several weeks later in which it confirmed her dates of service, dryly adding, "In your own interest we have refrained from adding comments to the certificate regarding conduct and performance."[56]

Turner, however, would not be so easily defeated. In November, Braasch reported to the HGA, Turner had approached a personnel employee and demanded to know the grounds of her dismissal. He had cited §4 of the BBG—"political unreliability"—but had refused to let her see her file. Turner had apparently pursued the matter with an employee of the city's central personnel administration, who had called Braasch the next day and ordered him to let Turner see her file. Ever since then, Braasch complained, Turner had been showing up in the institution and turning certain former colleagues against those nurses who had testified against her before her dismissal.

Braasch succeeded in having her banned from the institution's grounds, but he was also concerned about avoiding such problems in the future. If former employees were able to see their files and stir up trouble among staff, he noted, women in particular would be reluctant to testify against "workers hostile to the state." In January 1934, interestingly, the Office of the Mayor stood by the right of employees to see their files. "A different procedure would open the way for a system of informers."[57]

That this official and Braasch entertained very different ideas on the subject of denunciation is revealed by the latter's eagerness to pursue Turner's ruination more than three months after she was gone. Her file contains yet another statement from Nurse L.F., who testified again in January 1934 allegedly in response to a charge that she had made her earlier denunciation under the influence of a colleague: "Nurse T[urner] was a member of the SPD all the way until February 1933. She was not, as she maintains, merely in a formal relationship with this party, but rather was imbued by the Marxist idea. That's the only way I can explain to myself her enthusiasm, . . . her joining of the SPD, and her attempts to convince us of the falsity of the National Socialist idea."[58] Nurse M.M. added, "I worked several years together with Nurse T[urner] in House 6. Miss T[urner] was dues collector for the union and completely Marxist in orientation. One day in February 1933—I'm sure that it was after the *nationale Erhebung*—I was busy in the bathroom of House 6 when T[urner] came to me and informed me, beaming with delight, that the Nazis would now be thrown out. When I then told her that she could also include me, because I also belonged to the National Socialists, she turned away from me and ignored me thereafter. . . ."[59] The mayoral official's attempt to counteract such behavior notwithstanding, Turner's case leaves little doubt that at Wittenau, denunciation provided a convenient and highly effective tool for pursuing private agendas and venting personal animosity. And this, recent research suggests, was very likely no anomaly; denunciation for nonracial "crimes" was not only common in National Socialist Germany but indeed an important source of fodder for the Party's disciplinary apparatus.[60]

FORMER SPD members, however, were in general not treated nearly as harshly as was Nurse Turner. Nurse Jürgen Lorenz, in contrast to his colleagues with former KPD affiliation, sailed

fairly gracefully through the BBG review process despite his earlier SPD membership, demonstrating that this "lesser evil" was
something administrators were, theoretically, prepared to forgive.[61] Lorenz, who had worked at Wittenau since 1926, admitted to having belonged to the SPD for approximately a year between 1930 and 1931 and again from autumn 1932 until March
1933. But, he explained rather cryptically, he had joined only
under the "force of circumstance" and had never engaged himself politically or financially in the activities of the party. Moreover, he continued, "I can maintain in good conscience that I
have always been patriotically inclined. I can supply proof for
this by noting that in 1928 I hosted the National Socialist H.B.,
[who] was at that time politically persecuted, for ca. 6 weeks."[62]
He referred administrators to his formal exit from the SPD in
February 1933, in which he stated, "I vow to devote all my energies to the service of the NSDAP henceforth."[63]

This was evidently enough to save Lorenz from a §4 dismissal.
Braasch, however, wondered whether dismissal was possible on
the grounds that, according to his supervisor, Lorenz's behavior
on duty was almost "childish and impertinent."[64] Nothing came
of this, however, because over the following weeks Lorenz
shaped up, prompting the supervising doctor to conclude that
"a dismissal does not seem justified."[65] That was the final word
on the matter, and Lorenz remained at Wittenau until May 1941.

Nonpolitical Housecleaning: §6 as Administrative Blank Check

Nurses Lorenz and Turner were both former SPD members,
yet only Lorenz survived the BBG. He was able to convince administrators of his political reliability, whereas Turner's defense
collapsed by virtue of the damning allegations of her colleagues.
In addition, Braasch went to great lengths to argue that she was
an administrative burden, a claim which was by no means incidental to the BBG review process. While in her case it merely
solidified a case for dismissal already made quite soundly
through allegations of hostility toward the National Socialist

State, in other cases patently nonpolitical factors were the very foundation of BBG dismissals.

This was made possible, and in fact encouraged, by the sixth paragraph of the decree, which applied to Wittenau's non–civil servant nurses, as stated in the Second Implementation Ordinance:

§6

(1)

To simplify administration or management, persons signed up for public service can also be terminated if termination was not permitted per contract permanently or for more than a year, or *[if it] was tied to the existence of an important reason.* The position may not be filled again.[66]

To be sure, the intent of this paragraph was a point of confusion among Wittenau and city of Berlin administrators. Nurse Minna Weinz, for example, listed no prior political affiliation in her BBG questionnaires,[67] but Braasch prepared the paperwork for a §6 dismissal with the explanation that "for a rather long time, Nurse W[einz] has been absent very often on account of illness. Among other things, between January 2, 1930, and January 18, 1933, she was absent on eight [separate] occasions with a total of 286 days sick."[68]

The Office of the Mayor protested: "Nurse W[einz] by her own account did not belong to a political party. Political unreliability is neither charged nor proven. Frequent illness should not be a reason for dismissal in the spirit of the law from April 7, 1933. Dismissal on these grounds can follow on the basis of the contract."[69] The mayoral official intended to forward the matter to the HGA with a recommendation for dismissal on the grounds of a contract violation.

Dr. Lippert, acting as a Party intermediary agent (*Vertrauens-mann*), stepped in to clear up the matter, stating that "§6 is precisely the 'unpolitical' paragraph of the BBG, whereby the administration should be given the opportunity to dismiss unsuitable workers without tiresome proceedings. I . . . consider the case at hand as typically suitable for applying §6."[70] After another protest from the Office of the Mayor, Weinz was dismissed at the end of December 1933 as planned.[71]

DESPITE Lippert's straightforward and quite correct interpretation of §6, however, it is interesting to note that administrators went to great lengths to preserve the discursive apparatus already employed in the dismissals of "politically unreliable" nurses. We see this in the case of Inge Rupenthal, who began to work at Wittenau in 1923 and by 1933 had built up a history of frequent absences and debts. She reported no political affiliation in her questionnaires, yet the NSBO representative reported that "Nurse I[nge] R[upenthal] has . . . not . . . demonstrated through her personal behavior that she can participate in the construction of the state in the spirit of National Socialism and is suited to do so, since [she is] often sick!"[72] Nevertheless, Wittenau's administration sent Rupenthal a memo instructing her to produce a statement from a member of a pro–National Socialist organization attesting to her political reliability.

Nurse Rupenthal attempted to explain the legitimacy of past absences and added that she enjoyed taking part in NSBO activities. The Office of the Mayor even accepted her explanation and attempted to defend her before local Party officials. Party Member S., he wrote, confirmed that the Rupenthal family had not been politically active; moreover, Rupenthal was responsible for financially supporting her family. In light of this, he felt, no problems should be created for her at work. In any case, Rupenthal was not eligible for dismissal under §6 of the BBG on account of absenteeism; the only possible ground for dismissal was a contract violation.[73] Lippert stepped in once again to insist that frequent illness was indeed an appropriate basis for dismissal under the "unpolitical" §6,[74] and Nurse Rupenthal was dismissed on March 31, 1934.[75]

This case documents the emergence of an ominous linkage in administrative politics: health as a barometer of civic value. Nurses were to be kept or dismissed according to whether they had demonstrated that they were both willing and *suited* (*geeignet*) to support the National Socialist State; and suitability was construed in terms of health (among other things). While Wittenau administrators were very likely simply looking for a convenient way to rid themselves of the sources of extra paperwork, the fact that Party bureaucrats wove this linkage of health and civic value into the decree's fabric of possible interpretations, along with the fact that this reasoning became part of routine personnel management, reveals that an administrative "politics of exclusion" took shape in 1933 which discursively paralleled the "exclusion" of patients from the realm of the mentally healthy *Volk* and, eventually, their exclusion from the human community itself. This observation is in no way intended to trivialize the far more serious implications of exclusionary politics for patients—whose very lives, after all, were at stake—but rather to begin to illuminate a more general characteristic of institutional life whose implications we shall explore in the following chapters.

FOR reasons that are unclear, not everyone who was recommended for §6 dismissal was dismissed on those grounds, but the law seems to have been a catalyst and tool for identifying "problem" employees, even if they were eventually dismissed because of a contract violation. We see this in the case of Edith Martin, who entered general nursing following her 1920 divorce and held a variety of short-term positions before joining the Wittenau staff in late 1925.[76] She was a problem employee, administratively speaking, because she was frequently late for work and absent on account of illness. Losing patience in April 1931, the administration remarked, "As revealed in the personnel file, she has been absent frequently in past years on account of illness. It seems questionable whether she is still suitable for service in nursing."[77] No steps were taken until 1933, however, at which point administrators fell over themselves to have her dismissed.

Nurse Martin appears to have been well aware of impending doom when filling out her BBG questionnaire. In response to the all-important inquiry about previous (left-wing) political activity she answered with a "No!" in large letters, adding that "I did not belong to a party, but since January 1930 I have voted National Socialist."[78] The NSBO representative deemed her politically reliable. In September, however (and possibly on administrative request), her supervisor submitted a report on her professional performance that characterized her as "at work not always reliable, and she is sick rather often."[79] That same day Braasch drew up the paperwork for a §6 dismissal (which, it was hoped, would take effect "as soon as possible"). While acknowledging Martin's established political reliability and the NSBO representative's favorable evaluation, the administration deemed her unsuitable for further service at Wittenau on the grounds of her history of frequent absences and a total of five disciplinary warnings she had received since 1927.[80]

Once again challenging Wittenau's liberal implementation of §6, the Office of the Mayor responded that Martin was not eligible for dismissal under §6 of the law because she had not yet been in service for ten years. (For reasons left unelaborated, her work in nursing before 1925 did not count for the purposes of the law.) The only permissible route for dismissal lay in a violation of her contract. This was in the end the route taken; in mid-October Martin was issued a dismissal effective March 31, 1934—a dismissal that she unsuccessfully appealed in person in November and again in March. The administration claimed to sympathize with her ailments, which apparently stemmed from the 1912 birth of her daughter; "The fact of many absences, however, remains, as well as the not particularly outstanding performance."[81] Her dismissal was therefore not overturned, and Nurse Martin left Wittenau in March 1934.

WITTENAU'S administrators, then, rationalized the use of §6 with reference to an employee's propensity to create extra headaches and paperwork. Moreover, as in cases of politically "unreliable" nurses, we see that they allowed themselves a considerable degree of latitude in deciding what constituted a "problem" employee. They did not simply arrive at their decisions by adding up sick days; after all, Edith Martin, who had been absent 13 times since 1930, was dismissed just as eagerly as Erika Macher, who had missed 286 days in the same time span. In some cases the exact number of sick days was not even specified in Wittenau's explanation for a dismissal on account of absenteeism. Clearly, there was no specific formula involved; rather, absenteeism was a *formal* justification for a *subjective* decision based on considerations that often were not even addressed by the BBG. These "unofficial" considerations, the following case suggests, were frequently at the heart of the matter, and administrators exploited the decree to do away with the source of the problem.

Anja Reuter was a single mother who became a nurse at Wittenau in 1921. In 1933, she was affirmed by the NSBO representative as politically reliable after declaring no prior political affiliation and adding, "[I] have spoken with my son about politics because he always was a loyal supporter of the National Socialist Party." She added that he belonged to the Hitler Youth.[82] Yet, in spite of this, Wittenau proposed a §6 dismissal on the grounds that she was often absent on account of illness and had three thousand marks' worth of debts "which create a great deal of paperwork, etc., for the administration." Moreover, Braasch continued, she had shown herself to be "unsuitable for service in psychiatric care. R[euter] has a work ethic that lacks every sense of duty."[83]

To be sure, Reuter had been disciplined for insubordination during her service as a kitchen worker from 1919 to 1921.[84] Braasch, however, referred explicitly to personnel file pages 161 and 162 in justifying this evaluation, which read in part as follows:

> 1. On June 9, 1933, the patient Mrs. E.V., née W., died here in House 10. Nurse A[nja] R[euter], who had a shift that day on the upstairs station, spread the word among the patients, in particular to the patient Mrs. G.H. (a morphine addict), that Patient V. had not died a natural death, as the administration had told the relatives, but rather had actually hanged herself. "The people out there just have to know what's going on here in the institution."

2. Nurse R[euter] became excited about the way the patients are cared for and as breakfast was served said to the patients, among other things, "Now this one here is getting topping at public expense," so that the patients complained to the senior nurse.

3. Another time a patient explained to the senior nurse that she couldn't sleep at night because Nurse R[euter] was loudly recounting her entire private affairs during night duty.

4. On June 21, 1933, the patient Miss A.S. approached the doctor crying and said that the nurse on night duty, Nurse A[nja] R[euter], said the following to her on mornings when she had spent the night unable to sleep and plagued by pains: "Those are all hallucinations. That's how mental illnesses begin."[85]

These violations, reported to the administration by the senior nurse of the house in which Reuter worked, could not be proven with certainty because Reuter denied every charge except the last (to which she only admitted after initially lying). Her behavior, she explained, was a result of "nervousness" produced by domestic concerns; she promised to pull herself together in the future. The administration issued a warning, which the employee council supported after speaking with Reuter's colleagues and determining that "such statements are completely trustworthy." She was to be threatened with dismissal in the event of a repeat performance. That was the end of the matter until Reuter's BBG paperwork was processed over the following two months. The incident was used to render the case against Reuter beyond the shadow of any doubt: she was not only an administrative problem but also lacking in a "proper" attitude toward her work. She was thus to be dismissed on the basis of §6 at the end of June 1934.

Shortly before this date, Reuter wrote to the administration asking for a postponement of the dismissal until January 1, 1935. "As grounds for my request," she wrote, "I would like to mention that my son is still in training. I also ask on behalf of my elderly parents, [who] both receive thirty-seven marks pension per month and thus depend on their children. If I now have to leave my job, I cannot face my parents [and] my son and would be brought to the edge of desperation. Mit deutschem Gruß, A.R."[86] Reuter's on-the-job performance, to be sure, had improved in the meantime, but Wittenau was not in a position to help her. She should have filed such a request sooner; as it was, she would have to leave and then pursue a rehiring with the Office of the Mayor.[87]

Approximately one week after this decision, however, Nurse Reuter found another solution: she attempted to kill herself with gas. As the police reported, "A suicide note left behind states that she was terminated on October 1, 1933, and dismissed on July 1, 1934, from her post as a nurse at the Wittenauer Heilstätten, where she worked fifteen years, on the basis of the Law for the Restoration of the Professional Civil Service. R[euter] took this circumstance to heart and claims on that account to have been moved to the suicide attempt in desperation."[88] It is likely, however, that another factor contributed to her desperation. Reuter could have appealed the §6 decision back in October of 1934 and had been advised of this possibility.[89] She had not done so, she explained in a letter of application eighteen months later, because she had intended to marry. "Unfortunately my plans were thwarted, insofar as I had fallen into the hands of a man who was already married but had always kept this from me."[90]

Thus, faced with shattered hopes of marriage and the impending loss of her job, and already deeply in debt, Reuter had found herself on the verge of personal, professional, and financial catastrophe by mid-1934. After gaining only a temporary two-month position at the Herzberge institution during the summer of 1935, she renewed her appeals to the administrators of the city of Berlin at the start of 1936, reminding them of her broken heart, financial responsibilities toward her family, and the fact that other nurses dismissed under similar circumstances were currently being rehired.[91] This and another request for work in 1938 were turned down, ostensibly because of a lack of available positions.[92] But in fact she had little chance of being hired for anything more than temporary substitute positions; the Herzberge administration, after reporting favorably about her performance there in 1935, entered in her file an advisory against permanent employment on account of the incidents reported on pages 161 and 162.[93]

The four violations of mid-1933 were, then, taken seriously by administrators. Disturbing patients' sleep by talking about her private affairs, failing to take a patient's physical pain seriously, and calling patients freeloaders reveal the different "faces" of a woman whose personal and financial difficulties had rendered her frustrated, introverted, and impervious to the needs of others. She proved herself unable and unwilling to devote the necessary emotional energy to her patients—voicing, to the contrary, dismissive prejudices to the effect that patients were "useless eaters." Later developments notwithstanding, this was by no means acceptable language coming from a professional whose job consisted in part of dispelling precisely these kinds of views.

It is likely, however, that the first violation was particularly disturbing to administrators. Whether, according to relatives' belief, a patient died by natural causes or from suicide was by no means a minor issue; it determined whether those relatives would accept the death without incident or pose uncomfortable questions about why the patient hadn't been adequately supervised, and, worse, initiate unpleasant and damaging lawsuits. Nurse Reuter was reported for articulating what was supposed to be hushed up. By disclosing the patient's true cause of death, Nurse Reuter demonstrated a lack of allegiance to the institutional establishment and, more specifically, a failure to respect the institution's self-appointed right to regulate its own public image. The BBG provided a convenient pretext for thwarting this kind of independence.

SCHEINLEGALITÄT AND THE POWER OF DECEPTION

It is abundantly clear by now that although the Party issued the BBG "from above," it extracted cooperation in part by offering Wittenau's administrators a piece of the pie—by allowing them to pursue their own managerial agenda in the process. Administrators and government officials shared power by virtue of a decree whose euphemistic title and legalistic design seemed to promise fair and impartial implementation. The result was a complete emasculation of laws as reference points in the mediation of human relationships and their redeployment as a smokescreen for administrative opportunism: left to their own devices, administrators could interpret the provisions of the "law" as they saw fit; when questioned by those who were victimized in the process, they could take refuge in the decree's supposedly ineluctable binding force. They could, in other words, abdicate responsibility for their actions at the same time as they single-handedly and arbitrarily ended a person's career. At once confusing people about the intentions of the BBG and soliciting the potential victims' voluntary compliance in compiling personal histories, the Party headed off resistance and opposition before the victims could grasp what had happened. Indeed, securing the appearance of legality (*Scheinlegalität*) through the involvement of existing state bureaucracies was undoubtedly more effective to this end than any open and firm display of power by the Party alone would have been.[94]

We see just how ruthlessly the decree's enforcers exploited this situation if we follow Erika Macher's story to its end. Following her §4 dismissal in 1933, she attempted to appeal the decision. The process apparently became bogged down by more confusion about the BBG's application and was not resolved until early 1935. The exchanges during the intervening months are not in Macher's file; we know only that, in the end, the Ministry of the Interior informed her that the dismissal actually did not follow from §4 of the BBG but rather from §6, "in the interests of the business [of the institution]." "Your appeal is thus rejected," the official continued. "This decision is final."[95]

To be sure, Wittenau had told her in September 1933 that she was dismissed in compliance with the BBG §4, so no response other than appealing on that basis would have made any sense. Macher's appeal was, by any sensible reckoning, logical. She lived in a world, however, where the only logic that mattered was a primitive form of administrative metaphysics: one may not appeal a §4 dismissal if a §4 dismissal does not exist. This logic rendered her appeal an absurdity—something indigestible by the prevailing administrative system. If the BBG was a kind of blank check from the administrative point of view, allowing for the most absurd defenses of a decision, it was an impasse for nurses who were prevented at all turns from availing themselves of its redemptive possibilities. Like a window that allows one to see without being seen, the decree allowed administrators insight into what was going on and the freedom to do what they wanted, while nurses on the "receiving" end remained in the dark.

IT SEEMS superfluous, at best, to problematize what was at stake for nurses in the wake of an extended discussion about firing people. But if we want to understand the psychological implications of the BBG, we must do so; for it was a question of losing not simply a job but also one's place in the social, economic, and political order of things. The National Socialists romanticized work as a source of civic virtue as well as the foundation of future national greatness. Being deprived of one's job—or the possibility thereof—in this kind of political climate thus had profound psychological implications: shame, loneliness, helplessness, uncertainty, and disgruntled confusion are only a few. The BBG, moreover, targeted those who were civil or public servants—whose work was defined in terms of its high social value and rewarded accordingly. Exclusion from the army of the employed—and from this privileged group in particular—entailed the loss not only of financial means but also of the more general psychological comfort afforded by the certainty that one belongs to a group and has something to offer it.

On this note, it is no contradiction to repeat that—in comparison to what psychiatric patients, Jews, and other pariah groups of National Socialist Germany would soon endure—it was, after all, *only* a job that they lost. Wittenau's files do not tell us what eventually happened to many who were dismissed—whether, for example, Turner escalated her anti-Nazi agitation elsewhere and was sent to a concentration camp. But generally speaking, it is important not to exaggerate the injustice suffered by those

dismissed by the BBG in such a way that we lose perspective on
the far more serious implications of 1933 for people whom the
National Socialists would kill or maim within the next twelve
years. The purpose of identifying a "politics of exclusion" in institutional life is not to imply that nurses were subject to the
same degree of terror and persecution as all other inhabitants of
Germany at the time. Rather, it is part of an attempt to reconstruct their experience on the basis of the documents remaining.

In that vein, it is likely that in 1933 there was ample evidence,
for those who paid attention, that something had changed in administrative jurisprudence, and that nurses' careers hung pre-
cariously in the balance. Nurses Blau and Turner seem to have
understood that in order to have the slightest chance to "survive," they would need to dispense with the hope that any former or residual left-wing sympathy would be tolerated. Rather,
they would have to distance themselves as much as possible
from their formal affiliation by denying emotional commitment.
Their task was simple and at the same time nearly impossible:
they needed to convince administrators that their left-wing affiliation had simply been a formal matter—at best a temporary
mistake—and that they had supported everything that National
Socialism stands for, if not the Party itself, all along.

Macher, by way of contrast, openly verified her hostility toward National Socialist enthusiasts under interrogation, which
suggests that she had not yet grasped the uncompromising and
spurious fashion in which the decree would be applied. This is
not necessarily surprising: after all, the criteria for dismissal and
retention seemed clear—indeed, were codified in a "law"—and
she may have believed that without formal left-wing affiliation,
she was safe; or she may have presumed goodwill on the part
of the persons who received her testimony. The decree, as noted
above, was designed to deceive, and deceive it did.

In fact, her story would likely have demonstrated to other
nurses that although one could survive the process, one could
not be too sure of success if bad luck or a cranky colleague cast
one into the administrative spotlight. In practice, the criteria of
retention and dismissal remained obscure enough that one

could not really be sure how a decision had been made, and thus, if one survived, how decisions would be made in the future. The presence of National Socialist enthusiasts among their colleagues and the fact that denunciation was greedily received by administrators would very likely have cast a cloud of uncertainty and fear over those nurses who survived the process, didn't oppose National Socialism, but weren't fanatical supporters either. Perhaps it would be best, they may have thought, to keep quiet and stay out of other people's way in the future.

6

Reeducating Nurses in the Spirit of the Times: Geisteskrankenpflege *in the Service of National Socialism*

I̶N NOVEMBER 1933, nurses who remained at their posts might have come across an issue of *Geisteskrankenpflege* featuring a long pro–National Socialist article on the necessity of racial purity, followed by these remarks, made a century earlier by Hermann Groß, on the spatial organization of institutional psychiatry:

> A complete institutional separation of healing and care of the mentally ill is, considered in a narrower sense—and it may not be considered any other way in its nature—throwing out the baby with the bath. Even considered in a wider sense, care without a cure is like a tree trunk with limbs bound together, and also the other way around, a cure without care, like a chatterbox [*Ankedotenkrämer*], who only draws attention to himself so long as he does not become boring, but rather remains brief and interesting;—admittedly, here a kind of care must be understood that the mentally ill often need for years at a time until their recovery. Care is therefore a necessary condition of curing: and a reasonable person understands that the socialization of an unreasonable person, of an unhappy person, is not the work, not the cure of an illness, which is decided upon on the fifth, seventh, ninth day, and which often leads to recovery with the help of the doctor.[1]

Here, Groß touched upon ideas that had earlier been hailed as the practical and ethical foundation of Weimar psychiatry: that psychiatric illness does not lend itself to quick and easy solutions; that curing an illness cannot be managed and carried out like work on an assembly line; that institutional arrangements should accommodate themselves to the needs of the patients, and not the other way around. Psychiatric care, in short, must not get so caught up in professional and economic efficiency that it loses sight of its underlying purpose.

One may reasonably wonder what such remarks are doing in a psychiatric nursing journal in the first year of a dictatorship that did not even pretend to take such ideas seriously. In due time, psychiatric patients would be divided into categories of curable and incurable within institutional walls, if not in separate institutions, and their murder would be made viable through precisely the kind of thinking behind such separation: We need to focus our attention and resources on those with the best chances of recovery. Those "chosen" ones, moreover, would be subjected to precisely the medical impatience depicted above, reflected in increasingly aggressive treatments designed to "work" more rapidly than previous methods. This assertion of ethical continuity in institutional psychiatry, in short, seems to have very little to do with the grim realities of everyday life.

Be this as it may, it is probable that the inclusion of Groß's remarks was neither a mistake nor merely an attempt, in the midst of palpable institutional and moral deterioration, to give an otherwise inhuman agenda a patina of respectability. Rather, it was typical of nursing literature under National Socialism, which retained a remarkable degree of its former theoretical, practical, and ethical orientation. We can begin to understand the source of this apparent paradox if we remind ourselves that institutional psychiatrists and nurses were sandwiched between a fascist regime which regarded their patients as "worthless" lives *and* a vast pool of Germans for whom those same patients were cherished parents, children, brothers, and sisters. Pleasing the National Socialists was not their only concern, nor was it always easily reconcilable with their professional self-esteem and the wishes of the public sector—which they confronted directly and on whose "business" they relied. The result, for psychiatric nurses, was a body of literature with the most unlikely conceptual mixtures: "love" and threats, moderation and veiled aggression, patience and impatience.

Closer inspection of this assortment of ideas, however, reveals that these texts were not simply the result of a confused attempt to serve two masters; they had the potential to be highly instrumental in the professional (re)socialization of nurses along National Socialist lines. They thus provide a window to the discursive and rhetorical strategies that rendered National Socialist policies palatable to those, like nurses, who were enlisted in their support.

INSTITUTIONAL PSYCHIATRY, 1933–1939

Weimar psychiatrists, as we have seen, confronted a crisis of legitimacy on two fronts: First, the public continued to associate their profession with detention. Second, in light of ongoing economic crisis, state funding of institutional care came under fire and was drastically reduced. Psychiatrists faced considerable pressure to appear as medically successful as they were thrifty. Their solutions, as we have seen, entailed rejuvenating decades-old therapeutic experiments in occupational therapy and outpatient care. When these approaches failed to alleviate the demographic and financial pressures generated by the Depression, their therapeutic interests shifted from treatment to prevention.

The pressures from without changed in 1933: strategies of eugenic management suddenly became the cornerstone of a new authoritarian regime. The Law for the Prevention of Hereditarily Diseased Progeny of 1933 (*Gesetz zur Verhütung erbkranken Nachwuchses* or GVeN) foresaw the sterilization of all German citizens suffering from at least one of the following illnesses: "feeble-mindedness," schizophrenia, manic-depressive illness, epilepsy, Huntington's chorea, and hereditary blindness, deafness, and physical deformity. In addition, those suffering from chronic alcoholism could be sterilized.

Some authors contributing to psychiatric journals expressed relief at these developments because, enjoying the state's blessing, they would no longer be pestered by either legal problems or ethical questions that had heretofore beleaguered them in eugenics debates. As one wrote, the sterilization law "presents the German doctor, namely, the psychiatrist, with new tasks and frees him in the realm of eugenics from the emotional difficulties that we have found more and more embarrassing over the last ten years."[2] This freedom soon manifested itself with regard to euthanasia: after praising plans for voluntary assisted suicide in England, one *Psychiatrisch-Neurologische Wochenschrift* contributor added that "in my opinion, it can be considered a serious gap in the English draft of the law that the possibility of being permitted to kill incurable mental patients—and indeed on account of the state—has been entirely unconsidered; precisely this question demands a solution."[3]

Psychiatrists embraced the opportunity to promote National Socialist eugenic measures by participating in a massive campaign of public "enlightenment" on inherited mental illness.[4] In 1935, the Rheinland Provincial Administration reported that its institutions had "eagerly and willingly undertaken this task, which is not always easy, realizing that such enlightenment is of the utmost importance in the interest of the eugenic and population policies of the state, which are just in their infancy. . . ." One of its institutions had processed over 2,000 visitors that year.[5] At the Eglfing-Haar institution in Bavaria, tours of over 100 people were regularly conducted from 1934 onward, and by 1945 over 21,000 people (more than 90 percent of whom were men) had taken part in its 195 courses.[6]

A considerable number of visitors were members and officials of National Socialist organizations; but teachers, lawyers, doctors, and nurses were included in their ranks as well. Indeed, one psychiatrist detected an opportunity to use institutions not only as theaters for propaganda but as sites for nurses' formal training as well. Even general nurses needed to have a glimpse into the causes and nature of psychological illnesses in order to be in a position to handle those receiving outpatient care and to assist doctors in the implementation of the GVeN. Many nurses who had been instructed in heredity lacked the "vivid view" necessary for such assistance. "But if they have experienced the

mentally ill themselves, then the significance of these genetic illnesses will dawn on them, and if there have been religious reservations up to that point, then it is to be expected that they will
begin to waver from this experience, and that the actions of the
state will be recognized as a virtue."[7]

The point of such "experience" was, then, to convince nurses
of the "necessity" of eugenic measures—an idea that was amply
reinforced by a steady flow of official propaganda from government and Party circles. In a 1935 article in Nuremberg's
Fränkische Zeitung, for example, Party Member Götzinger reported on his visit to regional psychiatric institutions and described the horror he had felt upon discovering the "immeasur-
ability of human suffering" to be found within their walls.
"Here, living beings vegetate *without hope* and *without sense*. . . ."[8]
It was horrifying to think that the children in such institutions—
"these idiotic, imbecilic and half-imbecilic creatures, these animal-like, disfigured children[—]are supposed to be human beings." It was also horrifying to think that they were forced to
bear the burden of their parents' "sins of blood and race." Thank
goodness, the author concluded, that the Führer had created
laws "which finally are bringing about the containment of this
madness and are supposed to do away with the unconscious
distress of the physically, mentally, and spiritually disfigured
children[—]for the good of Germany, indeed for the good of
humanity."[9]

Nursing such people was portrayed in official propaganda as
an exercise in misdirected and fruitless martyrdom. "It remains
astonishing to us," Götzinger wrote, "how much evenhandedness, calm, and industriousness the doctors and nurses devote
to their duties. . . ." Some nurses even worked in such institutions over twenty years! "They actually protect the healthy people around them from the danger of the genetically ill. But what
[great] value could such love achieve in the genetically healthy
community of our *Volk*?"[10] The periodical *Neues Volk* published a
photo in 1934 depicting a young, handsome male nurse standing
behind a seated, frowning patient with half-clenched fingers.
The caption read, "This nurse, a healthy, robust person, is only

there to care for this crazy person [*Irren*] who is a danger to the public. Shouldn't we be ashamed of this picture?"[11]

It was precisely this kind of propaganda that breathed new life into the idea that psychiatric nursing was essentially concerned with detention rather than care of the sick. In 1936, one psychiatrist lamented that as a result, mental ailments continued to be neglected in general nursing training. He bitterly recalled that a local sport association had asked him if his senior male nurses wished to partake in a jujitsu course, and a matron of a large nursing organization had told him that even if a nurse had worked ten years in a psychiatric institution, she could not become a general nurse (*Schwester*) in just one year.[12] These kinds of attitudes found legal expression in the 1938 Law for the Reorganization of Nursing (*Gesetz zur Neuordnung der Krankenpflege*), designed to regulate training, certification, and professional activity of nurses and to assure a satisfactory supply for the war to come: psychiatric nursing was not considered "real" nursing and was thus excluded.[13]

Sterilization and Institutional Life

Statistically speaking, the GVeN played a smaller role in institutional psychiatry than has been assumed.[14] Although institutionalized patients constituted 30–40 percent of those sterilized between 1934 and 1936, the percentage decreased thereafter owing to a combination of factors: the progressive exhaustion of the "pool" of candidates, the expansion of sterilization to non-institutionalized categories of genetically ill, and, eventually, the decision to kill patients.[15] The majority of those sterilized came from the category of patients who underwent the operation as a condition of their release. (Patients eligible for release had the "choice" of either submitting to sterilization or paying for further institutionalization themselves.)[16] But because increasing numbers of patients were chronic cases, the GVeN did not enable psychiatrists to increase release rates as much as they had hoped.[17]

The law affected doctor-patient relationships in palpable and sinister ways. The frequent result of the be-sterilized-or-pay policy, for example, can be summed up by what a former patient was told by his doctor in 1935: "If you sign this [registration form], you will be released in fourteen days."[18] The main concern of compliant institutional doctors and administrators was to ensure that the GVeN was implemented with as little internal disruption and public alienation as possible. Ideally, they could best achieve this in the course of fulfilling their *Aufklärungspflicht*, or duty to ensure that patients understood what was going to happen to them: eligible patients, it was hoped, could be persuaded to initiate sterilization proceedings themselves.[19]

This, alas, did not prove successful nearly as often as hoped, which led very quickly to the discovery that bullying or deceiving patients into "volunteering" was much more effective. A Stuttgart medical officer, for example, reported that mentally deficient young people were not capable of applying what they were told about the operation to the designated purpose and tended instead to conclude that in the future they could carelessly sleep around. It was easier simply to have them sterilized without knowledge of what the procedure entailed.[20] Some patients suffering from "feeblemindedness" or schizophrenia refused to acknowledge their illness by signing a form on which the diagnosis was written; one doctor reported that in such cases he simply filled in that line later and did not let the patient see the paperwork thereafter. In any case, when patients did not cooperate, the director or medical officer in charge submitted the application.[21] These were not isolated incidents but rather part of a general phenomenon whereby "voluntary" applications for sterilization (*"Selbst"-Anträge*) of allegedly genetically ill people were obtained under duress, concluded after a candidate failed to protest, or obtained as a result of confusion and misunderstanding.[22]

Presenting releasable patients with the choice between submitting to sterilization and financially burdening their families was only one of a series of measures designed to cast patients into an increasingly isolated, and thus particularly desperate, situation. The reporting and evaluation procedures were in and of themselves flimsy, devoid of due process, and scientifically unsound.[23] A May 1934 ordinance stipulated that court appointments could be transferred from the usual official locations to the institutions themselves.[24] That same month it was decreed that applications for the sterilization of institutionalized patients should no longer be submitted to the court of the patient's town of residence but should rather go to that of the institution's. These measures doomed any outside support to failure and spared psychiatrists unpleasant encounters with relatives—a move that they welcomed.[25] One year later, in June 1935, patients' time for appealing a decision to sterilize was reduced from one month to two weeks.[26]

In light of this, it is perhaps not surprising that between 1934 and 1936 7 to 9 percent of all sterilization candidates had to be brought into the operating clinic by the police.[27] In 1934 three girls institutionalized at Hadamar who were slated for sterilization escaped but were caught and returned; a Cologne chief doctor reported that "revolts, incitements, and escapes" were difficult to prevent.[28] The Party's attempts to present compliant sterilization candidates as martyrs to the *Volk* remained small comfort.[29] Doctors paid the price for their complicity in the form of a distinct loss of public trust and, in some cases, boycotts.[30] One doctor reported in 1937 on the increasing alienation of relatives—one of whom, unwilling to cooperate in the collection of personal information, maintained that "he would now have to consider the doctor his enemy."[31]

Hunger, Crowding, and Violence in Everyday Life

Alongside these developments, demographic pressures and underfunding produced a rapid deterioration of institutional living conditions during the 1930s. The number of people treated in psychiatric institutions reached unprecedented levels; the number of long-term and chronic cases also continued to rise.[32] Although actual amounts spent on psychiatric institutions went up, expenditures per patient continued to be cut and "rationalization"—i.e., institutional consolidation—meant that doctors and nurses had to divide their time among more and more patients.[33] Supervisory shortages caused work therapy to be reduced in favor of bed-treatment, whereby patients spent days in crowded, poorly ventilated rooms.[34] Eichberg patients lived primarily on root vegetables.[35] (As we shall see, conditions continued to worsen after the outbreak of war.) As one might expect, the regime was not deemed responsible for this state of affairs; one administrator writing for the *Psychiatrisch-Neuro-logische Wochenschrift* blamed everything from the First World War and the Versailles Treaty to the Bolshevik Revolution for high costs and the deterioration of conditions in psychiatric institutions.[36]

In addition to this generalized misery, patients suffered from abuse masquerading as "sedation." One former patient in the Rheinland reported that after being incarcerated in a cell in the high-security ward with six other patients, he told the doctor, "You are a doctor; then why don't you behave like one." The doctor left and sent two nurses to wrap the patient's entire body as tightly as they could in wet towels, leaving him to scream in agony for at least one and a half hours thereafter.[37] This was hardly an isolated incident; patient records from the Hadamar institution suggest that the use of such "cold packs" was a routine method among nurses for immobilizing recalcitrant patients, in addition to administering large quantities of medicinal sedatives.[38]

This fusion of "sedation" and abuse in everyday life is one factor that loosened the lid on violence and afforded it a certain degree of legitimacy; the increasingly aggressive nature of therapies is another. As institutional conditions worsened and sterilization proved unable to reduce the number of institutionalized patients, psychiatrists suddenly "discovered" around mid-decade that certain new therapies being tested in Austria, namely, insulin and cardiazol shock therapies, were not as bad as they had originally imagined, and proceeded to deploy them as examples of cutting-edge science.[39] Some patients, indeed, reported being cured, and psychiatrists hailed the new treatments as medically beneficial and economically sound (the more people cured, the less money spent).[40]

One former Wittenau nurse did not give such a rosy account of these developments, telling an interviewer that "shock treatment was horrible for the patients. Real dramas took place. The patients had to be lifted by four nurses out of bed, into which they crawled with all their might. They were brought individually into the room for shock treatment. One nurse standing behind the patient held the gag to prevent [the patient from] biting the tongue; a doctor standing in front of the patient applied the anodes."[41] Indeed, the new therapies were drastic and life-threatening measures designed to shock the patient into a state of calm by generating a feeling of immanent death.[42] Insulin therapy resulted in (among other things) loss of muscular control, spasms, disorientation, and a feeling of hunger.[43] Shock therapy was particularly traumatic, generating a feeling of dying, intense fear, and frequent injuries and bone breaks.[44] In the context of these therapies, the concept of "healing" took on new dimensions; the patient was increasingly seen as the "bearer of a disturbance," and the goal of therapy was to eliminate that disturbance—to shock him or her into a state of "sociability."[45]

Psychiatrists did not see a great ethical problem here, arguing that they, like surgeons, sometimes had to take risks so that patients could get well.[46] That the "risk" to life and limb posed by schizophrenia in no way compares to that of a cancer in and of itself renders such logic absurd; but in addition, the new therapies ultimately made little difference in the number of patients who could be sent home healthy, and institutions remained overfilled.[47] Even worse, as psychiatrists pointed triumphantly to the relatively small number of success stories, the patients for whom they could do nothing loomed large and drew attention to their ultimate helplessness in the face of demographic pressures.[48]

The nagging presence of these patients side-by-side with the more hopeful cases fueled a discourse of medical and moral polarization. An administrator of the Kaufbeuren-Irsee institution, for example, wrote that most institutionalized patients were indeed curable and would sooner or later be released. "It would be untrue and irresponsible to characterize them as members of human society who are worthless and not competent [*tüchtig*] for life." It was unfortunate, but for technical reasons necessary, that the "idiots and people completely incompetent for life, as well as asocials and people who were a security risk," were also to be found, but their presence in no way detracted from the institutions' essentially medical character.[49]

This discourse had its roots in post-1929 Weimar psychiatry, which proposed various schemes for housing and treating patients as cheaply as possible—schemes that entailed categorizing them *medically* as curable or incurable. The preceding quotation raises the possibility that the addition of moral categories had a particular function: namely, it enabled psychiatrists to deflect official and popular contempt onto the incurable patients. Having done this, they could and did maintain that they still had the detentional function of protecting the public from dangerous and "asocial" patients; and for those national comrades (*Volksgenossen*) with more favorable prognoses, psychiatry still had a medical function to fulfill. As Peter Stolz has argued, they proceeded to oscillate between the two: "If therapeutic activity that did not hold much promise was questioned, they insisted on their task of upholding public security. If public assaults on the violation of their policelike security duty followed, they referred to their medical task."[50]

For the mentally ill, so it seemed, the days when they were innocent by definition and regardless of how they behaved were over: moral polarization, and with it the logic of selection, emerged as organizing principles of institutional life.

CONTINUITY AND BURIED TRANSFORMATIONS

The Nazi Seizure of Power and the Specter of Irrelevance

Psychiatrists under National Socialism seem to have realized that complicity and smooth transitions are best assured through the dampening of people's sense of alarm; for in the midst of

National Socialist consolidation in 1933, they began downplaying the seriousness of recent political developments. No, nurses were assured, psychiatry was definitely *not* sowing the seeds of its own oblivion by supporting compulsory sterilization. It would *not* wind up doing its job so "well" that psychiatric patients as such would eventually cease to exist and psychiatry would become obsolete. "[Psychiatric institutions] will never become superfluous."[51]

There were several reasons for this. Not all of the mentally ill fell under the purview of the sterilization law; those patients whose illness stemmed from physical injury or illness were exempt, as were chronically ill people who would never be released and, thus, would never have the chance to procreate. Moreover, the possibility remained that genetic mutations could produce as-yet-unknown forms of psychiatric illness.[52] Psychiatry would thus always be needed to provide long-term care and deliver cases of inherited illness up to the sterilization bureaucracy.

In addition, sterilization by no means cured patients and rendered them immediately eligible for release; many remained mentally ill and in need of institutionalization. Automatically releasing all sterilized patients would produce a security risk and deprive society of the labor of those family members to whose care they would be consigned.[53] Finally, even if current developments were to produce progressive decreases in institutional rates, Germany could not hope to "solve" the problem of "inherited inferiority" anytime soon even under optimal conditions; it would take generations, since some parents carrying inferior genes did not appear to be ill.[54] Thus, any way one looked at it, psychiatry's medical and detentional functions remained more or less as they had been before.

The ideal psychiatric nurse thus remained as indispensable as before; as Nurse Georg Roos wrote, "Psychiatrists and nurses are now called upon to do everything they can to protect the mentally ill from infirmity, to lighten their great burden, and to see to it that they can again be integrated into the German national community."[55] Nurses, in his view, were hardly of secondary importance in this process; rather, the nurse-doctor relationship was a "balanced relationship of two partners who are called upon to help sick national comrades and to promote their health. . . ."[56] While it was certainly true that the nurse's job was *subordinate* to that of the doctor insofar as it entailed carrying out his orders, "the work of the nurse is not worth less because of this."[57] Nurses' subordination, in short, was a necessary, and hardly degrading, dimension of the medical division of labor. Nursing was a suitable profession only for those motivated enough to carry it out in spite of its challenges and difficulties; only then would it offer the satisfaction necessary for the sustenance of professional enthusiasm.[58]

Mental Illness and the Human Community

The idea of mental illness as an "illness of the brain" continued to appear in nursing texts. The patient, one nurse wrote, "is just as sick as someone with an ailment of the heart, lungs, or liver."[59] This biological metaphor, combined with increasingly aggressive legal and therapeutic measures to "control" psychiatric illness, was undoubtedly the source of anxiety over whether mental illness could be contracted through contact with patients. In some texts, the answer was the same as in the previous decade: strictly speaking, "induced mental illness" could befall someone with (a) a predisposition to mental illness and (b) a close relationship with a mentally ill person of similar psychological makeup, such as a family member. Since only nurses from mentally healthy families were employed, and nurses themselves were not emotionally "close" enough to patients to enable contraction of a mental illness, the possibility was virtually eliminated.[60]

Nurses were nevertheless reminded of their *theoretical* vulnerability to the fate that had befallen their charges. "The nurse should empathize with his patients, [mentally] put himself in their place, and not forget that this tragedy could sometime happen to one of his dear relatives or even to himself."[61] This kind of empathy was, to be sure, mainly of *practical* importance; that is, it could help nurses discover and respond to the needs of their patients on an intuitive level. (One nurse argued that just as healthy people needed some kind of occasional change from the everyday routine, "the patient also needs a certain variety in his already inherently unhappy existence." For example, patients enjoyed the anticipation and celebration of holidays—including, "with pleasure," Hitler's birthday—and should be provided the opportunity to do so.)[62]

The implications of this idea are nevertheless startling, since proffering a shared human experience as the basis of psychiatric care was not even remotely consistent with Nazi ideology and, in certain ways, threatened it. But it was not unique. In 1937, for example, *Geisteskrankenpflege*'s editors published the article of a deacon who maintained that "I regard the patient as a human being just like every other and like myself." Nurses sharing this empathy had the potential to be more successful than they would be if they mechanically followed regulations: "No rules, no scheme, no requirements and bans, no force and violence will ever achieve what we can give of ourselves."[63]

The theme of shared humanity among staff and patients was particularly evident in a 1935 *Geisteskrankenpflege* article written by a doctor who had himself been a patient in a psychiatric institution. The very publication of such an article suggests that the editors were attempting to dissolve the pariah syndrome surrounding mental illness, along with the notion that the mentally ill were somehow fundamentally different. The content, however, pushes this farther: for the author, Dr. Bruckner, reported an unexpectedly high degree of self-control, patience, and sociability among his fellow patients. When an anxious patient paced back and forth in the dayroom, he heard hardly a sound of irritation from other patients. When the occasional complaint surfaced, it was met with a chorus of reproaches that this was a *sick* person who couldn't control his annoying behavior. "On these occasions I have sometimes had to ask myself," he wrote, "how long such a patient would be tolerated on the 'outside' and treated with forbearance and understanding! And who on the 'outside' would not immediately call for the 'book of complaints' if the food were to arrive cold on the table, while 'among us' such an occurrence is at the most only completely inciden-

tally commented upon."[64] If the editors of this journal had been
fully saturated with the National Socialist brand of contempt for
psychiatric patients *as such*, it would be difficult to understand
what interest they could possibly have had in publishing this
doctor's report. But it is indeed the case that many psychiatrists
involved in constructing an "image" of psychiatry in the National Socialist era took great pains to defend patients against
prejudice, even if, as we shall see later, their words obviously
cannot be taken at face value. In a curious way that runs counter
to all expectation, to National Socialist ideology, and to the
realities of institutional life, publishing psychiatrists and nurses
portrayed psychiatric patients as rightful members of the *Volksgemeinschaft*. This impression is only strengthened by the instruction that their caretakers must never simply allow mentally
incurable patients to die when physical illness befell them; and
nurses were to prevent suicide irrespective of the patient in
question.[65]

The Persistence of Orientation and Technique

The point of stressing the behavior-as-symptom principle to
nurses, as we have seen, was to drive home the message that
patients were not responsible for what they did.[66] This principle
was intended to enhance psychiatry's image as a medical (rather
than detentional) enterprise, but also, in a more specific sense,
to enable nurses to uphold moderation and humanity, as well
as discipline, during the stress, violence, and unpredictability of
everyday life. This principle continued to be articulated during
the National Socialist years; nurses were instructed to remind
themselves that patient violence or disruption was "the result of
hallucinations and crazy ideas of unpleasant content and the result of mistaken identity."[67]

Moreover, publishing psychiatrists and nurses continued to
insist that, as a result, every single person in their care, no matter
what they did or had done in the past, was a patient and to be
treated as such. As Dr. Hürten proclaimed, "mental illness is
fate, not guilt!"[68] Even institutionalized criminals were often

simply people whose illness rendered them vulnerable to temptation; "indeed, through their ability to be easily influenced," one nurse wrote, "they . . . first succumbed to temptation and became a criminal."[69] Accordingly, another nurse wrote that "these patients cannot be made responsible for what they say and do."[70] Returning any display of violence with violence was out of place on both moral and practical grounds: "That would be inhuman and also is never approved from a medical standpoint."[71]

Ideally, Dr. Wickel wrote, a nurse should attempt to prevent disturbances through activity: "The more we understand how to distract the patients from their hallucinations and crazy ideas through occupation, to socialize them through speech and example, the quieter they will be."[72] If a disturbance did arise, the nurse should attempt to calm the patient verbally. As a last resort, a patient would have to be physically restrained, "even though it unfortunately does not sound so nice." He described permissible restraint methods in great detail, specifying possible forms of patient injury that were to be avoided in the process.[73] Once pinned down to a bed by several nurses, the patient would be given a sedative by a doctor. If the anxiety persisted, the patient would have to be isolated, for no more than two hours, in a room that was neat, clean, and warm enough. After fifteen minutes the patient was to be checked. "Most of the time he will immediately be quiet, finding the room and solitude pleasant. . . ."[74]

"THE human mind is like a field; the less fruit that is planted in it, the more luxuriant the weeds grow."[75] Thus attempted Dr. Kesselring to convey the logic of *Erziehung* at a conference for matrons in 1935. Indeed, the Simonean approach, which sought to salvage and cultivate what was left of a patient's mental capabilities, remained at the forefront of psychiatric discourse during the National Socialist period—even though the insulin and cardiazol shock therapies were lauded as "quite effective and welcome from a medical standpoint."[76] Psychiatrists thus continued to portray psychological healing (and its necessary counterpart, the maintenance of discipline) as best achieved through staff members' verbally soliciting the cooperation of the patient. "The occupation of patients must be tried and tried again. . . . One goes farthest by speaking [to them]. If one succeeds in drawing a patient into activity, then the first step to recovery has sometimes been achieved."[77] Nurses were central to success, since they spent the most time with patients, and experience showed that "now and then the mentally ill confide something to the nurse that they do not want to tell the doctor."[78]

Indeed, successful *Erziehung* continued to be understood as a function of language technique, and the rule of thumb here was to remain calm, accommodating, and friendly. Nurses were never to insult, and thus possibly excite, a patient: "One should never mock, tease or aggravate the patients. . . ."[79] Rather, tact and empathy were required "to protect the legitimate feelings of our *Volksgenossen*."[80] Commands were to be avoided.[81] Nurses were discouraged from using colloquial, demeaning language when referring to their patients, particularly the word "crazy" (*verrückt*): "This word is not nice. Since we never impose an un-friendly word on a physically ill person, we should not do so on the mentally ill either. It is, after all, already sad enough for the patient himself and for his relatives that he has fallen sick. They deserve our sympathy."[82] Nurses were again discouraged from overestimating the reasoning capacity of patients and discussing their illusory or "crazy" ideas; they should instead attempt dis-traction. They were not to underestimate it, either, by casually discussing the escape or suicide attempts of other patients; "They think then of themselves, and already a good many have then attempted and carried out suicide or escape."[83]

Nurses were also reminded never to lie to patients: "Never lie to the patient, no 'white lies' either!!"[84] When collecting a patient at home for transport into an institution, for example, "one may never tell the patient something that is false. One should tell him, one has doctor's orders to being him to the hospital, his nerves need to be treated. When he is no longer sick, he will be released again. In the majority of cases the patient then goes qui-etly along."[85] These assorted language rules continued to aim at helping nurses cultivate a "friendly decisiveness" in their treat-ment of patients: "The psychiatric nurse should if possible spend his time among his patients as a pleasant companion. Without a doubt, friendliness and pleasant conversation have a quieting effect in the mental patient's clear moments and awaken a certain trust."[86] They were to *appear* to return such trust, but never to compromise their authority by doing so sincerely: "One should never. . . . become friends with a patient, always call the patients *Sie*, never allow intimacy to develop, and favor no patient. One should be equally friendly to all patients. But however friendly the nurse is, the patient must always have the feeling that the nurse is the authority."[87] Thus the tension persisted between the effectiveness of emotional proximity and the necessity of keeping a safe emotional distance—a tension that required nurses to be motivated in a general sense by "brotherly love" but prepared, in an emergency, to demonstrate "cold-bloodedness."[88]

A by-now-familiar facet of this code of conduct was controlling how the patient felt and perceived the intentions of others—controlling *appearances*. Particularly important was sustaining the appearance of the absence of coercion; but it was also particularly difficult because coercion often characterized the patient's first experience of institutional life. "This intrusion upon the freedom of the personality is in most cases bitterly felt, and a great deal depends on eliminating this feeling of having been violated." Thus nurses were to ensure that immediately upon arrival, the patient sensed that "he [would] be granted all the respect and love to which he is entitled both as a human being and first and foremost as a patient."[89]

This principle was to be upheld whenever possible for the duration of patients' institutionalization, especially since after their arrival they were installed in another situation that was often perceived as coercive, namely, occupational therapy. "Free time should awaken the feeling in the patients that at least during this time they can pursue their personal interests and inclinations. . . ."[90] In this context, nurses were also expected to give patients the feeling that they were quite happy to work on Sundays and holidays and took great pleasure in organizing patients' free time and thereby contributing to their mental recovery.[91] It would then be the case that the patients themselves "do not dread free time anymore; rather they look forward to it, recover more quickly, and perhaps take home with them whatever enthusiasm [they have acquired] for a sensible arrangement of free time as a permanent gain for their future life outside the institution."[92] The importance of boosting patients' moods was not limited to the most hopeful cases; the emotional comfort of more seriously ill patients mattered as well. "One may not take away the hope of recovery from a patient," one nurse wrote, and relatives were to be encouraged to observe this rule as well: "The patient, who sees relatives without hope standing beside his bed, is only made anxious. . . . Our wonderful task is to relieve the burden of the hard-tested, poor patients and to soothe their anguish. Our ambition is not only to nurse a patient back to health but also in case of emergency to make the last hour easier."[93] From the moment of institutionalization to the day of release or death, nurses were to cultivate an atmosphere charged with optimism, enthusiasm, order, and discipline.

While decreasing funding for psychiatric institutions resulted in the fact that the appearance of patients increasingly corresponded to, and thus reinforced, Nazi portrayals of "stupefied, unclean, virtually animalistic psychiatric patients,"[94] it is interesting to note that *Geisteskrankenpflege*'s authors were not unaware of the connection. For instance, according to one nurse, patients should be neatly dressed prior to work precisely to avoid this: "One should not mark out the patients, who as a result of their mental defect are often only externally conspicuous, as fools, insofar as one lets them go around in ill-fitting or even torn clothes."[95] This rule applied especially when visitors were expected: "The visitor judges the quality of the institution from the appearance of the patient. . . . Face, neck, and hands, and between the fingers must be washed."[96]

Sterilization, Complicity, and Moral Polarization

We see, then, that familiar themes received familiar treatment during the National Socialist years. The major novelty of the era, compulsory sterilization, also received extensive treatment; and alongside the rather predictable expressions of approval, we find psychiatrists again emphasizing the persistence of humane intent. Indeed, since one often finds references to sterilization as a punishment in historical scholarship,[97] it is especially important to emphasize that, however the matter appears to us now, Party officials and psychiatrists strenuously denied any connection between eugenic measures and personal guilt. Although today it is abundantly clear that cynicism, mercilessness, and prejudice abounded in the implementation of the GVeN, it is nevertheless revealing to explore the articulation of their alleged purpose: to apply "scientific" knowledge to social policy for the purpose of racial purity—unemotionally and without spite. In their attempt to sustain a sober, nonjudgmental discourse, psychiatrists presented themselves—and, by extension, nurses—as morally untainted agents in the whole affair and thus did away with the need to think a great deal about the significance of their own complicity. The discourse itself, however, wound up invoking National Socialist imagery of the noncooperative, nonconformist, asocial person and thus undermined their otherwise adamant insistence on all patients' intrinsic innocence.

There was no question in the minds of *Geisteskrankenpflege*'s contributors that proposed eugenic measures, and especially sterilization, were necessary and justified. They realized, however, that their enthusiasm was not universally shared, and went to great lengths to defuse any negative emotional impact of recent social and political developments. Psychiatrists reminded nurses that absolutely nothing had changed on the scientific front; eugenics was not an intellectual fad but rather a decades-old *science* whose "significance" had finally been recognized and incorporated into state policy in the service of the *Volk*. "If it is so that in past years and under the old regime everyone was talking back and forth, and one could not and did not want to decide on ideological grounds to do something to protect the eugenically valuable family lineages in our *Volk*, then we must be thankful that Adolf Hitler's ingenious insight and infectious energy have shown us a way to avoid the certain decline of our *Volk*."[98] Eugenic measures, psychiatrists repeatedly suggested, were not drastic and were hardly a reason for apprehension or alarm; they simply entailed "measures for grading fertility according to racial value."[99] Just as the prevention of infectious diseases was obviously preferable to treating them once they had appeared, preventing the spread of genetic deficiencies by taking analogous steps was a matter of common sense.[100]

There was, to be sure, a variety of possibilities for achieving the desired ends: "positive" eugenic measures such as marriage loans for nonpredisposed partners were undoubtedly useful for filling the gene pool with racially pure and healthy offspring; but, as Dr. Hoffmann insisted, positive measures could not work without "negative" ones which would ensure that undesirable elements tapered off and eventually disappeared.[101] One could, of course, attempt to "enlighten" predisposed people as to the need to refrain from reproducing and even forbid them to marry; but there was no guarantee that they would heed such advice, and, being irresponsible types anyway, they would have no qualms about producing illegitimate children. Incarcerating such people was too expensive, so sterilization was in fact the only viable choice.[102]

This kind of language notwithstanding, they insisted that sterilization was not a punishment. Its codification in the form of law was not intended to brand genetically ill people as criminals or asocials, but rather simply to protect everyone involved: "Sterilization must be legally regulated, on the one hand, because an unconditional granting of it could give occasion for abuse; and, on the other hand, [it must be regulated] so that the doctor carrying out eugenic sterilization does not run the danger of making himself guilty of grievous bodily harm [*Körperverletzung*]."[103] A law sanctioning compulsory sterilization also "spared" Catholics unpleasant conflicts of conscience.[104]

Moreover, psychiatrists reminded nurses, sterilization itself was not as traumatic as one would think. It was a simple, ultimately harmless procedure that had no effect whatsoever on the person's health: "The sexual drive and the ability to copulate are preserved in the sterilized person; solely the fertility is taken from him [or her]. On humanly understandable grounds, one cannot emphasize this point enough."[105] The violation of bodily integrity and the prospect of a childless future, psychiatrists apparently assumed, were not so bad so long as everything still "worked." (That the procedure was, to the contrary, a considerable risk to the physical and emotional welfare of the patient was not only unacknowledged but denied.)[106]

Once these points had been established, the moral legitimacy of specific eugenic measures was assumed to follow as a matter of course. But if it did not, psychiatrists could resort to stressing the urgency of the genetic "problem." The latter strategy often entailed citing birthrates among the "inferior" and the amount of money they cost the state, but psychiatrists also exploited preexisting prejudices and graphic anecdotal "evidence." Dr. Hoffmann, for example, argued that it was precisely because Germany was a "civilized" country that "inferior" people reproduced so quickly; completely lacking any sense of social or individual responsibility, they reproduced willy-nilly without asking themselves whether they could care for their offspring. Over the years, they had adopted the strategy of claiming, "The state must feed me and my children."[107]

Women, in Hoffmann's opinion, were a major source of the problem. As "proof," he cited a graphic report of a welfare department official (*Wohlfahrtsdezernent*) at length:

> I see standing before me this mother squealing on account of every little triviality. Wilted, ugly, badly clothed. Hair matted. Face ravaged by wrinkles. Hands dirty, knobby. Clothes torn, full of patches. Socks badly darned. Shoes worn out. A figure to pity. A cloud of bad smell behind her. Enough to make one vomit. They say she has always squealed so, smelled so. And indeed she has borne five children. Five times she has become a mother. Don't know by whom. A girl of fifth-rate [quality] and even so five times mother. She frequented the worst locales, drank, smoked. Got venereal disease, was in the hospital. Got well, in order to pursue her vices again. Became a mother again, her worms burdening [the child] with afflictions.[108]

This, Hoffmann noted, made clear "to every serious reader . . . how terribly necessary eugenic action is."[109]

Be this as it may, this discursive elision of "genetically ill" and "asocial" produced more than its share of problems in the implementation of the law. By 1938 Dr. Enge was attempting to bring his readership back into the fold by arguing that although such "asocials" were a significant source of the problem, they constituted only a subgroup of genetically defective persons, among whom many "mentally and morally fully worthy people" were to be found. Indeed, he continued, in 1935 the Reich minister of propaganda had asked the Association of German Newspaper Publishers (*Verband der Deutscher Zeitungsverleger*) to avoid using the term "inferior" (*minderwertig*) in connection with genetic illness. "Only the pronounced pests, asocials, and criminals are to be characterized as inferior."[110] This undifferentiated social and personal degradation was even more inappropriate because many genetically ill persons voluntarily applied to be sterilized after making the "painful" realization that producing children would be an injustice vis-à-vis the *Volk*. This display of martyrdom was hardly a sign of inferiority; it was rather an indication of "moral high quality" (*sittlicher Hochwertigkeit*).[111]

Thus psychiatrists portrayed themselves as humane and, above all, by no means vindictive; they were simply fulfilling their duty to the *Volk*, a duty that was particularly difficult precisely because it often meant anger and sorrow for the afflicted. Considering the above discussion carefully, however, we find reason to qualify this conclusion: their allegedly humane impulses were not directed at everyone but rather *reserved for the compliant*; asocials were asocials, just as they had been before.

The genetically ill did not constitute a homogeneous and uniformly stigmatized group, then, but rather two morally divergent ones: the "good" ones demonstrated their sense of responsibility by volunteering to be sterilized, while the "bad" ones reproduced with abandon. All were subject to sterilization, but through a clever rhetorical twist, psychiatrists generated pressure to conform by identifying and stigmatizing an "other" within that group, thus presenting the remaining members with the choice of "sinking" to the level of the asocial or rejoining the ranks of the respectable. They exploited the desperation that moves people to salvage what can be salvaged in a hopeless situation—to retain some dignity in the process of being robbed of their dignity.

Particularly important in the current context, however, is the potential result of this entire discussion in the minds of nurses. As we have seen, psychiatrists maintained that compulsory sterilization was not an issue worthy of great moral concern for nurses because it was not a punishment and had no lasting effects on health. At the same time, they spoke about sterilization candidates in connection with personal irresponsibility and guilt. The insistence on psychiatry's moral "neutrality" in the whole affair combined with imagery of the asocial enabled nurses to deny punitive *intent* and yet subscribe to a punitive *way of thinking*—namely, that some people in fact "deserved" it.

Fellow Human Beings and Emotional Proximity

Thus we see that in the process of denying malicious intent, psychiatrists adopted a language which, for the unlucky or uncompliant patients, was riddled with contempt. This phenomenon presents us with the possibility that the rules and messages proffered by psychiatrists cannot be taken at face value, and we must examine the arguments *behind* these rules for further insight into their meaning and into their potential to transform ways of thinking. As the above example suggests, we cannot simply ask ourselves what rules governed nurse-patient relationships; we must also ask ourselves how the rule in question affected the moral status of patients.

If we return to the subjects of premature death and suicide, for example, we find reason to qualify our previous impressions regarding the status of all patients as "fellow human beings." In psychiatric circles, the GVeN prompted the rather predictable question of "what next?" Would euthanasia follow? Indeed, as early as October 1934, Dr. Wittneben of the Hessian Brotherhouse at Hephata reported that, particularly among district committees (*Kreisausschüsse*) weary of financing institutional care, the law had raised the expectation that the "extermination of life unworthy of living" would soon follow. He categorically rejected this idea, asserting that in times of physical illness, psychiatric nurses must provide the same care for the most unresponsive, hopeless cases as they would for more hopeful cases with prospects for mental, as well as physical, recovery.[112]

This, of course, is consistent with the above-mentioned ban on allowing premature death and suicide. But if we read on, we find reason to question the extent to which this rule is truly an affirmation of the "rights" of the patient and thus an implicit critique of National Socialist attitudes toward the mentally ill. In fact, Wittneben defended this position with reference to none other than the Führer himself, who allegedly declared in a September 1933 speech that "the Creator has planted the drive of self-preservation inside all living things!" Wittneben, missing the point, understood this "drive" to be the equivalent of an "immortal soul" that, in his experience, sometimes made itself known from the depths of the most unresponsive, corpselike patient just minutes before death. "He who experiences something like this," he maintained, "will not dare to exterminate 'life unworthy of living.' "[113] "Of course" this did not mean that a dying patient should be kept alive—only that we as mortals were not in a position deliberately to shorten it; that "we as earthbound human beings ultimately cannot solve the body-soul problem, that we have, rather, a particular responsibility for these souls who are bound to the fragile body[;] as Roseggers says, 'Help the poor man carry his sheaf; otherwise he will go to the Lord and complain about you!' "[114] In the eyes of some believers, the existence of a soul rendered deliberate killing of any person, "useful" or not, contrary to God's will.

A similar kind of modesty underpinned the imperative to prevent patient suicide. Rather than arguing that no one should be killed because "mortals" were not justified to make such decisions, Dr. Donalies argued that no patient should be allowed to commit suicide because *nurses* were not in a position to make such decisions: "It is . . . not permissible to allow for deliberations which—in themselves and in other contexts perhaps debatable—are foreign to the purposes of sick care; we mean here deliberations such as whether suicide constitutes a form of desirable self-selection in the sense of preserving the species, etc."[115] Even if it was clear in the case of a "worthy" person that preventing suicide was desirable, "it [was] not acceptable to make distinctions in a particular case on the basis of this standpoint."[116] There were administrative reasons for this: psychiatrists, after all, had to look after the reputations of their institutions and were responsible for explaining the circumstances of death to relatives. More significant, however, they wanted to avoid the even more potentially dangerous consequences of nurses' taking such matters into their own hands.

What are the implications of this? We seem to have discovered a repetition of the requirement of humility vis-à-vis patients that we encountered in Weimar nursing literature. In the National Socialist State this was not, however, a collectively shared humility based on an acknowledgment of the essential vulnerability of *all* human beings—a humility to which *everyone* subscribes in order to create a psychological bulwark against the exploitation of the weak. The kind of humility being proffered was that of the herdlike masses who have resigned completely from the business of thinking critically and hand that business over to someone else. Nurses were encouraged to consider the question of a patient's social or moral "worth" irrelevant in their professional context—at the most, a private issue best kept behind closed doors (although Donalies did not squander the opportunity explicitly to call the worth of such lives into question). Thus it is not necessarily the case that the rules concerning death and suicide were an affirmation of the patient's integrity as a fellow human being, nor were they intended to enhance nurses' emotional proximity to their patients. Rather, they tended to encourage *abstinence from thinking about the moral status of the patient in the first place*. This abstinence, as we shall see, was far more useful to the Nazis than the most rabid fanaticism.

PROFFERING moral abstinence on matters of life and death was one strategy for discouraging nurses' interest in the fate of individual patients; another was insisting on the absolutely secondary nature of the individual patient's welfare vis-à-vis the social whole: "We must give up the orientation toward the individual person who has fallen ill, which has almost become a tradition, and turn our attention to the far more important problem of considering the entire *Volk*."[117] Success in this mental realignment was a matter of simple enlightenment: "If the nurse knows the laws of heredity, he will never again see the individual sick being in this patient; rather it will become clear to him that this patient is only a link in the chain of sickly 'hereditary lines,' and thus he comes to that "contemplation of the whole" which opposes the individualistic-Marxist worldview."[118] The already vague and limited rhetorical power of the individual patient's welfare in nursing texts thus received a decisive blow.

It would be mistaken, however, to exaggerate the intended effect of this "downgrading" of the individual. Weimar psychiatrists, as we have seen, implied that there *is* a difference on some level between the welfare of the individual and his or her social utility (reflected by their tendency to mention them separately). But their chief aspiration, which underpinned every therapeutic innovation, was to demonstrate that what was good for the patient was also good for society; thus there was no apparent need to discuss potential conflicts between science and ethics, and no need to worry a great deal about the possibility that psychiatry would diverge too widely from its essentially "humane" purpose. Indeed, all that was supposed to change was nurses' *perception* of patients in relation to other human beings, not their *treatment* of them: "The care of the pitiable patients should not be diminished. But from an understanding of the connections comes an understanding for the welfare of the whole."[119]

Thus, as in the sterilization discussion, nurses were presented with a professional image of themselves as caring and impartial—an image, in short, which was essentially identical to that of the previous decade in terms of ethical orientation. They were provided with explicit reassurance of their own moral innocence—indeed, moral virtue—at the very moment when the interests of the individual patient effectively lost their remaining integrity. The intended effect was complacency and self-satisfaction in the face of political developments, not the kind of contempt that might have instigated maltreatment or dismissive talk about "lives unworthy of living."

Nurses armed with such "understanding," it was expected, would serve as propaganda instruments for enlightening patients' relatives and identifying potential sterilization candidates through the reporting of genetic illness. In this capacity, they were to be mouthpieces and nothing more. They were not to bring mitigating circumstances to bear on their report or bother themselves with the question of whether a patient fell under the purview of the law. That was the doctor's task. For them, participating in the enforcement of the law was a simple yes-or-no affair: Did the patient suffer from one of the eight conditions or not? Nurses were not to dismiss the significance of a single episode of mental illness, such as a manic-depressive attack. "It is only a question of whether the patient just once in his life has suffered from a condition of that kind."[120]

THIS brings us to a final example of the reinforcement of nurses' emotional distance, namely, the finer details governing language between nurses and doctors—in particular, the nurse's daily report. It was on the occasion of the doctor's daily visit that nurses were to make such reports, and "at the bidding of the doctor. The nurses should not lead the conversation in the presence of the doctor." The report was to be limited to facts alone: "The report should never contain one's own opinion [but] rather only a simple description of what actually was observed or experienced. The doctor wants to form his own opinion about the patient's condition."[121] A motivated and competent nurse, therefore, was controlled at the very outset by the rule not to speak unless spoken to. Although a seemingly minor point, this rule was significant enough to warrant mention in more than one context.[122] As for the report itself, we learn that nurses' critical skills were to be fully concentrated on making a report as concise, objective, and *devoid* of judgment as possible.

It would be a mistake to interpret this state of affairs simply as a lesson in *Kadavergehorsam*. After all, in other contexts nurses continued to be encouraged to take intellectual interest in their profession and initiative in their daily activities; in fact, this was the surest way to achieve satisfaction in the profession they had chosen: "If [a nurse] has the internal compulsion to work on his further education, to raise himself above the average of his professional colleagues, *not simply to wait for instructions from his superior* but rather to make observations himself, to devote himself entirely to his patients, then he will seldom find a profession which can offer so much inner satisfaction as that of the psychiatric nurse...."[123] This, of course, sounds very impressive indeed, but closer inspection reveals that this comment is not at odds with the advice above. A good nurse did not remain *passive*, simply waiting for instructions; but what did he or she do instead?—made *observations*, which we have just seen described as ideally devoid of judgment. The emphasis on taking initiative obscures an underlying psychological pressure to think in an objective, not subjective, mode, and to reveal those thoughts on cue. It was not, ultimately, rules from without that were supposed to "control" nurses; rather, rules were designed to regulate thought and action from within.

We must remind ourselves that in their substance, these articles did not greatly differ from commentary on this point during the Weimar Republic. What had changed is the potential *implication of these rules under changed circumstances*. Although a harmless enough attempt to order professional relations in the course of relatively "normal" daily activities during the Weimar Republic, explicitly limiting the scope of critical thought to the execution of a static set of technical responsibilities takes on a new significance when patients mysteriously begin to disappear and rumors about killings start to circulate. The evidence that nurses were not "truly" bound to an ethic of obedience during the "euthanasia" program is by now widespread and persuasive; but these details of their dealings with doctors suggest that such claims of rigidified subservience may not have been products of false consciousness or outright lies either. Here, we gain some insight into why it may very well have *appeared* to nurses that it was not their job to trouble themselves, let alone comment, about the fate of their patients.

Therapy, Conformity, and the Loss of Innocence

Work therapy, as we have seen above, retained both its therapeutic and its economic importance in nursing literature of the 1930s. If one looks closely, however, one begins to detect a shift in psychiatrists' attitudes about what kind of work was done by whom—a shift that reveals the erosion of medical integrity and the increasing determination of therapy by the dictates of utility.

Weimar psychiatrists attempted to downplay the economic importance of what was done in the course of occupational therapy; for them, what mattered was that *something* be done. In the 1930s, this notion came to be treated as outdated. Some patients, one senior nurse wrote in *Geisteskrankenpflege*, had made small playthings or models with great enthusiasm in the past; "but in the end it was after all only an activity that would appeal to a child, but not to a healthy, grown-up person."[124] While it certainly made sense to have the more serious cases start with easy tasks, another nurse noted, more capable patients were to be promoted to increasingly useful activity: "We must turn our attention to bringing the patient from simple forms of work to ones of progressively higher value, and ultimately helping him work on his own."[125]

The importance of progressively more complicated and "useful" occupation was more explicitly formulated by Dr. Wittneben, who championed the achievements of his own institution. The staff's therapeutic efforts on behalf of their "feebleminded" charges were directed at the mastery not of abstract skills such as spelling or counting but rather of concrete skills that would make them "competent" (*tüchtig*) for life. "It is far more important to us that a patient learns to chop potatoes correctly [or] to dig over a field than that he can recite poems or songbook verses, or that he knows where Constantinople is."[126] Reading figured into this process only insofar as it served the purpose of communicating values that would fuel productive activity. Patients were first educated in simpler values such as helping others or being kind to animals; they then would be taught the "higher" ethics of honor and loyalty to the Fatherland; they would learn that the industrious person gets more than the lazy person, and that striving for property is a good thing; they would be shown how to use money.[127] Psychiatry could not work wonders; but it could at least salvage the patient's feeble mental capacities, transform them into modest but sufficient performance, and thus prevent the mentally ill from becoming a "burden" to society at large.[128]

DURING the National Socialist years, occupational therapy had an additional and equally important function. As one nurse wrote, it provided a context in which patients could feel that they were "members of the human society . . . who are still useful in life."[129] "Imbeciles" in particular lacked a "feeling for order and community"; through work, they would learn "to control themselves and to suppress that which is not helpful for collective life."[130] Through occupational therapy, patients learned the virtues and "necessity" of conformity within a group.

Nonconformity, that is, disruption or bad habits, signaled that "therapy" was not working; nurses were thus to act as corrective influences. Particularly with criminal patients, the nurse "must work with great decisiveness against all bad habits and when necessary make clear that he is not willing to accept ill-mannered conduct, mean-spirited behavior, and offenses against the community and the house rules."[131] This is a point that we have encountered in the writings of Weimar psychiatrists: since psychiatric illness could be "seen" only through behavioral symptoms, the alteration of those symptoms was a subject of increasing therapeutic interest. *Erziehung* aimed at the alteration of behavior in such a way that it would increasingly conform to the virtues associated with *Sittlichkeit*. During the 1930s, *Erziehung* continued to be explained in terms of cultivating the remaining "healthy" parts of the patient's mind, while mental health and illness corresponded, for all intents and purposes, to the presence or absence of *Sittlichkeit* in the social "world" of the institution.

There is, however, a subtle and highly significant difference: the relation between work and sociability was articulated in language that suggests an increasingly rigid mapping of mental health and illness onto the value system of *Sittlichkeit*. Although a stated goal of *Erziehung* continued to be the extraction of patient cooperation through language, the kind of behavior expected was highly specified. A common metaphor, for example, was getting someone "on the right track": "In some cases a bad habit of a patient can lead to a good result if one understands how to cleverly lead them onto the right track."[132] Occupational therapy's success was partially ascribed to its helping overactive patients channel their energy onto a "social course" and thus allowing "no room for wrong actions."[133] A decade earlier, order and discipline characterized a favorable environment in which a patient could be socialized; but *during the National Socialist years, they increasingly constituted not part of the therapeutic "background" but rather the goal of therapy itself.*

The result of this was a "bending" of certain rules in the interest of order and discipline. In 1940, one nurse wrote that it was useful to respond to a patient's "crazy" ideas with a "harmless joke . . . so that the patient notices that he is not taken seriously." This was intended to prevent the patient from sinking deeper into his or her illusions. "With irascible people," he continued, "it is, however, better to appear to go along with their ideas."[134] Apparently the demand for nurses to remain truthful had become less important than keeping the peace.

This development is most vividly seen, however, in commentaries on handling discipline from the National Socialist period.

To be sure, we saw in the above discussion how little had changed from a decade earlier; most important, the behavior-as-symptom principle and patients' unaccountability for their actions continued to underpin the ban on nurses' returning violence with violence. Cracks in this humanitarian edifice, however, appeared at least as early as 1935 in Dr. Kesselring's above-mentioned speech before a conference of hospital matrons. Although familiar, his advice reveals that the emergence of order and discipline at the forefront of psychiatric praxis had distinct consequences for the moral status of patients.

Waxing philosophical, he told the matrons that the human mind reflected nature: it consisted of creative and destructive forces. Human history showed that even among "normal" people, it was difficult enough to keep the destructive forces tamed; but among psychiatric patients, the task was even more formidable and the results potentially catastrophic: "Anyone can best judge what an unhealthy spirit in institutional life means if he observes how a single excited patient is able to arouse and upset an entire ward, how such a patient is in the position to poison all pleasure in work with his remarks about 'exploitation' and 'improper unreasonable demands,' how he destroys every community by generating hostilities and through mutual suspicion, how he ruins the appetite of the others at mealtimes through his eternal grumbling. We absolutely must protect our patients from this kind of harm."[135] The disruption produced by patients' spiritual chaos was highly contagious, but, thankfully, so were the virtues of order and discipline. Nurses were charged with a kind of collective spiritual realignment whereby the destructive impulses of their charges would be snuffed out and a "healthy" spirit would prevail. "The helpful and loving spirit that must manifest itself in every good institution will come to life only when every employee is so imbued with it that he radiates it directly on the entire environment and carries the others involuntarily along. The finer and kinder the tone that emerges from the personnel, the less the primitive person will try to assert himself with crude and rough methods."[136] This is the demand for "managed appearances" writ large: nurses were not simply in charge of creating an environment in which things went smoothly, interpersonal harmony prevailed, and patients could go about the business of "healing" under optimal circumstances. Rather, they were responsible for giving life to a "spirit" that spread like smoke through the institution, permeated all its inhabitants, and eliminated every imaginable reason for disciplinary problems.

The glorification of this "spirit" was not unique to Kesselring; Dr. Hürten used a similar metaphor, writing that "a correcting principle must fill the entire house as the prevailing spirit, draw each phenomenon and course of daily events inside the house into its track, [and] obligate the doctor, nurse, and patients [*Insassen*] in the same way."[137] We have now reached the heart of the matter, where the prerequisite or "background" of the healing process had turned into its very goal. While order and discipline had originally been seen as a necessary pre- and corequisite of successful *Erziehung*, increasing the likelihood that patients would be *drawn* to cooperate in their treatment and *voluntarily* behave, coercion reentered psychiatric discourse through the back door, so to speak: the "correcting principle" was to prevail in everyday activity, and patients, just like mentally healthy doctors and nurses, were subject to a "duty" to follow it. Those who were institutionalized precisely because of their inability to play by the same "rules" as mentally healthy people were subjected to those rules as part of their treatment. They were thus expected to display the very capacities that they were there to acquire, and those who did not had to learn quickly indeed.[138]

We see this in Kesselring's rules for handling deviance. Not bothering to trouble himself with reminders about what nurses should think in such circumstances (i.e., remind themselves of the behavior-as-symptom principle), he proceeded straight to the techniques of crisis management. In the spirit of Simonean work therapy, nurses were to extinguish any disruption of order immediately in order to succeed: "One of his most important principles is that for every disruption, for every inconsiderate act vis-à-vis other patients, a reaction which ends the disruption must immediately and inexorably follow."[139] Patients were to be constantly reminded to be considerate of others around them; and "when direct, friendly advice does not suffice, the necessity of the required consideration is emphasized in the presence of others."

At this point, Kesselring began a subtle slide from explaining "friendly decisiveness" vis-à-vis an essentially innocent person to the verbal coercion of a guilty one: the failure to extract conformity through peer pressure was to be followed by threats behind closed doors: "He who is too hard of hearing for these requirements is to be 'confidentially' advised by the personnel that unpleasant measures should be expected if he continues to offend against the required decency."

But, Kesselring continued, "the methods are by no means exhausted yet. . . ." Threats were to be carried out if the patient continued to resist cooperation: "When the patient is immediately and automatically taken out of the community after each inconsiderate act and transferred into an unpleasant environment, a better adaptation to the desired spiritual atmosphere tends to follow very soon. It is important that in the process one does not moralize, that the measure does not take on the character of a punishment, which in such cases only has an upsetting effect, but rather that it is simply declared to be a necessity and carried out with an expression of regret, but mercilessly."[140] Again, Kesselring's references to the power of suggestion, the necessity of firm and immediate reaction to disturbances, and the occasional need for isolation echoed Dr. Wickel's advice above. But his attempts to echo him in spirit failed in the face of logical contradictions. How could he advocate a patient repetition of the rules as the precursor to isolation and then maintain that conformity was best achieved by "immediate and automatic" removal of the patient from the group following each episode of inconsiderate behavior? If isolation was truly not a punishment, but rather an attempt to distract and remove the patient from the source of anxiety, why did the isolation environment need to be "unpleasant"? If patients had only limited control over their behavior, why so much emphasis on threats?

An answer to these questions might read as follows: it was not only the welfare of the well-behaved patients that was at issue when a patient became violent, but also the legitimacy of the entire psychiatric enterprise. Nurses were entrusted with building a "world" permeated by friendliness, politeness, industry, and self-discipline; any alternative interpretation of everyday realities tore at the edges of their carefully constructed picture of the way things were. Moreover, there was no *logical* reason for complaints or alternative interpretations. Behavior that did not conform to the prevailing procedures and attitudes proffered by nurses (even a plausible critique of work therapy as "exploitation") thus had to be dismissed as the nonsense of a "primitive"[141] and contrary person. It is this subtext that constitutes the reintroduction of coercion into the theoretically noncoercive practice of *Erziehung*.[142]

The result, Kesselring's commentary suggests, was the emergence of a politics of everyday life where lines were drawn not only between nurses and patients but also between well-behaved patients and hell-raisers—the "disruptive and antagonistic elements."[143] Although he promoted the same techniques for crisis management as had Weimar psychiatrists—techniques that were grounded on the essential innocence of a mentally ill person—Kesselring explained the logic behind those techniques with a language which suggests that, on some level, patients were in fact deemed responsible, to *some* degree, for their deviance.

The question of patients' intrinsic guilt or innocence was thrown into relief during the National Socialist years by the presence of institutionalized criminals. This subgroup of patients bore, by definition, *factual* guilt, insofar as they had committed a crime. The problem for psychiatrists concerned whether such people also bore *moral* guilt and should be stigmatized as a consequence. Weimar psychiatrists, as we have seen, had little difficulty maintaining the moral innocence of their "factually guilty" patients in nursing texts. It seems, however, that the Nazi regime's merciless campaign of aggression against "asocials" and various other "enemies" of the regime put psychiatrists in an awkward situation—after all, it would be highly impolitic for them to continue to maintain the absolute inno- cence of such people, if they had ever truly believed it in the first place. The result was an attempt to find some middle ground.

Dr. Hürten discussed criminal patients at length and, as we have seen above, declared that "mental illness is fate, not guilt!" In doing so, however, he dodged the essential question, which was not whether people were guilty for being mentally ill, but rather whether mental illness rendered them unaccountable and thus innocent in a moral sense. On this point he was ambivalent, writing that the occupants of the high-security ward (*Bewahr- haus*) were "pathological people who *through their own guilt and strange fate* were torn away from the correct path in life and from the circle of their relatives, criminals who are shut off from human society and ostracized. . . ."[144] Luckily for all involved, however, the question of moral guilt or innocence was not a crit- ical one for nurses anyway, since their caretaking and socializing responsibilities were not past- but rather future-oriented. Their chief concern was working with what mental "material" they had and cultivating mental health from there. In the Simonean tradition, Hürten advised nurses to keep in mind that such pa- tients, whatever they had done, "still have not only bad charac- teristics but also frequently a shred of a feeling of selflessness that wants to work itself out somehow."[145] By doggedly cultivat- ing what little remained of a patient's virtues, a nurse could arouse feelings of responsibility and respect. The centerpiece of treatment and discipline was bringing the patient to trust the doctor as someone in whose hands his or her fate lay.[146]

This, in the end, was the real concern of Hürten's article, not the assertion of the essential educability—and redeemable social worth—of patients. He was attempting to motivate staff, who worked with a stigmatized group of people, to assume leader- ship roles and demonstrate their *own* social worth. Indeed, the more mental illness was equated with moral degeneracy during the National Socialist years, the more strenuous were the efforts to puff up the egos of nurses—particularly those nurses at- tending to criminal patients:

The correct conduct with the unsociable, criminal, mentally inferior [people], [people of] defective character, and mentally ill people requires personnel to have, in addition to a keen instinctive sense for every readiness to react among the patients [*Insassen*], a high degree of tact, zeal, circumspection, and a ready courage[—]in short, personality values that correspond in particular to the manly virtues. The nurse should be not only a nurse but also a respect-inspiring socializer [*Erzieher*], lively role model, sincere adviser of the patients, and the intermediary agent between patient and doctor, whose skillful and conscientious colleague he is in every endeavor.[147]

That the moral and potential social "worth" of patients was by no means affirmed in this article is further suggested by Hürten's agreement with critics who opposed expenditure of public funds for the care and detention of "elements that are biologically inferior and harmful to the *Volk*." Future "organizational" changes would attempt to reduce nurse-patient ratios in the high-security wards—without, of course, compromising therapeutic effectiveness or the security of their inhabitants.[148] Thus Hürten left the question of guilt unclear and implicitly affirmed public contempt for such people—contempt that certainly was not reserved for criminal patients.

Be this as it may, Hürten had no interest in undermining the moral status of criminal patients *too* much—since they, along with their fellow noncriminal patients, gave rhyme and reason to the entire psychiatric enterprise. Moreover, he was not alone in claiming a rightful place for them in institutions. Dr. Bücken, for example, realized that criminal patients were increasingly unwelcome in the eyes of some doctors and nurses, but he attempted to change their minds. Although he could sympathize with such feelings, criminals should nevertheless be treated without exception with the same decency as other patients: "I know that it is difficult for some nurses to see the patient in a schizophrenic murderer, and not the murderer. . . . On the other hand, if we know about the great devastation of the personality that can be caused by mental illness and the other previously mentioned disorders, then it will not be impossible for us to separate the criminal element from the illness and to behave in a humane way."[149] To keep them on the straight and narrow in this respect, he urged nurses to avoid speaking of patients as dangers to the public.

Bücken's advice sounds ludicrous indeed if we consider that it appeared during the fifth month of the T4 program. It may, however, have had (intentionally or not) specific psychological effects on its readers. First of all, it reiterated humanitarian sentiments that had been at the very foundation of psychiatry's self-understanding for years, namely, that anyone in their care was to be treated as a patient—and, by extension, nurses were better off not thinking about guilt and innocence (just as they were not to think about whether to allow death or suicide). Second, nurses were told that the legal and medical systems were working together to ensure that these people were treated fairly, with goodwill, and with special attention to their "medical needs" while also protecting the community at large.[150] Thus they as nurses need not worry about the fate of patients because the "experts" were looking out for them and had everything under control.

The Transformation of Responsibility

During the National Socialist years, there was great emphasis in *Geisteskrankenpflege* on the already-widely-proffered idea that a willingness to assume a tremendous amount of responsibility was essential for a psychiatric nurse. Although, as we have seen, nurses were explicitly excluded from assuming moral responsibility in matters of life and death, their technical responsibilities were manifold: since many patients could not speak or otherwise express physical pain or illness, only nurses, who observed them around the clock, were in a position to notice changes and alert the doctor accordingly; in this sense, they bore responsibility for the day-to-day welfare of the patient and for the evolution of his or her condition. Nurses were also partially responsible for the success of therapy insofar as they served as role models

and enticed patients to work. Last but not least, they were responsible for preventing suicide and escape—protecting, that is,
patients from themselves and society at large from patients.[151]

After "euthanasia" measures and the war began, however,
psychiatrists began to radically downgrade the degree of responsibility doctors and nurses could reasonably be expected to
assume in their detentional and therapeutic capacities. A Mar-
burg psychiatrist, for example, wrote a three-part article in 1943
that emphasized the limited ability of institutional staff to prevent patient injury or escape. While of course negligence and
inattentiveness had no place in psychiatric care, it was nevertheless the case that "in practical psychiatry—as everywhere, in the
end—a certain moment of danger has to be accepted . . . , a certain moment of uncertainty always remains, [and] in deciding
the guilt or responsibility question in a particular case it is not
always easy to find something that is completely fair for *all*
those. . . . who are affected."[152] As an example, he recounted an
incident in which a patient had died after eating over one and
a half pounds of poisonous berries while on a wood-hauling
mission with fourteen other patients and one nurse. The state's
attorney had dropped charges against the nurse but lodged
them instead against the doctor on duty, on the grounds that
perhaps this particular patient's condition spoke against his
being sent to work with a group under the supervision of only
one nurse. The author reported having submitted an expert's report in defense of the doctor, after which the charges were
dropped. "In this sad incident we were dealing with an unlucky
coincidence, as can happen sometimes in occupational therapy
and in modern treatment of the mentally ill in general, without
their application therefore having to be regarded as questionable."[153] With this example, one can detect a hint of unconditional exculpation—a deferment of responsibility in such a way
that no one is, in fact, responsible. The most radical expression
of this psychological and moral bailout, of course, was the simultaneous participation of institutional personnel in murdering allegedly "incurable" patients. Although they could hardly
take refuge in "unfortunate accidents," many psychiatric staff

maintained after the war that responsibility for their own complicity lay elsewhere. Although a full discussion of the origins and dynamics of this psychological accommodation must be deferred until chapter 8, let me note here that the process of reconceptualizing "responsibility" in nursing texts entailed first *partially* dissolving it: as we have seen earlier, the responsibility of patients for their own behavior was no longer completely rejected; and here we see that the responsibility of staff for patients' behavior was no longer unconditionally maintained.

The notion of responsibility that crystallized from these shifting attitudes privileged the *Volk* as the primary object of moral concern. In addition to emphasizing nurses' diminished responsibility in the area of detention, psychiatrists frequently discussed nurses' responsibility in the area of institutional economy—a phenomenon rendered increasingly logical and necessary by wartime scarcity of goods. Alongside their caretaking activities, nurses were told, sensible and thrifty consumption of resources in daily institutional life was an important duty. "In the National Socialist State," wrote one local official in this context, "this kind of behavior, sustained by a consciousness of responsibility, must be demanded from all members of the state—even from the smallest."[154] Even the seemingly trivial practice of sending dirty articles of clothing to the laundry without trying first to brush out the dirt was, under current circumstances, nothing less than "irresponsible" behavior.[155]

Discussions about thrift before and during wartime drew on the rhetorical power of machine analogies: nurses were encouraged to think of themselves as parts of a great institutional machine that could function properly only through the cooperation of everyone. Although occupied in just one sphere of institutional life, they should not proceed with blinders on, liberally using up resources on their patients without regard for established rules. Administrators, they were reminded, were charged with keeping expenditures within strict limits—and they were legally responsible for financial trouble, even when caused not by themselves but rather by wasteful staff. Thrift in the usage of medication and supplies was thus not only essential from a practical standpoint but also a moral virtue—an expression of camaraderie and responsibility.[156] Deviation was not only impractical and futile but also contrary to the social norms of institutional life, in which everyone had certain technical responsibilities whose fulfillment demanded cooperation and goodwill. A wasteful nurse, in this social environment, was *asocial* and subject to the exclusion that such a characterization brought.

It is, of course, well known that it was not a question of saving a few marks here and there in psychiatric institutions of the 1930s and early 1940s, but rather of catastrophic underfunding and overcrowding. Still, the message was clear: whatever their views on cost cutting, nurses were in no position to change policies, and there was no sense in trying since scarcity was presented as a fact that was beyond even administrators' control; moreover, the prospect of ostracism by professional peers rendered any deviation from the norm less appealing. Familiar, human impulses—the desire to get along with others, to contribute in a positive way to a cooperative effort—were activated for the purpose of cultivating acquiescence in a patently inhuman state of affairs.

The welfare of patients themselves was not often discussed directly, unless the author happened to be engaging in self-congratulatory praise of recent therapeutic "advances."[157] They were not directly spoken of as "unworthy life" either; *Geisteskrankenpflege* articles tended to direct attention, rather, to facilitating a process as economically as possible; the fact that this "process" concerned human lives was, generally speaking, a side issue.

This reconstituted notion of responsibility that emerged around the time of the war's outbreak discouraged nurses from thinking not only about individual patients but about *themselves* as well. Nurse Roos, for example, described nursing in autumn 1940 as a profession demanding first and foremost selflessness— by now a familiar idea. But he did not speak of selflessness in the sense we have encountered earlier, as a virtue connected with a willingness to work a few extra hours, to listen patiently to the illusions of a patient, and in general to offer one's best care to people who were stigmatized by the public. It was, rather, a virtue whereby one contributed to a collective effort (in this case the maintenance of the institutional machinery) without heeding one's personal desires or inner voice. Anything less than full commitment to the cause was a sign of crass egoism: "One may not cling to his own ego year in and year out," Roos reminded his colleagues. Selflessness was no longer an emanation of the self but rather a *negation* of the self.

To drive this point home, Roos attempted to effect an absolute mental separation between professional and private selves. A nurse had many duties, of course, both on the job and in private life. The latter, however, came a distant second. "Attending to the nursing profession and to private interests are two completely different things that can never be fulfilled together, because no one can serve two lords. There is no golden middle way to be found that enables the nurse in equally satisfactory ways to devote himself to nursing and simultaneously to serve himself."[158] The point, of course, was to reconstruct the motivational apparatus surrounding nursing—to turn nurses' attention away from their patients and toward abstract notions of their "duty" that were deliberately vague and thus always subject to revision. Nurses could certainly gain satisfaction from their work when they saw that "joy radiates from the eyes of the patients and a happy ray of hope is on their faces."[159] But personal satisfaction was by no means guaranteed and was thus a wholly insufficient motive for anyone's undertaking the profession to begin with. "Brotherly love" and a keen sense of the need for technical competence were indispensable: "The smallest omission or the smallest oversight can become the patient's undoing. Even with these trifles it is a question of the health and the life of the patients. Reliability and absolute loyalty are in order, if we want patients to be placed in our hands for care."[160] At a time when psychiatry was effecting its own practical and moral annihilation, killing or knowingly delivering often desperate and resistant patients to certain death, Roos deftly remained consistent with a discursive tradition over twenty years old at the same time as he redefined the implications of its central concepts (duty, responsibility, compassion) in a way that made them instrumental in murder. It did not matter that at the time he wrote this article, the lofty ethical foundation of nursing to which he refers had in practice been reduced to rubble; he needed only to drive home the far more welcome point that one cannot serve two masters—and after many years of dictatorship, it was abundantly clear which master was to be served. In wartime, and at the bottom of an institutional hierarchy, nurses were thus provided with the kind of psychological reinforcement that eased the journey down the slippery slope from treatment to complicity in murder.

Politics and Professional Life
under National Socialism

Alles neu
Macht der Mai—
Klingt's in schöner Frühlingszeit
Wenn im neuen, grünen Kleid
Prangen Wiese, Wald und Flur.
Ew'ges Wirken der Natur.
 Doch mehr noch als die Lenzeskraft
Alljährlich neue Wunder schafft,
Mehr fortgeweht was morsch und alt
Als Frühlingssturmes Urgewalt
Hat eine Kraft die noch nie war:
Das erste deutsche Hitlerjahr!
 Es hat vernichtet, was doch schon verloren
Doch mehr an Gutem und Neuem geboren.
Er hat als Größtes der Schöpfermacht
Den Menschenfrühling uns gebracht. . . .[1]

THESE VERSES, which were composed in 1934 for the Berlin-Buch staff's special "evening of camaraderie" (*Kamaradschaftsabend*), suggest that the political changes of the previous year had generated a spirit of newness and optimism in the institution.[2] Nationwide formal changes in institutional organization and practice offer further indications that nurses' daily life was heavily punctuated with rituals of National Socialist "camaraderie": the introduction of the "Hitler Salute," obligatory membership of personnel in the NSBO, and obligatory participation in parades and festivities united administrators and nurses in a collective adventure of "national renewal."[3] As a reward for their dedication, some nurses could look forward to a copy of *Mein Kampf* in honor of twenty-five years' service.[4] It would seem that, ideally, nurses' professional life—and their own thinking—was to be politicized along National Socialist lines: they would embrace the regime's patronage of politically acceptable *Volksgenossen*, its hostility toward suspected left-wing critics, its antisemitism, and its contempt for psychiatric patients; they would manifest these standpoints in daily practice, and they would be rewarded for doing so.

Closer inspection of episodes from the daily administration of Wittenau's nurses in the 1930s reveals that this was by and large not the case. Although there is much to suggest that personnel management and arbitration of disputes in many ways ran parallel to the aims of the Party—after all, officials in both spheres often cooperated in hiring, firing, and arbitration decisions—specific cases of administrative divergence from fundamental National Socialist principles reveal other or additional criteria that were involved. These examples not only prompt us to question the influence of Nazi politics and ideology on professional activity inside psychiatric institutions; they also provide clues enabling us to construct a more comprehensive interpretation of administrative behavior and, by extension, to understand how National Socialist principles were incorporated into nurses' lives.

This chapter pursues such understanding by looking *behind* the facade of political and professional harmony created by Party functionaries and sympathizers, and it does so quite literally with the aid of accounts that were reserved for administrative eyes only. The stories to be found there suggest that Wittenau administrators' willingness to do the Party's bidding found its limits in (among other things) their desire to retain their professional autonomy—that is, to assess and meet their own personnel requirements as they saw fit. Their fixation on fulfilling certain technical responsibilities—on keeping the wheels of institutional life turning—is the factor that brings politically inconsistent acts under one roof. Of final and ultimate interest will be the effects of this fixation—both real and potential—on the atmosphere in institutions and on nurses themselves.

THE POLITICIZATION OF PROFESSIONAL LIFE: WITTENAU'S ADMINISTRATORS IN THE SERVICE OF THE PARTY

There is much to suggest that hiring-and-firing decisions during the National Socialist years hinged primarily on the political profile of nurses. The priority that NSDAP-affiliated applicants enjoyed is demonstrated by the case of Anton Harz, a Party member who was hired at Wittenau in 1934 on the recommendation of the local *Sturmführer*. No pretenses were made about the criteria for employment on either side: without wasting a word on the candidate's interest in or suitability for the job, the *Sturmführer* instead described him as a long-standing, dedicated Party member who had suffered extraordinarily under the "terror of the Marxist staff" at work in the late 1920s. He had been unemployed since 1932 and was "willing to take any job, just so that he can finally once again work at all and not burden the state as a parasite."[5] Braasch met Harz personally, deemed him suitable for the job, and favored hiring him "out of consideration for his brave defense of the National [Socialist] State, for his family, and his long unemployment. . . ."[6] So much for the golden rule of psychiatric nursing, whereby "he who seeks the job for money should look elsewhere."

These examples multiply[7] and include BBG victims who were considered for reemployment in 1935 when the provisions of the law began to be rolled back. The cases of nurses who availed themselves of this opportunity suggest that here, too, personnel policy followed the dictates of Party policy—that is, the administration's "value" system entailed assigning priority on the basis of political criteria.

Peter Winkler, as we learned earlier, belonged to the KPD from January 1 to February 15, 1933, and, despite having joined the NSDAP two months later, was fired on the basis of BBG §2. He attempted to rejoin the nursing ranks at Wittenau several years later and supported his case with reports on his praiseworthy performance in the service of the Party.[8] The NSDAP personnel office manager maintained that Winkler had joined the KPD under pressure from his colleagues. Since joining the NSDAP, he had "behaved irreproachably in every respect and [had] tried to atone for his mistake through voluntary services and financial donations of every kind."[9] The German Labor Front also spoke about his performance in glowing terms.[10]

Braasch jumped on the bandwagon, writing to the HGA in late 1936 that Winkler had performed admirably during his nineteen years of service at Wittenau. Although he had been compelled to support Winkler's earlier dismissal on the basis of BBG §2, the former nurse's sparkling performance in the service of the Party made it impossible for him to continue to hold this position. He henceforth supported rehiring Winkler at the first available opportunity.[11]

This willingness to rehire continued to prevail in the Office of the Mayor as well, although Winkler would have to wait until 1940 for a job (at Berlin's Wuhlgarten institution) owing to a lack of positions.

Violence, Arbitration, and Ideological Sympathy

Administrators also demonstrated their ideological sympathy with the National Socialists in their role as arbitrators. In 1939, for example, Wittenau patient S. claimed that Patient C. had been given a black eye by Nurse Roland Eichel, an active SS-man and veteran Party member (that is, a member of the so-called Old Guard). Eichel maintained that he had never struck a patient, and a colleague supported this claim, adding that Patient S. was an "educated Jew, who often has quite a bit of nerve and claims special rights. As a result he is from time to time shown his limits by the nursing personnel. It is therefore possi-

ble that, for this reason, he wanted to avenge himself on E[ichel]
and simply accused him of abusing Patient C."[12] Braasch concluded that there were not sufficient grounds to initiate disciplinary action against Eichel. Besides, he added, "in my opinion
less worth may be given to the testimony of the mentally ill, especially since we are talking about Jews, who actually have a
predilection for untruth."[13] Wittenau's administration also expressed sympathy with Nurse Flora Lenz, who insisted after a
1938 clash with Jewish relatives that it was extremely difficult
for her to treat Jews the same as other national comrades.[14]

Correspondence of other institutions suggests that this kind
of dismissiveness regarding the welfare of abused patients was
not limited to Wittenau. For example, a 1936 episode of patient
abuse at the Weißenau institution prompted discussion among
Württemberg psychiatric administrators and government and
Party officials about revising—that is, softening—the existing
punishment of dismissal. Of course, the Winnetal Directorate
agreed, deliberate abuse should continue to be punished thus;
but it was also the case that nurses sometimes simply lost control
of themselves, which was "psychologically understandable" in
light of daily provocation in the form of insults, spitting, and
attacks. Surely, it was more appropriate to issue a warning with
the proviso that a second offense would result in dismissal.[15]
Commenting on the same case, the German Labor Front agreed
that, although such "derailments" of course warranted the "se-
verest punishments," a warning should precede dismissal. If this
were not enough to demonstrate that the welfare of the patients
in question was quite distant from the thoughts and concerns of
the participants in this debate, it may be added that both parties
expressed concern for the innocent victims who would be unjustly penalized by dismissal: the *families* of nurses fired for patient abuse.

To be sure, the Directorate of the Weinsberg institution opposed changing the regulation; but here too the welfare of individual patients was apparently not its central concern: warnings
and fines were already routine disciplinary responses in cases of
abuse that were not particularly grave, and more serious abuse

was and should be met with dismissal. Tampering with this informal arrangement was a bad idea: "The reputation of the institutions would greatly suffer if the public found out that a nurse who severely abused a patient unjustly is allowed to remain at his post. There is already a widespread opinion in the public that patients in the institutions are beaten. . . ."[16] It thus continued to be the case that, as we have seen earlier, there was room to negotiate how seriously rules concerning the treatment of patients should be taken. So long as "official" rules remained credible in the eyes of the public, some administrators were willing to tolerate deviations—even when those deviations involved abuse.

As a final example of the degree to which administrative attitudes toward patients dovetailed with National Socialist propaganda, it is instructive to consider a complaint by the Berlin-Buch institution's Director Bender to the HGA in late 1939. At his institution, he wrote, there were approximately one hundred criminals who were an extraordinary burden; they were uncooperative, and their care was unnecessarily expensive. He wanted to have them sent someplace else where they could be more "appropriately" accommodated. In early 1940, the HGA reported that it was working on the problem, prompting Bender to reply impatiently that

> it has been proven that a selection of criminal addicts, despite repeated and lengthy stays in institutions, again and again have relapses and commit further offenses. These people are inappropriately accommodated here. They are a bad example to the cases with a more favorable prognosis, and their care here is too expensive. The "purpose of institutionalization [*Unterbringung*]," about which, experience shows, the court inquires again and again, will never be fulfilled because the prognosis of these cases is completely unfavorable.
>
> I request that you consider whether the institution could be freed of the unnecessary burden of these people.[17]

He did not need to trouble the HGA a third time, commenting several months later that "the matter is not to be further pursued, since we can assume that it will be taken care of in the course of measures, arranged by the interior minister, for the methodical economization of the psychiatric institutions."[18] The T4 program, which Bender had in fact been enlisted to help plan,[19] would quite literally eliminate the source of the problem.

PERSONNEL MANAGEMENT AT SECOND GLANCE: THE PRIMACY OF INSTITUTIONAL ORDER

These anecdotes are part of a much longer, gloomy story of the psychiatric establishment's support for National Socialist attitudes and measures against the Jews, the regime's critics, and the mentally ill. It would be a mistake, however, to conclude that administrative behavior was guided exclusively—or even primarily—by political loyalty. Administrators sometimes disagreed among themselves on the extent to which National Socialist principles should be translated into practice, and they continued to discipline nurses for abusing patients. Wittenau's Karl Braasch sometimes made attempts, albeit feeble ones, to support nurses who had been placed *outside* the sphere of politically acceptable *Volksgenossen*, and he did not *necessarily* esteem nurses who were NSDAP sympathizers or even Party members any more highly than nonmembers. Although willing to assign Party members priority at hiring time, he did not prove to be such a willing agent of political favoritism—and persecution—when he made decisions about retaining reliable nurses and ridding himself of intolerable ones. It would seem that administrators had their own specific criteria for organizing and managing professional activity in their institutions, and the following discussion attempts to discover them in episodes from everyday life.

In Defense of Patients? Administrative Discord and the Punishment of Abuse

Despite official propaganda and its appropriation by numerous exponents of institutional psychiatry in the 1930s, it would be mistaken to conclude that unmitigated contempt for patients was universal or that the existence of such contempt meant that violence against patients was openly advocated. The Directorate of Eichberg, which would later be instrumental in the murder of thousands of patients, was dominated by senior district official [*Landrat*] and wily NSDAP enthusiast Fritz Bernotat—a man who made no secret of his contempt for psychiatric patients and clogged the gears of the Nassau district's bureaucratic oversight machinery in the 1930s so that reports on the miserable living conditions of Eichberg's patients would remain unheeded.[20] He was no friend of Dr. Hinsen, who resigned as director in 1938: at a conference of directors in the mid-1930s, Hinsen would report after the war, Bernotat had announced to the gathering that if he were a doctor, he would "do away with these patients." "I told him publicly in the same forum," Hinsen said, " 'German medicine can congratulate itself that you are not a doctor.' After that there was a pregnant silence."[21] Professor Karl Kleist, who inspected institutions in Hesse-Nassau and the Rheingau in 1938, found Bernotat a thoroughly offensive character as well: speaking constantly of unworthy lives and asocials, Bernotat was not in the least troubled by the appalling living conditions and minimal medical or therapeutic activity that prevailed in the region's institutions. Not all patients were incurable, Kleist maintained, but even in the case of chronic patients, "expenditure on these unfortunates should not fall below a tolerable minimum."[22]

Also contrary to the impressions generated by the first part of this chapter, abuse of patients was not officially promoted in spite of prevailing ideological trends. Throughout the 1930s, and even in the course of the "euthanasia" program, nurses continued to be discouraged from such behavior and disciplined for it. Eichberg nurse and longtime Party and SS member Norbert Gelsen, for example, was reported in late 1937 for having beaten up a patient who accused him of stealing cigarettes from an examination room. Director Hinsen wrote in his file: "I have sharply reprimanded G[elsen] in the presence of all the doctors, said to him that violence against patients, even if they are otherwise a bad lot, is grounds for immediate dismissal, and threatened him with criminal proceedings . . . in the event of a repeat performance."[23] In addition, Berlin-Buch nurse Eva Felmann was dismissed immediately for patient abuse in January 1936, took the city of Berlin to the Labor Court, and lost two months later. When she appealed the decision that summer, the court recounted the charges at hand: striking a patient in the face with her slipper and striking another in the face with a wet towel while holding her by the hair. In addition, Felmann was reported by other witnesses to have a history of abusive behavior involving slippers, wet towels, and her fists. The court deemed the witnesses credible and saw no reason to alter the prior verdict. Felmann was eventually not only dismissed but sentenced to four months in prison.[24]

Even in 1939, when six years of National Socialist propaganda against the mentally ill had had ample opportunities to secure widespread sympathy, the administrator overseeing psychiatry in the Rheinland (*Psychiatriedezernent*) informed institutional directors that there had recently been a number of cases of abuse by nurses on wards for violent patients. Some patients had been physically injured, and one even died after a heavy male nurse attempted restraint by lying on the patient and crushing his ribs. In several cases severe punishments had been required. Institutional directors, he advised, should attempt to avoid further incidents of this nature through training, keener supervision of nurses' activities, and the introduction of nightly inspections.[25]

Finally, it is instructive that Eichberg nurse Andy Gibbon was disciplined for abusing a patient in spring 1941, in the midst of the T4 program. A senior nurse reported: "On an inspection round this morning I heard a patient loudly screaming as I entered the upper section of the ward for unruly male patients. I quickly went over and saw how Nurse G[ibbon] continually struck Patient E., who sat in the bathtub, with a wet shirt. The face and right eye were deeply reddened from the blows. This episode is one more piece of evidence that G[ibbon] does not possess the suitability to be a nurse, despite plenty of instruction and warning."[26] Dr. Mennecke, in consultation with Bernotat, wasted little time having Gibbon dismissed.[27]

These cases notwithstanding, the punishment of abuse during the National Socialist years is not as paradoxical as it may seem. After all, the previous chapter has already suggested how discouraging abuse could fit in very nicely with a more general program of aggressive treatments, substandard living conditions, and muffled contempt for patients: at issue was not the welfare of patients but rather the absence of disruptions of daily life. Gibbon's case raises a further consideration, namely, administrative opportunism: according to a later statement by Mennecke, Gibbon was unpopular with his colleagues;[28] he apparently was not particularly liked by Mennecke either. It could well be the case that some nurses who were fired or disciplined for abuse had fallen from administrative grace for some other reason. Punishing abuse, then, not only discouraged nurses from disruptive behavior; it could also serve as a convenient pretext for dismissing nurses whose prior misdemeanors had not sufficed to warrant their removal.

Political Fanaticism as Administrative Problem

A more substantial case is made for this argument by the story of Wittenau nurse Lena Holstein. Despite loud proclamations of her nationalist sympathies and long tales of the price she had paid for this during the Weimar Republic, she made a permanent nuisance of herself and was promptly dismissed after crossing the line between disruption and abuse. Her story not only demonstrates the close connection between punishing abuse and upholding order; it also introduces the Wittenau administration's rather remarkable indifference to "correct" political views.

Born, raised, and trained as a nurse in Bavaria, Holstein took up her first Berlin position at the General Hospital of Berlin-Buch in 1926.[29] In 1927 she was transferred, at her own request, to the Berlin-Buch psychiatric institution.[30] The six years that followed were not happy ones; as she would recall years later, her nationalist inclinations rendered her a fish out of water in that hub of left-wing sympathizers, Berlin. "I was this dirty-minded

woman [*Mistfink*]! And I was hounded! Hounded from one institution into the other." She would later report having been
snubbed by her Berlin-Buch colleagues for wearing a Bavarian
dirndl in her free time.[31]

The following year, Holstein became involved in a dispute
with a fellow nurse and assaulted her. Shortly thereafter, and
very likely as a result of the incident, she was selected for a
nurse exchange with the Herzberge institution—an exchange
that she vigorously, but unsuccessfully, protested.[32] Some years
later she would maintain that "I was arbitrarily transferred from
the Berlin-Buch psychiatric institution not because there had
been an open, honest report about me, but rather because
the[—]at the time all too left-leaning[—]staff councils and the
Central Health Office fancied it."[33] During her three-year tenure
at Herzberge, insubordination and mistreatment of patients be-
smirched her record. But here again, Holstein's account was
quite different; she had been mercilessly harassed on account
of her nationalist sympathies. "One day," she confessed, "I lost
my head and punched a KPD doctor, a very young man, in the
face." The only way to spare herself dismissal in the wake of
this incident, she explained, had been to join the SPD, which
she had promptly done. (In fact, Herzberge recommended her
dismissal in May 1932; it was the HGA administration that
commuted this to a transfer to Wuhlgarten with a warning that
any repeat performance of her past behavior would truly be the
last straw.)[34]

Holstein was involved in more personnel shifting in 1933,
when she was temporarily sent to Wittenau to relieve a staff
shortage. Several months later, when asked to take her back,
Wuhlgarten refused on the grounds that it had a surplus of
nurses. The personnel manager, however, could not resist adding that he was pleased to be rid of Holstein, who got along neither with her colleagues nor with her patients.[35]

Once at Wittenau for good, Holstein's behavior was apparently acceptable until December 1935, when a minor dispute
with the senior nurse about a shift assignment on the eve of Holstein's vacation ended in her transfer to another house in the

institution.[36] (It was in defending herself on this particular occasion that she poured forth her tales of political persecution during the Weimar years.) Four months later, an accusation of abuse started the administrative machinery rolling again; Holstein was reported to have struck a patient in the face while uttering, "You damned ass, you intransigent liar, I'll give it to you!" Finally pushed to the limit of its patience, and with a doctor's affirmation of the patient's credibility in hand, the Wittenau administration saw to it that she was dismissed.[37]

If this sounds like a rather unspectacular story of the "problem employee," in which administrators (predictably) shied away from the uncomfortable and burdensome process of actually *firing* someone, it was, as we have seen, a highly dramatic and tragic story in the eyes of Holstein—a story of rampant professional and political persecution. In the course of her career, she wrote a number of letters aiming to convince administrators that she was a helpless victim of incompetent and mean-spirited colleagues, and to awaken their pity.[38] She never failed to add that she had also suffered greatly before 1933 on account of her nationalist disposition, carrying her level of detail and hysteria on this point to an unprecedented pitch after her dismissal in a letter that she submitted to the National Socialist periodical *Der Schwarze Front*.[39]

It is instructive that the Wittenau administration, despite its own National Socialist sympathies, does not appear to have been swayed in the least by these arguments. On the contrary, after the 1935 insubordination incident Braasch defended the character and prior conduct of Senior Nurse B. and added that "it seems peculiar when Nurse H[olstein] maintains in her report ... that she was transferred from Buch to Herzberge because the Marxist staff council of [the Berlin-Buch institution] and the left-leaning Central Health Office did not like her, and when one later must determine from the files that she issued complaints to the Communist staff council at Herzberge and bragged to the station doctor that [it] would protect her. ..."[40] In any case, at the heart of the matter was Holstein's disruption of daily life through her confrontations with other staff members, and on this point Braasch insisted that "Miss H[olstein], like every other staff member, must adapt herself to the institutional discipline and maintain an appropriate tone vis-à-vis her superiors and colleagues."[41] Two months later, after Holstein had committed the far more serious violation of abuse, Braasch and the HGA had no reservations about having her dismissed.

This should not, however, lead us to misinterpret their intentions, which were revealed after her dismissal. Holstein took the HGA to the Labor Court and demanded a financial settlement and a "respectable certificate"; she did not want to return to her hometown in disgrace.[42] This was granted, since in the court's opinion abuse was not proven, and Holstein's insubordination was due to her "pathological condition" rather than malice. The court secured a compromise: the HGA would withdraw the charge of abuse as unproven, and Holstein would take back what she had said to and about the senior nurse with her apologies. Her certificate was to be free of any reference to insubordination or abuse; it was to state, rather, "Employment in public service ended by mutual agreement on March 31, 1936."[43] At issue in these proceedings was not any kind of restitution on behalf of the abused patient or, for that matter, Holstein's colleagues but rather the simple elimination of an administrative nightmare.

SIMILAR measures seem to have prevailed in cases of disruptive Party members, even though for obvious reasons it was more difficult to dismiss them. Nurse Flora Lenz, a militant NSDAP supporter and member of the "Old Guard," was by no means revered at the Berlin hospitals in which she worked, nor at Wittenau, where she landed in 1937. To the contrary, administrators did everything possible to have her taken off their hands. The tension between the privileges of Old Guard status and the frustration of administrators resulted in a desultory career for Lenz within Berlin's city limits: ineligible for dismissal, she was simply transferred from one hospital to another (and within hospitals, from one station to another) during her years of employment up to 1940.

In the early 1930s, Lenz nursed at several hospitals without incident. At the end of September 1934, she was transferred from the Rudolf Virchow Hospital to the Berlin-Buch psychiatric institution—a transfer that she bitterly resented; she had, after all, been trained as a general nurse (*Krankenpflegerin*), not a psychiatric nurse (*Irrenpflegerin*).[44] She was absent, allegedly on account of sickness, for seven days shortly thereafter and upon her return was reported for abusing a patient. She once again maintained that she was a general nurse and simply did not know how to deal with psychiatric patients, leading Director Bender to comment that "it seems highly doubtful that she can remain in psychiatric nursing."[45] She was soon transferred to the Ludwig Hoffmann Hospital.

This arrangement was by no means acceptable to her, however, because she immediately found herself in the psychiatric ward. This prompted a letter of protest to the HGA in which she explained how happy she had been in a previous position at a Berlin convalescent home. "Without reason or cause . . . ," she continued, "I was transferred to a psychiatric institution on October 1, 1934. I am certified in general nursing [*Krankenpflege*], and psychiatric care does not matter at all to me . . . in this occupation I am emotionally destroyed."[46] Her request was heeded, and she was transferred to the Rudolf Virchow Hospital.

Once in her new position, she immediately proceeded to continue her already long history of insubordination and noncompliance with whatever orders did not please her, often threatening to report the colleague to hospital and Party authorities. These were not idle threats; in late 1934 she reported a colleague to the hospital's staff council for calling her a Communist. She had never belonged to the SPD or KPD, Lenz maintained—but the council might be interested to know that "Nurse M. doesn't seem to know anything about the Hitler Salute. I was asked by Patient B. where a complaint could be made about the fact that Nurse M. enters a room and says, 'Good day.' "[47]

It is instructive that Lenz's attempt to curry favor with the hospital administration had precisely the opposite effect. After a year of in-house transfers and no end to the problems in sight, an administrative officer presented her with various statements and damaging reports of her prior performance in an attempt to bring her to reason. He later reported: "I have also deemed it impertinent that at every opportunity when she receives orders she does not like, she threatens to report the matter to the Party and the Labor Front. I have suggested to her that, as a member of the Movement and as a National Socialist, she set a good example for her colleagues in integrating and subordinating herself vis-à-vis others and in executing her assigned duties. It should not come to pass that nonmembers of the Movement make such a Party member out to be a repulsive example."[48] Nurse Lenz promised to try to do better, but within a month new complaints had rolled in.

The administrator clearly could not continue to leave his employees at Lenz's mercy; but, as he reminded the HGA, trying to dismiss a Party member was not a good idea. The latter, thus, resumed its search for a suitable place for her and was curtly rebuffed by Hufeland Hospital's administrative director, who noted that she had already been dismissed from their hospital "because she constantly caused strife and was known among the nurses as a troublemaker." If her current coworkers could not favorably influence her behavior on the job, there was not much chance of a behavioral metamorphosis at their hospital, which was undergoing consolidation and staff displacement. In conclusion, he dismissed the argument that as an NSDAP member she deserved special consideration. "This fact can only work to her disadvantage in the judgment of her case, since members of the NSDAP are instructed again and again to set a good example at all times."[49]

The HGA's investigations turned up nothing; Lenz was to circulate for another year between the quarantine, gynecology, urology, and children's stations of the Rudolf Virchow Hospital. Complaints ranged from insubordination to negligence and malicious treatment of patients.[50] A particularly revealing testimony concerning Lenz's attitude toward patients came from Senior Nurse S., who reported the following remarks of Lenz to a senior doctor in February 1937:

1. It would not be in the spirit of the Führer to allow Patient K., who currently is still receiving inpatient treatment, to listen to the Führer's radio speech with us, since K. was released from prison. (Medically speaking, there were no reservations concerning risk of infection.)

2. "A psychiatric patient should not be given a cardiac drug to preserve her life." Nurse L. added that she would report these facts listed under (1) and (2) to an office of the NSDAP.[51]

Lenz flatly denied the second charge and, as for the first, admitted to saying only, "Patient K. has headphones, why is he listening in with us?"[52]

In light of this, it is amazing indeed that the HGA's next transfer initiative in September 1937 deposited Lenz back at the bedside of precisely those patients for whom she had so blatantly expressed her contempt. To her, however, her transfer to Wittenau was incomprehensible for other reasons: "I am not aware of any misdemeanors on the job, have behaved respectably and properly, . . . and have always fulfilled my duty conscientiously. I do not know what I have allegedly done wrong, nor why I have received a warning."[53] Lenz was the object of considerable administrative restraint at Wittenau, despite the fact that the old problems of staff rabble-rousing resurfaced immediately. By February 1938, the senior nurse's evaluation of her performance had declined from "suitable as a nurse" to "not very suitable for psychiatric nursing." Even so, the administrative director tried to subdue tempers by speaking to Lenz's colleagues and reminding her supervisor that she was a veteran, and thus privileged, Party member. Thus the senior nurse should "always try . . . to make clear to her what she has to do on the job and that she should also be concerned in every way not to provoke Nurse L. to resist"—as though Lenz's behavior were a matter of simple misunderstanding.[54]

Behind the scenes, the administrator's frustration over the situation came to the fore. In a letter to the HGA, he wrote that since 1933 "a great number of nurses, among whom several members of the Old Guard were to be found, have been transferred to [this] institution because they were not usable elsewhere. On occasion they had had confrontations so that they could no longer remain at other institutions." He had tried to reintegrate them into the work process, most of the time without success. "It is," he continued, "extraordinarily difficult for a senior administrative official when he tries to integrate this kind of *Volksgenossen* into the work process, and, when [this attempt] completely fails in spite of the efforts of superiors, measures other than those suggested by the institution are taken."[55] Lenz's case, he felt, demonstrated exactly the kinds of difficulties that arose when personnel decisions were made by the HGA. Institutional administrators should be making these decisions, with the labor courts and Labor Front waiting in the wings to handle appeals.[56]

The patience of the Wittenau Directorate reached its end in spring 1939, when Lenz refused a senior nurse's order to help carry a stretcher; it insisted that "under no circumstances can she be further employed here." There was little cause for worry, because within a year Lenz would be spirited off to Hadamar to serve in the first phase of the "euthanasia" program.[57] This would undoubtedly have been music to administrators' ears: The T4 program would finally free them of a persistent and incorrigible troublemaker.

It is therefore mistaken to assume that a pro–National Socialist administration such as Wittenau's esteemed Party members in an unconditional fashion. It did not—and *could* not—because an uncritical pro-NS stance was not always compatible with the order and discipline of everyday institutional life that they were required to uphold.

We can better understand this dilemma if we return to Nurse Lenz's case. In 1938, as we have seen earlier in the chapter, Braasch defended her against charges that she had been impolite to patients' relatives. As it turned out, this had been the case only for the relatives of *Jewish* patients; and he could readily sympathize with her claim that it was terribly difficult for her to treat Jews the same as other *Volksgenossen*.[58] His *initial* response, however, was that "[i]n general, one here takes the standpoint that it must not matter for a nurse whether Jews are at issue or not." The point here, of course, was not to defend the Jews but rather to drive home a principle of great administrative importance: independent, disruptive behavior—even if it was praiseworthy from an ideological standpoint—threatened the smooth functioning of the institutional machine; it therefore had to be discouraged. In this respect, the "rules" inhibiting expression of opinions, which we encountered in the previous chapter's discussion of nursing texts, found reinforcement in the politics of everyday life.

Private Life over Political Correctness: One Party Member's Fall from Grace

Nationalism and Party membership, then, did not necessarily bring with them any guarantee of administrative favor if they were accompanied by disruptive behavior on the institution's wards. The case of Anton Harz pushes this point one step further: Party members were not necessarily the objects of administrative favoritism even when their transgressions were limited to the *private* sphere.

Anton Harz was an SA-member and father of three who, as we have seen above, was hired at Wittenau in 1934 on the recommendation of a *Sturmführer*. In 1935 it came to the administration's attention that Harz had considerable debts, and in 1936 he was forced to ask Wittenau for onetime financial support because, unbeknownst to him, his wife had spent all their money and gotten him into financial trouble. The family had been evicted from their house the day before, and his wife had run off with the money given to her by the local welfare office. If Wittenau would be so kind as to offer him support, Harz promised to handle the family's finances himself in the future and accept supervision from the National Socialist Welfare Agency (NSV). "Should [no solution] be reached," he added, "I intend to legally incapacitate [*entmündigen*] my wife or divorce her."[59]

The local NSDAP came to Harz's defense, promising to keep an eye on him and see to it that he stayed out of further financial trouble, but a day later the NSV submitted a long, detailed report on the Harz household that would cost him not only the temporary custody of his children but also his job. When NSV representatives visited the apartment, it was in an "indescribably neglected condition"—filthy and full of cobwebs. Harz's infant was found in the basement, lying naked and unclean in a laundry basket full of rags. His eleven-year-old son, also reported to be unclean, had a history of skipping school and performing poorly when he was there. The sixteen-year-old daughter was "completely decadent": she had a history of theft, lying, and having " 'intimate' relations with at least one young man." Harz's wife was described as "slovenly, uneconomical, and mendacious, also apparently mentally impaired"—a woman who had done her best to keep the dereliction of their children and the impending eviction secret from her husband.[60]

Even so, the report continued, Harz cannot have been completely unaware of what was going on; after all, the police had penalized him three times in connection with his daughter's failure to report to school. Moreover, when the eviction took place, Harz had become "impudent and abusive and [had behaved] like someone possessed." The eviction had required the aid of two police officers, one of whom Harz had come close to assaulting. He was, in short, apparently unable to control his wife and assume responsibility for his children; the NSV recommended initiating proceedings to revoke guardianship of his children.[61]

Despite signs over the following weeks that the situation in the Harz household had marginally improved,[62] Braasch sent the HGA a long letter recommending dismissal; Harz's further employment would gravely endanger the reputation both of the institution and of public service workers.[63] This request was heeded, prompting Harz to appeal the decision in Labor Court in late spring 1936. There, the relevance of private conduct in the determination of professional suitability was upheld: the court accepted the city of Berlin's argument that it could "not any longer be held responsible for entrusting the care of mentally ill and mentally handicapped persons to a staff member who cannot uphold order in his own house."[64] Party members were not exempt from compliance with standard rules of professional— and nonprofessional—conduct.

NS Policy in Administrative Hands: The Utility of Legal Loopholes

Just as Wittenau's administration attempted to free itself of disruptive or otherwise undesirable sympathizers of the Right, on at least two occasions Braasch supported *non*disruptive, reliable nurses belonging to politically persecuted groups who would otherwise have had no chance to gain or hold a position. To be sure, this support was feeble; but it lends credibility to the idea that a nurse's political or racial profile was neither the only nor necessarily the decisive factor determining how administrators treated nurses.

Robert Wendel, who was fired under the BBG for former KPD membership despite over five years of satisfactory service, reapplied for a nursing position at Wittenau in 1934. Braasch seemed amenable to the idea and indeed saw some hope of success since, according to the second implementation ordinance, former KPD members could be rehired *if* they had belonged to the party only a short time, their membership was a thing of the distant past, the candidate had not engaged in Communist activity in the meantime, and the candidate demonstrated that he or she had not "made the Communist worldview [his or her] own."[65]

Braasch thus asked the local administrative office of the NSDAP (*Gauleitung*) for a report on Wendel's recent political activities and was told that "after this time [of his 1920–1921 KPD membership] and in particular after his dismissal from the Wittenauer Heilstätten, nothing else unfavorable with respect to politics has become known about him." It had no reservations about his being rehired in case of staff shortages.

Almost a year later, Braasch got wind of the fact that Wendel had pursued his case with the Gestapo.[66] Apparently attempting to curry favor through denunciation, Wendel maintained that he had been fired unjustly at the prodding of those who had been the NSBO representatives at that time, whom he would characterize in a letter respectively as a homosexual who had made advances to a patient; a thief who had gone to jail for pocketing meeting dues; and a ruthless opportunist who had given up his KPD membership in 1933 in order to pursue a career in the ranks of the NSDAP.[67]

Interestingly, Braasch did no more than insist that Wendel had provided information on his KPD membership himself and had been dismissed solely on those grounds,[68] and all relevant bureaucracies agreed to keep Wendel in mind for a position should one become available.[69] By the autumn of 1937, however, the *Gauleitung* had changed its mind, writing that Wendel had "not yet provided evidence that he fully and completely approves of the National Socialist State," and refusing to support his reemployment.[70] Although the reason for this reversal remains uncertain,[71] Wendel undoubtedly did not help his case by accusing Party officials of what at the time was considered patently "asocial" behavior. His 1939 attempt to be rehired was also rejected, and Wendel would have to wait until April 1945 before Wittenau would take him on again. In any event, his case suggests that Braasch was prepared to exploit legislation that would enable him to reacquire a good, reliable nurse who happened to be an ex-Communist; but he was evidently not prepared to challenge the recommendation of the Party.

A second and even more remarkable example of this kind of administrative "mercy" concerns Peter Zewen, who was hired as a nurse at Wittenau in mid-1940 despite serious inconsistencies in the personal information he gave when accepting previous employment. (In 1937 he described himself as Catholic—the same year the NSDAP *Gauleitung* reported him to be a half-Jew—and in 1940 he reported himself as evangelical.) Zewen, by all accounts, was a good nurse. But his professional record was to receive a fatal blow in July 1941 when a patient, whom he had accompanied into town to pick up an artificial eye, got away from him. Braasch promptly gave Zewen his notice effective September 30.

We learn from Zewen's personnel file that the patient's escape was a mere pretext for dismissal: Zewen was actually to be dismissed because he was, according to a 1937 memo from the NSDAP (written when Zewen was substituting at Berlin's Horst-Wessel-Hospital), a half-Jew. (Why this suddenly became an issue in 1941 is not clear from the file; it is possible that the memo was overlooked when Zewen was hired or perhaps not considered relevant; an NSDAP representative had reported to Wittenau prior to Zewen's employment there that "there are no reservations on my part with respect to politics.")[72]

Zewen does not seem to have been aware that his dismissal was anything other than a punishment for the escape and sought to save his job with reference to mitigating circumstances. Of course he had made a mistake, he wrote to the Directorate, by going into a pub with a patient "to answer the 'call of nature' " and ordering two glasses of malt beer. But the patient had made secret preparations for escape and thus betrayed the trust that was bestowed upon him on *everyone's* part in the institution. Punishment through dismissal was therefore truly harsh.[73]

Braasch remarked in Zewen's file: "Certainly, the punishment is harsh; I would not have dismissed Z[ewen] if he were not a half-Jew. We are not allowed to employ half-Jews here. But if short-term employment is possible, I am willing to withdraw the dismissal."[74]

Zewen wrote a second long letter to the administration, this time seeking to direct their attention to the sorry state of his personal affairs. Since the end of 1940, he wrote, he had been confronted with one catastrophe after the other: illnesses of his three children, the deaths of his father- and mother-in-law, and the resulting financial burdens. "When now, after all these misfortunes, a person deviates somewhat from what has been prescribed to him, it is after all certainly not absolutely necessary from a humane standpoint to punish the person with dismissal, particularly since he has been punished enough by the misfortunes. . . . In spite of everything I have performed my duties as if absolutely nothing had happened, punctually and attentively. . . ."[75] This seems to have moved Braasch somewhat; he noted in Zewen's file, "Should employment as a *Mischling* be possible, and the doctor has nothing against further employment, I am prepared to do away with the notice."[76]

Unfortunately for Zewen, the doctor did indeed have reservations. He referred Braasch to 1933 and 1935 ordinances banning the employment of non-Aryan persons in public service. Zewen could therefore not be hired as a *Mischling*. He was willing, though, and legally permitted, to hire Zewen as a wage laborer (that is, as an *Arbeiter*, as opposed to *Angestellte*, or salaried employee).[77] There were no available positions in this category, however, and Zewen left public service in September 1941.[78] Once again, the administration was not prepared to ignore or circumvent the regime's regulations governing personnel decisions; but Braasch was apparently willing to interpret and deploy them in such a fashion that the reliable Nurse Zewen could be retained.

Protecting Administrative Autonomy and the Limits of Cooperation

The story of Wittenau nurse Eberhard Hartmann demonstrates that, also contrary to the impressions generated above, psychiatric administrators did not always work hand in hand with Party functionaries in personnel management. To be sure, Hartmann's personnel file does not initially suggest any hint of tension: Wittenau periodically gave him days off in the autumn of 1937 for military exercises, a *Reichsparteitag*, and a course in NS propaganda (*weltanschaulicher Lehrgang*).[79] The problem arose when Hartmann's activities began to impair his nursing performance: in spring 1938, he was caught sleeping on a night shift and was threatened with dismissal in the event of a repeat violation. Several weeks later, the district office manager (*Kreisamtsleiter*) of the NSV came to Hartmann's defense, informing the

Wittenau administration of his dedicated service to the NSV during his free time and requesting that he be exempted from night shifts for an indeterminate length of time.[80]

The administration rejected the request for an open-ended exemption as a matter of principle; "the night shift constitutes one of the most important obligations in psychiatric nursing." It would, however, make an exception in Hartmann's case by freeing him from the night shift for four weeks.[81] This was apparently not a satisfactory compromise; the NSV representative repeated his request one month later. He reminded Wittenau that Hartmann was an exceptionally dedicated NSV trainee whose success required the exemption. He also sent a copy of the letter to the district mayor (*Bezirksbürgermeister*) and extracted that official's assurance via telephone that his request would be honored. Braasch, he added, considered it "self-evident" that Hartmann should be considered for the shift exemption.[82]

That Braasch did not, in fact, consider the matter self-evident is indicated by the tone of his response in Hartmann's file: "As a concession I hereby declare that I agree to free Nurse E[berhard] H[artmann] from the night shift for the duration of one more quarter-year, at the most, however, until October 31 of this year, in order to leave him enough time to get used to the new work position there. However, at this time I want explicitly to call attention to the fact that a further exemption from the night shift beyond October 31 of this year is out of the question."[83] Hartmann would be given days off (vacation days) again in the autumn on account of NSV-related activities, and from December 1938 through February 1939 Wittenau granted Hartmann three months unpaid vacation so that he could work on a trial basis in one of Conti's district offices. Hartmann proved suitable for this position and left Wittenau immediately thereafter.[84]

The confrontation outlined above has very little to do with politics in an ideological sense; after all, we have seen in other contexts (particularly the BBG and hiring criteria discussions) that in this respect, Braasch and people like the NSV representative were birds of a feather. Rather, it was a struggle for control over a man with two identities, nurse and NSV trainee. Braasch was undoubtedly all too pleased to learn that Hartmann was active in Party exercises; but as far as he was concerned, Hartmann was subject to the same expectations and responsibilities as his colleagues. The NSV succeeded in weaning Hartmann away from his nursing job and extracting Wittenau's assistance in the process, but we nevertheless see once again that being "pro–National Socialist" in a general sense did not preclude conflict with the Party's adherents and representatives.

Policing Women's Political and Private Lives:
An Unaffordable Luxury?

The above cases suggest that Wittenau's administration was more concerned with acquiring and retaining reliable nurses than with promoting the National Socialists' political and racial agenda. Political consciousness seems to have been even less important to Wittenau's administration—or perhaps not taken as seriously—when female nurses were at issue. Nurse Agnes Jost, as we learned earlier, was fired in 1933 for her membership in the Communist-oriented RGO. When considering her for reemployment in 1935, administrators of the personnel bureaucracy were suddenly willing to accept her 1933 assertion that she had not been aware of the RGO's Communist orientation when she joined it.[85] Moreover, as Braasch added in a file note, "Mrs. J[ost] is a war widow. A son of hers has been with the police force since October 1, 1933. The NSBO already deemed her suited for participation in the construction of the state in the spirit of N[ational] S[ocialism] in August 1933."[86] They were willing to reemploy her as soon as a suitable position was available if she agreed to withdraw her appeal. For reasons that are beyond the scope of the current discussion, Jost refused to do so and was thus not reemployed;[87] but her case presents the possibility that by 1935, administrators were willing to excuse former Communist affiliation on account of naive ignorance *if* the nurse was otherwise reliable and likely to perform well. Although I encountered only one other similar case during research for the current study,[88] it is possible that women were more often eligible for this kind of administrative mercy because they were regarded as "naturally" less politically conscious, more gullible, and ultimately less responsible for "errant" behavior.[89]

This possibility is strengthened by the case of Wittenau nurse Emilie Fuller, who, like Harz, was an NSDAP member guilty of "moral" transgressions in private life, but whose political orientation never entered into the debate on how she should be dealt with.[90] The trouble started in 1936, when Fuller was reported for distracting a married office employee from his work.[91] Soon, the man's near-hysterical wife would be bending the administration's ear with tales of her husband's infidelity and demanding Fuller's dismissal.[92] Braasch forwarded the matter to the HGA, which concluded that the affair was not a sufficient cause for dismissal; there was no concrete proof, and even if there were, the blame rested squarely on the shoulders of the married man: "As a married man and father, G. should have summoned enough strength of character not to begin this relationship in the first place, let alone continue it." Moreover, firing Fuller would simply remove the final hindrance to the unfettered continuation of the relationship: their status as coworkers who were both subject to institutional scrutiny and discipline. The best solution for all involved was to transfer G. to another institution and to retain Fuller "under keen observation." Finally, Fuller was to be told that this kind of off-duty behavior was damaging to the institution's reputation, and that a continuance of the relationship would result in dismissal.[93] This threat apparently needed to be repeated a second time, but Fuller headed off any further administrative intervention in mid-1938 when she quit on account of marriage.[94]

It appears that not only an affair with a married man but even pregnancy out of wedlock was not necessarily grounds for women's automatic dismissal: according to a *Gemeindetag* questionnaire from 1936, only two out of twelve regional governments reported that unmarried nurses in their psychiatric institutions were generally dismissed when they became pregnant. The Nassau district reported that dismissing nurses on the grounds of pregnancy was illegal, and the other respondents reported that such nurses were generally permitted to resume their careers after delivery unless there were serious misgivings about their suitability for further employment.[95]

One must not overestimate the generosity of administrators, whose central criterion in judging "suitability" was the intrusive, and for their purposes irrelevant, question of why the woman was pregnant to begin with. (Women whose pregnancy was deemed the product of an "immoral"—or "notoriously immoral"—lifestyle were dismissed; those who performed well at work and whose pregnancy was an accident—a "onetime mistake in a lifestyle that can otherwise be described as respectable"—could be retained.)[96] Rather, they seem to have wanted to secure maneuvering room for themselves in staff management. In establishing hiring and firing criteria that were by and large matters of personal opinion, they could deploy traditional mores (in this case, the scandalous nature of pregnancy out of wedlock) as they wished or according to staff requirements.

Indeed, there are good reasons to suspect that this occasional willingness to tolerate women's political and private transgressions was conditioned not only by sexism but also by the pressures of staff shortages. It was particularly difficult to acquire and retain competent female nurses because they left when they married,[97] and many who remained were burdened with familial responsibilities. The difficulty was explicitly formulated by the Directorate of the Berlin-Buch institution during discussions about nurses' training in the mid-1930s. Even though its hiring policy stipulated that one-quarter of the institution's nurses (excluding supervisory nurses) could be hired without any particular training or experience, and that the rest should be certified "as much as possible,"[98] the problem of obtaining and retaining qualified female nurses had remained intransigent. In response, the Directorate not only sought to introduce in-house courses but also applied in 1937 (unsuccessfully) for the construction of its own nursing school. As grounds for its request, it cited continuing problems created by the marriage of young, competent nurses and their replacement by "older, completely wrung out, and hardly employable persons":

As nurses we have mostly divorced women and unmarried ones with one and several children. Almost all these nurses have their own household. They thus have double duties, first as housewife, insofar as they have to look after the household and children before their shift, and then the duty of carrying out their work as a nurse. That these people come to work already worked-out and cannot achieve as much as a single person who comes to work well rested, is obvious. As a result of overwork, these nurses are very often sick, very nervous, and thus . . . often hardly productive.

In addition, many nurses who had been transferred recently to their institution from the Hufeland Hospital were deeply unhappy with the assignment to psychiatric care; their performance was unsatisfactory, they were absent from work for the flimsiest reasons, and they pestered the HGA to return them to a general hospital. "These nurses are more a burden for us than anything else but by no means completely satisfactory nurses." In general, the administration estimated, 25–30 percent of their nurses were unsuitable for their work.[99]

But in what sense were they "unsuitable"? Part of their unsuitability, apparently, stemmed from age and single motherhood; but the Berlin-Buch administration cannot possibly have believed that training in psychiatric care could even begin to solve these more deeply rooted problems. What *could* be changed, and what administrators and bureaucrats had at least *partially* in mind when they drew up such plans, was work discipline. The HGA instructed institutions in its 1935 memo that "in these introductory courses the ethical ideas of the nursing profession are to be *especially* emphatically pointed out," as well as in supplemental training courses for experienced nurses.[100] We gain a glimpse into the intended meaning of "ethical ideas" later, when the Berlin-Buch administration asked its planning committee to design such courses to impress on nurses the idea, proffered by the HGA, that thoughtlessly calling in sick was not compatible with the "higher" professional ethics demanded in the nursing profession.[101] The ethic in question was very likely first and foremost a *work* ethic, and training courses were in-tended to be exercises in the installation of this ethic in the minds of nurses—exercises in motivation and self-discipline.[102]

Attempts to realize these aspirations at Berlin-Buch were not altogether successful. During its first year, despite general en-thusiasm on the part of participants, many were discovered to have a poor educational background and were lacking in the necessary discipline to master the material. Regarding nursing as a source of money rather than as a profession, the majority were simply interested in the more sensational aspects of the course and were unwilling to review at home what they were being taught.[103]

THE above cases shed some light on why administrators did not automatically tailor their personnel management to a crude pro-Right, anti-Left version of the National Socialist agenda: they had technical responsibilities whose fulfillment was not always compatible with a blind pursuit of that agenda. Indeed, in the face of problems on the scale described by the Directorate of the Berlin-Buch institution, it is hardly surprising that an obsessive preoccupation with nurses' political profiles was a luxury that could not be afforded. Rather, as we have already seen in our discussion of the BBG, administrators attempted to deploy their own political or personal convictions in a way that promoted stability and efficiency in daily life. Although they were very likely all too pleased to stock their nursing ranks with members of various National Socialist organizations, their primary con-cern was to ensure an adequate quantity of nurses who were reliable, discreet, respectable, and competent.

Even a National Socialist zealot like Bernotat occasionally showed signs of subordinating ideological rigor to adminis-trative sensibility. In autumn 1938, for example, five Eichberg trainees, two men and three women, appeared before an exami-nation committee consisting of two doctors, one administrator, *Landrat* Bernotat, and Deputy Director Friedrich Mennecke. The trainees, who had completed the written portion of their examination two days earlier, answered questions concerning anatomy, physiology, psychiatric illness, professional duties and legal provisions, administration, and finally "several questions concerning the history of the NSDAP and its structure." In this last category, Bernotat reported that the trainees—especially the female ones—showed that there were still gaps in this area. Still, however, the trainees had done a very good job indeed; Bernotat reminded them to pay closer attention to public and administrative affairs and sent them home with the result "fully satisfactory."[104]

A second example concerns a decree from June 1938 which required that Jewish patients be accommodated such that (a) the possibility of "racial defilement" was completely eliminated and (b) they occupied separate rooms from Aryan patients. In response to an inquiry from the *Gemeindetag*, Bernotat reported that the first requirement was met in Nassau's institutions; but the second, although desirable, was not possible because housing Jews separately in some institutions would require "disproportionately high expenditures" for structural changes and an increase in personnel.[105] One of the most notorious criminals to emerge from the war in connection with patient killings was not driven by the National Socialist ideal of racial purity to *such* an extent that he was willing to tax administrative resources beyond a point which he considered reasonable and necessary.

As Bernotat and the rest of Germany's psychiatric administrators would soon discover, there were other ways to achieve the same results. Herein lies the true catastrophe of psychiatric administration during the 1930s: administrators did not always follow the regime's precepts to the letter, but their divergence seems to have been the product solely of a desire for technical efficiency and, as in Bernotat's case, by no means incompatible with cooperation or overall agreement with the Party's principles and overarching aims. Ideological consensus between psychiatric administrators and the regime's representatives was helpful but not necessary to the viability of the National Socialists' increasingly aggressive and exclusionary policies.

Insecurity and Isolation in the Service of National Socialism

The evidence presented thus far does not lead us to expect that nurses' professional life was thoroughly politicized in the 1930s if we understand the term to mean blind patronage for the SS-man, on the one hand, and hostilities against Communists, Jews, and psychiatric patients, on the other. It is likely, however, that it *was* politicized in ways which were ultimately of more far-reaching consequence. Formal changes and rituals designed to promote National Socialist ideals cultivated an acceptance of structured authority, a readiness to contribute to a collective effort, and the habit of taking orders from superiors without asking for reasons. As we shall see in more detail in the next chapter, the internalization of *these* principles was ultimately all that was needed for National Socialist policies to succeed; even if institutional personnel failed to become supporters of the regime, they supported the regime anyway by taking their assigned places in institutional life and uncritically fulfilling technical responsibilities.

This development was aided by other aspects of institutional life that we have encountered in previous chapters: discouraged from establishing friendships with patients, powerless vis-à-vis administrative decisions, and surrounded by probing eyes and ears of potential denunciators, nurses who were not already National Socialist sympathizers were very likely intimidated into behaving as though they were. Despite propaganda and rituals designed to imbue them with a sense of belonging to a *Volk*, nurses seem to have been ultimately quite alone on the job and in the face of personal hardship.

Familiarity as Taboo: The Continued Priority of Professional Distance

Nurses continued to be discouraged from any kind of familiarity with patients. Eichberg nurse Karl Jelmann, for example, was strongly reprimanded by Director Hinsen in 1938 for chatting with a patient about the homosexual activities of two other patients and then failing to report these activities to a supervisor: "You have, contrary to institutional regulations and the necessary sense of tact for a nurse, discussed in-house gossip [*Anstaltsklatsch*] with a patient, and indeed with a known ... grumbler. This behavior is not worthy of a nurse and ... violates the basic principles of the nursing profession."[106] Jelmann was threatened with further disciplinary measures in the event of a repeat performance.

In summer 1936, Wittenau nurse Hartmann, whom we encountered earlier, went beyond informal conversation with patients; according to the senior nurse, he had been discovered playing cards with patients when he was supposed to be supervising them during their work, and using the informal form of "you," *du*, to them. Hartmann unsuccessfully attempted to demonstrate his innocence by arguing that there was no work to be done at the time, and that he had only been watching, not playing. He was given a warning and transferred from the high-security ward to another ward.

Hartmann was very unhappy about the transfer and took his case to the local Labor Front; he reportedly felt that his honor had been violated. The Labor Front asked Wittenau to reconsider the wisdom of giving Hartmann a "double punishment." It was this that prompted Braasch to articulate precisely what was at stake in the incident. Hartmann had violated spatial regulations, insofar as he had retreated with the patients into another room out of view for the game; he had violated professional regulations by doing something other than what was on the agenda, namely, renovative work, of which there had been plenty. In this connection, whether he played or simply observed the game was beside the point. Last, he committed a grave violation of the structure of authority: he said *"du"* to particularly unpredictable and obstreperous patients and thus "placed himself on familiar footing with them." Braasch added that the transfer was made simply because Hartmann had demonstrated that he was not reliable enough to work in the high-security ward; it was not a punishment but rather a measure in accordance with administrative responsibility.[107] Administrative responsibility apparently required separating Hartmann from patients for whom he was no longer an authority but quite possibly a friend.

Hands Tied? The Handiness of Administrative Duplicity

This discouragement of informal conversation with patients, if it was effective, essentially marooned nurses on their islands of authority; and if they could not develop personal contacts with patients, there was not much hope of their doing so with administrators, who were not only brief and bureaucratic in their written correspondence but, as in the following cases, duplicitous.

When administrators rejected nurses on political grounds in the years following the implementation of the BBG—be it through dismissal, failure to (re)hire, or failure to promote—they attempted to play down or deny the impact of political criteria in the decision. In mid-1939, an Eichberg station nurse retired, and Nurse Klara Keller, who had been substituting for her, asked the regional government to offer her the position permanently.[108] Eichberg's Directorate rejected the idea on the grounds that Keller was "in moral respects" unsuitable for the position. It nominated, in her stead, the competent and reliable Nurse Sara Huften, who was an engaged and enthusiastic Party member.[109] The government's representative in the affair accepted this and sent Keller a brief rejection notice. She apparently issued an appeal, because the representative mendaciously assured her several weeks later that "the promotion of S[ara] H[uften] to station nurse occurred not on the grounds of her NSDAP membership but rather in consideration of the fact that she is particularly suited to be station nurse."[110]

Administrators also distanced themselves from the political nature of their rejections when reemployment was at issue. Erika Macher, whom we encountered earlier as a BBG victim, attempted to be reemployed at Wittenau in 1935 but was refused. In an *internal* memo, the city administration referred to a lack of available positions and added that there were still plenty of "politically faultless" people in line ahead of her.[111] Macher was not informed of her politically based low priority in the rejection notice.[112]

Berlin-Buch nurse Georg Ertel's experience was similar. After being fired under the BBG for his KPD membership (1926–1929), he persistently sought reemployment during the 1930s and was the subject of regular reviews of his political reliability. Although Ertel claimed to be working for the NSV, the local *Gauleitung* wrote in 1936 that it could not guarantee Ertel's political reliability in light of his former KPD membership.[113] The Office of the Mayor told Ertel that there were no positions available, and that even if there were, numerous applicants were in line ahead of him.[114] The following year, NSDAP representatives upheld this judgment, adding that Ertel was now refusing participation in the NSV and behaving in a very unfriendly way toward political leaders.[115] One suspects that Ertel had given up his work in the NSV because he realized it would not help him get a job. In any case, the Office of the Mayor once again simply told Ertel that it was "not possible" for him to be rehired, without offering any further explanation.[116]

To be sure, even those whose reemployment was supported in internal memos had to wait years at a time for a position, so it may very well have been the case that there were not any positions to be had; the point, however, is that this was not the entire story. While administrators across Party and health care bureaucracies made an enormous collaborative effort to rank potential applicants according to the heinousness of the original "crime" and their degree of political atonement, nurses were simply told that there were no positions to be had—that, in short, the entire situation was beyond administrative control.

One can only speculate as to why administrators distanced themselves from their own political discrimination in this fashion, but a plausible explanation may lie in their desire not to flaunt Party patronage unnecessarily and thus antagonize its nonbeneficiaries; another may lie in their desire to avoid confrontations with the frustrated and disappointed recipients of their rejection notices. After all, an administrator who presented himself as someone who had made a reasoned decision—politically based or otherwise—invited challenges and demands for an explanation. Better to leave nurses thinking that they were at the mercy of a large, powerful bureaucracy whose workings were hopelessly complicated and mysterious. A nurse on the receiving end of these brief and vague messages would have been less likely to hold administrators responsible and more likely to resign him or herself to a general "situation" that did not seem to be alterable by anyone—at any rate, anyone in their immediate vicinity.

At least one nurse seems to have been thinking along these lines: Werner Sommer was fired from the Berlin-Buch institution in 1934 because he failed to report his Spartacus League membership from 1919 to 1921 on his BBG questionnaire and admitted to it only later during a discussion with the administrator in charge. This harsh treatment was followed by over a year of unemployment, until he was hired as a substitute nurse at Wittenau in 1935 and again in 1936. Plagued by health problems, he appealed to the wage contract office and to State Commissioner Lippert to be transferred to an office job. Finally, Sommer sought assistance from none other than the Führer himself.

> *Mein Führer!*
>
> The undersigned requests that you graciously take note of the following letter.
>
> I am 55 years old and have worked for 11 years with pauses as an office employee of the Berlin municipal authorities, now, however, as a nurse at the Wittenauer Heilstätten.
>
> My employment as a nurse has brought about . . . such a worsening of my heart and nervous problems that I must reckon with a breakdown on my part if I continue, especially since my wife has been mentally ill for years. In spite of great effort, up to the present time I have not succeeded in reacquiring an easier position as an office employee.

In my great need you, *mein Führer*, are my only hope of a change in my situation, insofar as you, *mein Führer*, provide me with your help.

So that I can once again be employed as an office worker with the Berlin municipal authorities. [*sic*]

Trusting in your great goodness, *mein Führer*, and in hopes of a favorable answer to my request, I close with a

Heil mein Führer,
W[erner] S[ommer][117]

It seems astonishing indeed that someone who had already tasted the bitter pill of political persecution, and whose situation had only gotten worse since 1933, would seek the help of the man who was responsible for his misfortune. But he was far from alone; at least one thousand letters and petitions were delivered to Hitler's chancellery daily, indicating that written correspondence had become an attractive form of citizen participation.[118] Sommer's letter is exemplary of an attitude that was instrumental in the process by which a basic consent to the regime was secured: the belief that Hitler would do something if only he knew "bridged the gap between, on the one hand, the need for uplift, security, and a positive outlook on the future and, on the other, the disillusionments of everyday Third Reich life."[119]

Hard Times and Married Life

This need for uplift existed among men who were trying to support families as well as among women, who generally continued to leave their jobs shortly after marriage in order to take up housekeeping under their husbands' financial "umbrella"—even when no such umbrella was there. The persistence of tradition in matters marital meant that women were handicapped in their ability to handle financial crises that might befall their families.

Wittenau nurse Anke Jahreis, for example, married an unemployed man in December 1933 and asked the Directorate three months later to hire her husband in her place, explaining that working and being a housewife constituted a double burden.

This request was rejected owing to lack of positions, but Jahreis left Wittenau anyway in May 1934, claiming the "transitional pay" (*Übergangsgeld*) due to her as a woman leaving on account of marriage. The sum marked a "transition" to nothing more than further hardship; five months later she reminded Wittenau once again about her unemployed husband. Braasch reported a continued lack of positions but promised to keep him in mind. Luckily for all involved, the matter was brought to a close several months later by his employment elsewhere.[120]

Herzberge's Nurse Lisa Biegel faced similar difficulties. She had a child in 1921 and fulfilled her child-raising and nursing responsibilities satisfactorily until her marriage to a nursing colleague in late 1935 and subsequent departure from her job. A few months later, her husband contracted tuberculosis, was unable to work, and eventually became ineligible for further pay. Biegel was rehired by Herzberge in a substitute capacity but, now a wife rather than a single parent, was no longer eligible to receive child and rent support. The Herzberge Directorate was sympathetic to her plight and persuaded the HGA to continue the support on a temporary basis. Offering a bit more in the way of financial security, such as giving the experienced and competent Nurse Biegel a permanent post, was apparently not up for discussion: a senior nurse noted that, although her work was satisfactory, Biegel was married and thus could be considered only for substitute positions.[121] It is not clear from her file when or if her husband returned to work, although one suspects that he did not: Biegel would spend the next eight years working steadily, but temporarily, in a series of four- to six-month nursing positions throughout Berlin.[122] Financial security thus remained out of reach.

NURSES facing financial stress in their private lives would likely have experienced another kind of stress at work, namely, the specter of denunciation. As one administrative employee from the Rheinland would remember years later, "People couldn't talk to each other anymore."[123] One doctor's reaction to an incident at the Berlin-Buch institution in early 1933 suggests that the psychological burden of this state of affairs would have been considerable. "In one case, 'Heil Moscow' was recently called out by someone in the institution. Such behavior gives grounds for suspicion of traitorous views and activities. In any case, a public nuisance is constituted implicitly in such cases and is to be prosecuted."[124] To be sure, it was not clear whether the exclamation had come from a patient or an employee; but in any case he would instruct all staff members that such incidents were to be reported to the Directorate, and he would see to it that the police were informed.[125]

How nurses adjusted to this state of affairs is largely a matter of speculation; but most likely they would have been inclined not to be vocal about their views but rather to keep a low profile. Nurses who felt a certain degree of solidarity with patients— or at the very least sympathy—would perhaps have encouraged patients to do the same. This was the case, at least, when Patient J. resisted pressure to sign his own application for sterilization, adding among other things, "Your leader is not my leader, my leader is God." Later, a nurse who was apparently familiar with his disposition advised him, "You mustn't speak so openly."[126]

Anecdotes like these do not lend much credibility to the notion that professional life for nurses under National Socialism was permeated by harmony, mutual trust, and unanimous loyalty to a higher cause. Rather, life seems to have been an exercise in fulfilling technical responsibilities and participating in political rituals while adding as little of one's own personal commentary as possible. The discouragement of informal conversation with patients, administrative duplicity, and the specter of denunciation would more likely have produced feelings of uncertainty and isolation than the kind of jovial solidarity that was promoted at the Berlin-Buch institution one winter's night in February 1935:

> *Beim Schaffen getrennt, doch eins im Denken,*
> *Als müßtest des andern Schicksal Du lenken,*
> *Als seist Du ich und ich sei Du,*
> *So meints die Kameradschaft der Heilbu.*[127]

8

War, Mass Murder, and
Moral Flight: Psychiatric Nursing,
1939–1945

If I had been told to hit a patient with a hammer on the head, then I would have known that it is murder, and I would have refused under all circumstances to do it.[1]

Nurse M.A.

IT IS NOT known for certain exactly how many people, both German and foreign, fell victim to the so-called "euthanasia" measures that were spread out in two phases over the course of the war years, although the figure probably lies between 150,000 and 200,000.[2] What is certain, however, is that these deaths were not the product of barbarous bureaucratic initiatives' being ruthlessly forced upon unwilling psychiatric staff; rather, staff members executed those initiatives efficiently and without organized protest. By war's end, the ultimate moral collapse had taken place: institutional psychiatry had shown itself to be fertile ground for ruthless and far-reaching exterminatory policies, after two decades of trumpeting its intentions and methods as "humane."

The methods of killing, as far as nurses were concerned, involved no violence and no blood; patients were sent away in buses, or, in the second phase, they fell into a sleep from which they did not awaken or wasted away from hunger until they died. Most nurses seem to have adapted to murder under these circumstances, with or without pangs of conscience. To be sure, our discussion of nursing literature has already identified rhetorical strategies for integrating a subdued contempt for patients into a superficially humanitarian agenda; we also encountered the implicit legitimation of violence against patients in the context of *Erziehung* and the treatment of violence as an administrative, rather than moral, issue in everyday life. Was this enough to desensitize nurses morally in the midst of mass murder? Were other, or additional, factors involved? Were nurses, in fact, desensitized? The following discussion seeks to investigate these questions by considering what nurses did, or more often did not do, in the course of the killing operations, alongside their own explanations of their behavior as they appeared in the Eichberg and Meseritz-Obrawalde testimonies (1945–1946 and 1961–1962 respectively).

INSTITUTIONAL PSYCHIATRY, 1939–1945

We have seen earlier that institutional living conditions in Germany deteriorated precipitously during the 1930s at the bidding of cost-slashing administrators like Bernotat and their superiors, and needless to say of Hitler himself, who stated that "the food supply does not allow for the incurably ill to be dragged through the war."[3] Not surprisingly, matters became worse during the war years. A 1941 report from the Düsseldorf institution read, "The patients complain of hunger, [and] weight loss is widespread. Many of the newly admitted die in the first days after admission or a short time thereafter."[4] This state of affairs was not attributable to wartime food shortages, especially in the fertile area surrounding Eichberg. Rather, with prompting from Berlin, the Bavarian Ministry of the Interior released a "Starvation Diet Decree" in November 1942 which stipulated that those institutionalized patients who performed useful work were to be "better provided for at the expense of the other patients." It was in all probability circulated to other provincial governments as well, but regardless of the absence or presence of legal blessing, rations had long since been reduced to starvation levels.[5]

The regime embarked on drastic consolidation measures after the onset of the war and "euthanasia" measures in 1939. In Berlin, for example, public psychiatric institutions began to be converted into hospitals one by one. Wittenau, perhaps on account of the excellent scientific and therapeutic reputation it had acquired in the 1920s and 1930s, was spared, and by 1943 it was the only remaining public psychiatric institution in the city. Be this as it may, consolidation and the loss of 350 beds in the wake of a bombing raid in late 1943 placed Wittenau administrators under increasing pressure to transport patients to provincial institutions, from which some were sent on to killing centers like Meseritz-Obrawalde. In addition, detailed examination of patient records and statistics has suggested that an indeterminable number of patients were killed in the institution itself through a combination of medication and starvation during the war years.[6] Of Berlin's 9,204 psychiatric patients in 1939, only 1,807 remained in 1945.[7]

While psychiatrists pursued shock treatments and other therapeutic "innovations" with more enthusiasm and optimism than ever,[8] life inside the institutions themselves acquired a brutish character. A 1940 *Gemeindetag* questionnaire on methods for containing patients reported that in Brandenburg's psychiatric institutions, some nurses were provided with guns to "prevent escape."[9] Meanwhile, two years earlier Waldheim male nurses had begun to be trained in shooting "with great enthusiasm" and "really good performance." This was ostensibly a preparation for war: in case of an air raid, the institution's 1938 report noted, assembling unruly patients in cellars was "out of the question." Therefore, "personnel must remain at their post in order to prevent under all circumstances—if necessary with a firearm—escape of patients."[10]

To provide a context for the following discussion, let us focus briefly on conditions in the Meseritz-Obrawalde and Eichberg institutions during the war years. On the basis of some testimonies, it could be said that these two institutions were not only geographical opposites (the former being in the east, the latter in the west of what was then German territory) but also opposites in terms of atmosphere before 1939. Conditions at Eichberg were deplorable; but, according to a former management employee who left Meseritz-Obrawalde in 1939, the atmosphere there was quite different: "Obrawalde was the second or third newest institution in all of Germany at the time, had modern equipment, and was run according to correct medical principles. Nurses and also other staff members very much enjoyed carrying out their duties in Obrawalde back then because Obrawalde was considered more or less a model institution[;] there was a very collegial relationship among the staff and also a very good relationship between the staff and the patients."[11] These "good relationships" were soon torn asunder, as Meseritz-Obrawalde was converted from a "model institution" for therapy into a model institution for killing. In 1937, it closed its nonpsychiatric facilities and thereafter functioned solely as a psychiatric institution; in 1939 it was placed under the direction of the provincial government of Pomerania.[12] Originally built with a capacity for 700 patients, the institution saw a patient population of 900 that year, which skyrocketed to approximately 2,000 in the following years, under the "care" of only three doctors.[13] According to a former patient, absolutely no medical treatment took place at Obrawalde during his time there in the last year of the war.

> The people lay in metal bed frames on top of each other, on straw sacks. The privy lay open between the rows of beds. All night long you kept hearing the sound of flushings. One was not supposed to be able to move and go along the aisle; that would have been a reason for someone to be selected [for killing]. Here there was only a minimum to eat. In the morning there was bread and coffee. At midday there was watery soup with a few globules of fat for the workers. If one was lucky, there were a few more globules, but it was all basically water, so that one could not be nourished by it.[14]

Those who did not work, he added, received "soup" consisting of potato peels in water. "The people were supposed to be made apathetic, so that they could be brought to death slowly." Relatives were forbidden to send food packets to the patients and were told by letter that the patients already had enough to eat.[15]

In the midst of this deliberate starvation, doctors and personnel killed about 20–50 patients per day in Houses 6, 9, 18, and the children's station with injections and orally administered sedatives.[16] By the end of the war, over 10,000 patients (according to some accounts, almost twice that number) would be dead, with a 97 percent death rate among incoming patients in 1944.[17] Under these circumstances, nurses' responsibilities were transformed: no longer were they providing care within the framework of a medical-humanitarian enterprise, even in the widest stretch of the imagination, but rather sustaining the *appearance* that such care still existed in the midst of systematic murder. Specifically, nurses lied to patients concerning what was about to happen to them, encouraging them to drink the bitter "medicine" if they wanted to get better.[18] Patients' well-founded suspicion did produce its share of recalcitrance: witnesses maintained that patients were brutally forced to take the deadly medication, either being hit in the face, dragged into the killing room, or having their mouths forcibly opened.[19] Nurses' testimonies suggest that when patients would not drink the bitter medicine, they were simply given an injection instead. In any case, nurses not only provided technical assistance with the killings. They also exploited, in the service of deception, that trust which sick, helpless, and often desperate people invested in them.

To facilitate the business of mass murder, Meseritz-Obrawalde was provided with its own fanatical autocrat: Walter Grabowski was made administrative director in November 1941 (the first director ever appointed there who was *not* a doctor)[20] and promptly rendered himself unchallenged leader through personnel changes.[21] Described by a former staff member as an "unbearable person and an absolute despot," Grabowski was rumored to have been involved in killing Jews in Kalisch before his arrival in Obrawalde. Grabowski's appearance lent a considerable degree of credibility to rumors of his brutal past. Although a short man, he was a physically imposing presence: he was remembered by several former colleagues for routinely parading through the institution in a hunting hat, carrying a walking stick, and accompanied by a large dog.[22]

EICHBERG, too, would spell doom for thousands of patients. In addition to serving as a layover institution for over 2,000 patients who would later be gassed at Hadamar during the T4 program, it became a center for "medicalized" killing in 1941; 2,722 adult patients died between 1941 and 1945.[23] Here, too, the fact that killing was by and large "medical" and thus "bloodless" in no way meant that patients were somehow spared suffering. Besides suffering from crowding and from lack of heat and proper clothing, many patients wasted away and eventually died of starvation.[24] Routine neglect was reflected in doctor-patient ratios, which worsened to the extent that one doctor was no longer responsible for 150 patients but rather for 300.[25] Patients' misery was compounded by the fact that for the duration of the war, visits from relatives were forbidden.[26]

To make matters worse, Eichberg's patients lived in constant fear of being thrown into the so-called bunker, a series of underground cells established at the beginning of the war to contain the criminally inclined. It was, in fact, routinely used for arbitrary and cruel punishment of any patient who had as much as gotten on a staff member's nerves.[27] A "sentence" there meant confinement in one of a series of dark, filthy underground cells without heating and toilet facilities, and with little or no food. Nurses reported that patients sometimes stayed in the bunker for six months or more, and throughout this time staff were not permitted to supplement the prisoners' meager rations.[28]

Abuse of patients seems to have been common, if not routine. Nurse Elsen, for example, was described by former patients as "anything but a nurse," a sadistic physical and verbal abuser. According to one, Elsen pulled her hair and beat another woman in the bathtub with a scrubbing brush so hard that it broke into pieces.[29] Another patient watched in horror as Elsen dragged a patient through the room by her hair when she asked for more bread.[30] Yet another former patient said that she had witnessed a murder in 1942: a nurse pulled the hair of an old woman when she did not direct her gaze properly. When the woman defended herself, the nurse pulled her down and repeatedly struck her head against the floor until the woman was dead. The patient never learned how the nurse or Dr. Schmidt explained the woman's death.[31]

Eichberg, too, had its own fanatical autocrat in the form of this Dr. Schmidt, who was, according to the almost unanimous testimonies of Eichberg staff and former patients, an unpredictable, violent man who abused alcohol as well as patients, throwing the latter into the bunker for the flimsiest of reasons.[32] Described by one colleague as a "hothead and a psychopath,"[33] he made his rounds wearing his SS-uniform and carried a pistol.[34] Schmidt expected his nurses to rule with an iron fist as well; when a nurse expressed his fear that a patient might be able to run away as he brought him to the bunker, Schmidt responded, "Then shoot him dead!"[35]

Schmidt surrounded himself with a small but loyal contingent of assistants. Senior Nurse Heidrun Seidel, for example, was described as one of Schmidt's right hands. Although she routinely assisted Schmidt in murdering patients, she reportedly attempted to hold at least one patient back from a T4 transport (the sister of a friend of hers) and claimed to have suffered so much from conflicts of conscience that she went all the way to *Landeshauptmann* Traupel in Kassel to try to leave her job.[36] Unfortunately, she had a deluded and unquestioning admiration for Schmidt, and in this respect the relationship of these two killers may have been on a par with that which Burleigh describes between Hadamar's Alfons Klein and Nurse Irmgard Huber: both seem to have been cemented by the woman's unflagging support of the man in question in spite of her own conflicts of conscience.[37]

Nurse Friedrich Golsmann was also described as Schmidt's right hand and "a fanatical National Socialist who bragged that he had been very active in the persecution of the Jews. He said he had given a Jew a good slap around the face."[38] He was on informal terms with both Schmidt and Director Mennecke and, to round out the picture, received a gun of his own to wield during his shifts.[39]

From Carers to Killers and from Killers to Carers:
The Correlation between Cruelty and Murder

Against this background, one is tempted to agree with Michael Burleigh that there is "no great psychological mystery about why these 'carers' became killers. . . . " Many psychiatric nurses, he argues, were tired, frustrated, and already desensitized to the suffering of others. Many had internalized common pejorative attitudes about the mentally ill and saw nothing in the patients in front of them to change their minds.[40]

If we consider the matter further, however, the participation of nurses in murder is not quite as transparent as this characterization suggests. To cite just one example, several of those former Eichberg patients who witnessed or experienced sadistic abuse at the hands of Nurse Elsen insisted that she was the complete opposite of one of the accused, Nurse Mathilde Frey, who by her own account gave injections on Schmidt's and Seidel's orders so that the patients "would die sooner."[41] In the eyes of these patients, Frey was an "outstanding" nurse with exclusively good qualities.[42] One patient who had been abused by Nurse Elsen considered her transfer to Frey's station a kind of small miracle: Frey often invited patients into her room to talk and to listen to the radio; she not only offered encouragement in times of crisis ("Don't lose courage" and "For you, too, the day of freedom will come again") but, in contrast to other nurses, upheld the small but significant habits of common decency, such as saying, "Good morning" and "Good night" to the patients.[43] These are not isolated accounts; Nurse Frey was also characterized by former colleagues as friendly, respectable, diligent, caring, adored and trusted by her patients. Her manner was similar to that of a mother looking after her children.[44] Elsen and Frey worked under the same roof, but it would be mistaken to describe their character, behavior, and motives in the same way.

It is not particularly hard to understand why people with a history of cruelty did not have a great deal of difficulty carrying on at a place like Eichberg and getting along well with people like Schmidt. More vexing, and ultimately of more historical importance, is the question of why people like Frey, who even by disinterested accounts treated patients with decency, may have been drawn into killing—and why people who were at the periphery did not feel moved by what was going on to such a degree that they protested.

Nursing at the Periphery of Mass Murder

In order to understand how nurses reacted to what was going on around them, we may usefully begin with testimonies from the early months of the "euthanasia" program's first phase (T4), from nurses at the "periphery" of the killing process, and work our way over time toward the "center"—namely, toward nurses who killed patients themselves during the second stage of *"wilde Euthanasie."* Although the discussion identifies a temporal transition from not-knowing to knowing about the killings, and draws various physical and psychological boundaries between assistance and direct participation, these categories are intended to be analytical rather than descriptive. That is, they are intended to facilitate an understanding of how nurses adapted themselves to killing as everyday practice, rather than to represent a general experience.

The T4 Program, Patient Transports, and the Acquisition of Knowledge

The T4 program (named after the program's administrative center in Berlin's Tiergartenstraße 4) began with a secret decree administered by Hitler on October 1, 1939, and backdated one month so that it would coincide with the invasion of Poland.

Reichsleiter Bouhler and Dr. Brandt were to be empowered to grant a "mercy death" to the incurably ill in consultation with doctors and after a "humane evaluation" of their condition.[45] Administrators of psychiatric institutions would be required to submit a questionnaire for each patient attesting to race, duration of care in the institution, current medical condition, whether and how often the patient received visits, and work capability. All questionnaires were to be sent back to the T4 central and evaluated by one of a number of special "experts" who reviewed the cases and designated those to be killed with a "+" and those to be spared with a "−."[46] On the basis of this "evaluation" alone—that is, without any personal examination of patients or consideration of their files—transport lists were compiled and sent back to the institutions, followed shortly by a team of specially selected T4 staff and nurses who collected and accompanied the transports, via a series of layover institutions, to one of six killing centers.[47] Immediately following their arrival, patients were undressed, photographed (again with the help of nurses), then killed with gas in rooms disguised as showers. Before Hitler issued his official "stop" to the T4 program in August 1941, over 70,000 people had been killed.[48]

Initially, the transports seem to have proceeded relatively smoothly. One former nurse described a transport to the Grafeneck killing center as follows:

The evening before the transport, we received a list with the names of the patients who were picked up. Early in the morning, the buses drove up, and the windows were painted gray up to the top. The patients received a slip of paper with a number. Then they filed by one by one, and we wrote the number on the bare back in ink. Because they thought that we were going to transfer them to another institution, they were generally quite calm. Indeed, they did not know what was going to happen to them. Then they were led into the bus, always seventy-five. A few weeks later the clothes were sent back from Grafeneck.[49]

As the purpose of the transports became known at various institutions, nurses could no longer depend on the ignorance, and thus docility, of the doomed. Patients screamed and bitterly resisted being loaded into the buses; sedation with injections became necessary. A Kaufbeuren-Irsee nurse recalled one patient in particular who called her and her colleagues "murderers" as she was loaded onto the bus. "It was the same with her as with the others," she continued; "they were picked up, on the next day they were dead and the relatives got news, dead of typhus or whatever, and it was all lies."[50]

A former T4 transport nurse noticed that the general atmosphere in these institutions changed palpably as the truth became known: "With the first transports, we were even warmly received and looked after well. But later this was different, after the institutions had somehow noticed or learned about the purpose of our transports."[51] It seems that when nurses at various institutions found out about the killings, they first reacted with horror, then carried on with their daily routines in a state of depressed resignation.[52] At the most, it seems, doctors and nurses tried when they could to have certain patients held back from the transports, and even then the morally redeeming value of this low-level sabotage was sometimes compromised by favoritism. Some nurses refused to bring patients into the buses, but sometimes they tried to send other patients in place of those whom they cherished.[53]

WHILE the T4 program was being organized and prepared in the Reich, the regime orchestrated a parallel killing operation in the East: the patients in Pomeranian institutions were evacuated to the newly occupied province of Danzig–West Prussia and summarily shot by SS units.[54] Since these killings were in many respects part of a larger effort to develop mass murder techniques for Jews, Sinti and Roma, and other victims, they were until recently only seldom discussed in connection with the T4 program. Yet, in addition to providing the context in which psychiatric nurses first assisted in the murders of their own charges, these episodes provide insights into how participating nurses processed knowledge that came their way about the killings. At times, they even point to a shared experience with participants in the T4 program farther west.

As the Lauenburg institution was being dissolved in January 1940, for example, Nurse Anke Sutte and several colleagues accompanied a group of patients to the Kosten institution. Initially, she noticed nothing particularly suspicious about the transport: the nurses carefully prepared the usual accoutrements and belongings for such a trip. When they had reached their destination, however, they were surprised to see the patients delivered into an empty room. The nurses, they were told, would arrive later. They stayed overnight at the institution; as they were leaving the next morning, they saw a military vehicle with soldiers in gray uniforms entering the institution's grounds. One nurse waved to the soldiers, who called back that she should stay behind with them. No, the nurse replied, if she stayed behind she would be shot.[55]

The nurse, Sutte explained, had simply been making a reference to the proximity of the Russian front and the possibility of being caught in hostilities; but when the group reached the train station, a military official approached and asked to speak to the nurse who had spoken of shootings. Only with great difficulty could the accompanying doctor and senior nurse free her from the situation.[56]

Sutte was transferred twice over the next several months; and even though she never found evidence of patients' actually being killed in the institutions themselves,[57] unsettling hints about their ultimate fate continued to come her way, and eventually the purpose of the transports became impossible to deny: patients struggled and screamed when they were collected and then transported away in these vehicles; they were sent with nothing but the clothes on their backs and jammed in so closely that they could only stand or crouch. She once saw two older women from the convalescent group, who were fully lucid, go to the window and say, "Come, let's look one more time at God's sun."[58] Sutte eventually succeeded in quitting, but only with "great difficulty" and the loss of eleven months' compensation to which she would otherwise have been entitled after thirteen years' service.[59]

Elfriede Dänemann also worked as a transport nurse in the East. In particular, she remembered a transport from Treptow to Lauenburg in 1940. She and her colleagues were told to leave the train in Lauenburg, and it continued on without them. She certainly thought that sending patients off unattended was strange, but she reported not having had any idea of what might happen to them, outside of the vague worry that the patients might not be in such good hands as they were with her. Everyone had thoughts about it, she noted, and "talked a little about it in intimate circles, but who would have dared back then to speak openly about such things."[60]

It must be pointed out that transports of patients were no invention of the Nazis, and for these young women the prospect of accompanying one meant, at the very least, a change from the normal routine and, at most, a small adventure. Martha Möll explained, "Happy to be able to make a trip into the occupied territory, we nurses naturally liked to participate."[61] It is plausible, in other words, that some nurses initially agreed to accompany such transports in ignorance of their purpose and figured out only gradually that patients were being transported to their deaths. The problem is that their testimonies offer little in the way of certainty about when the killings became knowledge as opposed to suspicion or rumor; there is always the chance that nurses deceived themselves about what they knew when.

It is precisely this latter point, however, that is most interesting and revealing about these testimonies. Sutte, after several experiences whose meaning must have been very difficult indeed to deny, reported having a "bad feeling"—yet this feeling was evidently strong enough to prompt her to remove herself from the action. Dänemann, in a similar fashion, reported feeling that transported patients would not be "treated as well" at their destination as heretofore and was not eager to muse with her colleagues about exactly how they might be treated. The point here is not that nurses knew about the killings but denied it to their interviewers, although this may very well be true; it is that they do not seem to have been eager to admit to *themselves*, let alone others, that they knew.

Avoiding the Unavoidable Truth: Nursing at the Layover Institution Eichberg

This response was not limited to nurses who worked only briefly at the "margins" of the killing process. We find similar language even among nurses at the Eichberg institution, who continually prepared transports to Hadamar over the course of eight months in 1941 and saw patients' clothes return a few days later—who heard and repeated stories about relatives who received two urns or a notice announcing the death of a patient who had already been sent home.[62] Nurses who had far more regular exposure to the signs of organized killing, and thus far more opportunities to find out the terrible truth and deliberate about their own participation, spoke in decidedly vague terms about how and when they acquired knowledge of the killings at Hadamar.

To be sure, many nurses, and even a senior nurse, testified that they were not told the truth about the destination or purpose of the transports. According to one nurse, Dr. Mennecke told assembled nurses and staff that in the current state of war, the institution might at some point have to be cleared quickly to create space for a hospital or to retreat from an approaching enemy. Therefore, the older patients were going to be evacuated immediately and a number of transitional patients would be arriving shortly for brief stays. "All the commotion would become very interesting and instructive for us, since we would be able to meet new patients and new cases, we would deal with other people, and a bit of variety would come into our professional life."[63] The nurses were instructed not to bother trying to hold back patients they liked or those who were useful, "since he alone would bear responsibility and would not like [people] meddling in his affairs."[64]

This explanation seems to have been accepted by some nurses, even those who worked directly with the doomed patients by marking their backs with blue numbers.[65] Others who were either more insightful or more honest, such as Senior Nurse Jürgen Haag, immediately suspected that something was amiss: "Although I did not personally know the purpose of the transports, I had an unpleasant feeling about them from the beginning, because I was aware from the speeches of the National Socialist leader and of influential personalities that the excessively high number of psychiatric patients was complained about again and again. This feeling naturally was fed anew by rumors that later came through to us."[66] It did not take long for this "unpleasant feeling" to acquire firm foundations: "When the clothes first came back, we could imagine nothing else than that the patients had been done away with there."[67] One veteran nurse noticed an orthopedic shoe apparatus belonging to a patient he had known. "I said to myself at the time that the owner of these shoes cannot work without this apparatus and thus must have been killed." He had given this patient a stamped postcard on which to report his safe arrival in Hadamar, and it was never returned.[68]

The return of patients' clothing was one factor that enlightened nurses about the purpose of the transports; rumors were another. Former nurse Jacob Schumann said that, although the nurses did not know at first what the "Hadamar Action" was, "later we learned that the patients who had been brought there were more or less brought to their deaths in an unnatural way."[69] Former nurse Johann Minden, who spent these months doing paint jobs together with patients, learned that the transports were going to Hadamar "after some time." "Later," he reported, "I heard outside of the institution that these patients were more or less killed there."[70]

Again, as with the transport nurses farther east, these vague references to "bad feelings" and the gradual acquisition of knowledge that patients were being "more or less" killed at Hadamar awaken skepticism—especially when viewed in conjunction with other testimonies such as "the expression 'they [the patients] are put on the grill' was generally used."[71] Surely, it seems, they *must* have known, and their vague language suggests that they did not want to admit the truth of the killings to themselves. They engaged, in short, in self-deception.

If we consider the matter further, however, "self-deception" does not entirely capture what was going on; for it implies that nurses had indisputable information about the killings and closed their eyes to the whole affair, saying, "That can't be true." Nurses, as we have seen above, did not say, "It can't be true"; but they *did* report that their information was vague and allegedly acquired painfully slowly, as if they were holding themselves in an eternal state of not-yet-knowing-for-certain and *preserving the fiction that it might not be true*. With few exceptions, this "having-grounds-for-suspicion-but-not-knowing-for-sure" was a perfectly tolerable state of affairs for carrying on with their daily routine—perhaps even an ideal one, under the circumstances. After all, working under this "umbrella" of rumors meant that they were exposed to information which was unavoidable anyway, but also conveniently protected from the kind of certainty that might set one thinking and perhaps produce a conscientious imperative to *do* something. This may explain why, again with few exceptions, nurses do not seem to have been particularly eager to inform themselves about their patients' fate by asking questions or investigating.[72]

As OBSERVATIONS and rumors piled up, this strategy of accommodation undoubtedly lost much of its utility, and Eichberg's nurses had to confront the fact that they were sending patients to their deaths. What then? Some nurses indeed felt compelled to do something: they attempted to leave their posts and, failing that, to have patients held back from the transports.[73] The majority, however, carried on as they had before because, they often argued, any alternative course of action was futile and forbidden. As one nurse said, "We could not revolt against it and were bound according to institutional rules and by the doctors to maintain the strictest confidentiality."[74]

In this vein, nurses reported having been subjected to vague verbal threats of punishment if they dared to even discuss the transports out of house.[75] After killings had begun at Grafeneck in 1940, and rumors made their way to Eichberg, Mennecke felt the need to issue another reminder at a staff conference: "It was being said again and again that patients were being killed in institutions. He [thus] had to bring it to their attention that anyone who maintained something like this, but could not prove it, would have to reckon with a prison sentence."[76] This statement, ironically enough, was recounted by an already suspicious nurse who took it as confirmation that the rumors were in fact true; but for those in attendance who were disinclined to challenge authority, or who were simply uninterested, Mennecke's warning may have preempted any inclination to act on behalf of patients before the transports to Hadamar had even begun.

Nurses at the "periphery," then, may have been trying to hold themselves in a state of uncertainty about the fate of the transported patients. Their testimonies leave the impression that rumors did not necessarily clash with the "official" explanation for what was going on; rather, their coexistence seems to have had a placating effect, with each explanation balancing the shortcomings of the other: if the "official" explanation seemed dubious, rumors provided a plausible account for what might be going on. On the other hand, one certainly did not want to have to believe that patients were being *gassed*; and here the "official" explanation and accompanying threats came to the rescue: they enabled those who did not want to believe rumors to sustain their belief that they were untrue.

MEDICALIZED KILLING AND MORAL FLIGHT: "WILDE EUTHANASIE," 1941–1945

The official "stop" of the gassing of patients in August 1941 marked nothing more than an interruption and redeployment of killing techniques in a more decentralized fashion. Children's "euthanasia" continued unabated, and adult patients were henceforth killed with hunger diets and overdoses of sedatives within the walls of ostensibly "normally" functioning institutions. This second phase of unofficial "euthanasia" (*"wilde Euthanasie"*), lasting from autumn 1941 through the end of the war, would claim at least as many victims as had the first.[77] In the context of this decentralized killing, nurses assisted in compiling lists of patients on their station to be transported. Some accompanied transports, and in the killing institutions themselves, as we shall see, they carried out a number of tasks to facilitate the slow, medicalized killing of their charges: they deceived suspicious patients about the purpose of the injections and drinks administered, transported patients into and out of the rooms in which they were killed, and sometimes administered lethal injections themselves.

The story of how nurses adapted to their new set of duties is a complicated one that requires analysis of a variety of ostensibly incidental comments they made about their professional lives during these years. But by way of orientation, a useful beginning is a brief survey of nurses' own explanations for their assistance or direct participation in killing patients.

"Discipline and obedience were the highest law . . .":[78]
Compulsion, Duty, and Psychological Entrapment

At first glance, the Eichberg and Meseritz-Obrawalde trial records suggest that nurses' complicity in murder was the result of inescapable external and internal pressures. A few of the more common arguments are as follows:

The imperative force of professional duty. Many nurses pointed to the fact that they had been trained to follow doctors' orders and were neither authorized nor qualified to challenge those orders. Nurse were, according to this reasoning, obligated to execute every order, regardless of its content.

The silencing force of confidentiality. Some nurses reported or suspected that those *directly* involved in killing patients were sworn to secrecy by their superiors.[79] Others who were either uninvolved or active in an auxiliary capacity could not remember being sworn to secrecy—but they noted that regardless of this, their professional code demanded the strictest confidentiality (*Schweigepflicht*).[80]

The displacement of moral and legal responsibility. Many said they believed that the killings were part of a larger, perhaps even organized but in any case "official," undertaking. One Eichberg nurse, for example, testified that he did not know whether Schmidt was acting of his own volition or on orders; but the killing of individual patients was *rumored* to have been ordered from Berlin.[81] Reflecting on his own participation in the deaths of two children, another Eichberg nurse said that he "had his thoughts" about it, but "since the order apparently went out from Berlin, and the measures were completely in the spirit of Dr. Schmidt [and] corresponded with his views, I felt in no way responsible."[82]

Many Meseritz-Obrawalde nurses, too, said they believed a law or special order from Hitler stood behind the killing operation. Who were they to question the wishes of the Führer? A law, however, was apparently not necessary so long as they could place responsibility for their participation squarely on someone else's shoulders: Margarete Göbel admitted to feeling "relieved" when Dr. Wernicke agreed to assume full responsibility for the killings.[83] Eichberg senior nurse Heidrun Seidel, who claimed to have had unbearable conflicts of conscience, also testified, "I tried to soothe my conscience by telling myself that the doctor alone bears responsibility."[84]

The immobilizing force of dependents. Some Meseritz-Obrawalde nurses reminded their interrogators of their familial responsibilities. Margarete Göbel was needed by her aging parents. Helene Koch was responsible for a three-year-old son, and her mother lived in Meseritz as well. Martha Möll, similarly, was responsible for her grandparents and had a son in January 1944.[85]

The immobilizing force of potential reprisals. Perhaps the most often-cited reason for nurses' participation is the fear of punishment. The Meseritz-Obrawalde testimonies, in particular, are rife with references to various forms of punishment and persecution to which Grabowski might subject those staff members who refused to participate in killings or otherwise fell from grace. One woman, who worked in the kitchen from late summer 1942 onward, said that "there was a rumor going around in Obrawalde that anyone who did not follow his orders would be sent to the Warthegau, the so-called danger zone."[86] Martha Möll also reported being told that a nurse was once sent away with a transport and never came back.[87] Some men in the coal yard, she added, said that Grabowski was very strict, ordering reduced food rations as one of his milder punishments. Another nurse, who told political jokes about Hitler and Göring while supervising patients in the fields, was told by a colleague that if Grabowski found out about this, he would send her to a concentration camp.[88]

Eichberg nurses, too, reportedly stood under threat of severe reprisals in the event that they as much as *talked* about the killings. When questioned about the deaths of a group of thirty to forty children from Hamburg, for example, Harald Donner said, "One certainly knew what had happened, but one could not say anything. *Landrat* Bernotat had once said at a staff meeting that if he heard even a hint that a male or female nurse spoke about the conditions here or, in particular, said something in public, he would make him or her accountable and stop at nothing [*über Leichen gehen*]."[89] Whatever anxiety Bernotat's potential reprisals engendered, the terrorizing presence of their more immediate superiors was reportedly sufficient to snuff out any thoughts of noncompliance. Anton Straub, who admitted to assisting Schmidt and knew that the patients in question were supposed to be killed, claimed, "I could not put up a fight against the tasks Schmidt assigned to me. Dr. Schmidt was a boor who would not have stood for refusal and undoubtedly would have ordered the most far-reaching consequences for me if I had refused."[90]

NURSES, the above arguments suggest, simply could not extract themselves from the grisly business of mass murder. Their accounts awaken a certain skepticism: the assertion that mere rules, laws, and precedents have the power to make people murder—allegedly against their will—is hardly convincing. Nurses' claim that they feared being sent to a concentration camp is somewhat more persuasive until one learns that there are no known examples of this punishment's actually having been meted out.[91] The accounts they gave as *defendants in criminal proceedings* cannot be taken seriously because they are nothing more than nurses' attempts to exonerate themselves of wrongdoing.

As far as the Eichberg testimonies are concerned, it is very difficult to disprove this argument. Not only were some nurses defending themselves against murder charges; a great many more were still employed at Eichberg in 1945–1946 when they gave their testimonies. The majority, in short, did not have a great interest in telling the truth about life at Eichberg, and this occasionally meant that some told patent falsehoods. According to one veteran nurse, for example, "With regard to the treatment of patients on the stations, I can only say for myself that it was strictly forbidden for nurses to hit the patients. This also did not happen and it is not known to me that Dr. Schmidt abused patients."[92]

The Eichberg nurses were also not in a particularly self-critical state of mind; comments about personal feelings and explanations for their own conduct were generally made only in passing and often contradicted the testimonies of people who knew them. We have seen above, for example, that Nurse Elsen was accused by former patients of abusing patients regularly. Yet she, of all people, testified that the *nurses* lived in a state of terror: "The nursing personnel could more or less give no positive details or had to keep quiet [with regard to the killings]; otherwise they would have ended up just like the victims themselves."[93] Thus a victimizer shamelessly presented herself as a potential victim.

Statements such as these should warn us to evaluate nurses' testimonies carefully and critically. They are not, however, grounds to dismiss the entire body of testimonies as mere excuses, lies, or attempts to rationalize moral cowardice out of existence. Certainly, rules do not "force" people to behave in a certain way, as though human beings are nothing more than passive vehicles for the translation of ideas into practice; people process explicit and implicit "rules" along with other circumstantial factors, and they decide to behave a certain way. The fact that nurses failed to make this distinction, however, does not in any way justify the conclusion that they were deliberately falsifying their own thoughts and behavior, and that they actually subscribed to the notion of "life unworthy of living."

The reasons for this become clearer once one stands back from the testimonies somewhat and reads *beyond* nurses' own explanations for their behavior. In doing so, we discover the possibility that these so-called excuses or rationalizations were not necessarily thought up after the fact and under the pressure of interrogators but rather played a role in their reasoning at the time. The catch is that *this role is not the role nurses ascribed to them.*

Rumors, Long Sleeps, and Suspicious Disappearances:
"wilde Euthanasie" at Eichberg

Let us begin once again with the question of how knowledge of the killings was acquired. A number of Eichberg nurses testified that they had no firsthand knowledge of Schmidt's killing patients but had certainly heard rumors to that effect.[94] As one veteran nurse stated, "It was generally known among the nurses and throughout the Eichberg [institution] that Schmidt killed patients. We just called him the 'mass murderer.' "[95] This nurse himself deduced from the increasing numbers of bodies he carried to the graveyard that this was no misnomer.[96] Nurse Gertrud Besier was similarly candid, saying that she and her colleagues noticed that patients would fall into a long sleep from one day to the next, and commented among themselves that this seemed unnatural. They did not know that Frey or Schmidt gave the patients medications or injections, "but it could not have been any other way."[97]

Still others simply happened to be around when Schmidt and his team were in action. From time to time, according to one male nurse, Schmidt appeared on the wards and said things like "What is he still doing here? I do not want to see him anymore." On cue, one of his close assistants would spirit the patient off to an examination room and, later, carry the dead body away.[98] The procedure was similar on the women's side: Schmidt came to one nurse's station and roared, "Nothing is being done on this station!" Thinking that this was a criticism of the untidiness of the ward, she approached him for clarification. As she did so, she was held back by Seidel, who explained, " 'Because the old people are still alive!' or something like that—because so few are dying—that is what Dr. Schmidt meant."[99]

THE Eichberg testimonies, then, introduce the idea that nurses who worked in institutions for medicalized killing, but who were not immediately involved in the killings, stumbled into knowing what was going on or drew their own conclusions from suspicious cases over time. At Eichberg in particular, it seems that a great many nurses remained in the position of relative "outsiders," insofar as Schmidt and his small circle of close assistants carried out the killings themselves, out of sight of other nurses. Whether or not this is true, the fact remains that the Eichberg testimonies do not offer many insights into how those nurses who assisted with the killings thought about their new roles. For a more detailed analysis, we must return to Meseritz-Obrawalde, where nurses were gradually drawn into the killing process and, twenty years later, offered a number of important insights into how it happened.

The End with No Beginning: Procedural Integration and Knowledge after the Fact

At Meseritz-Obrawalde, as well, nurses who were serving on stations reported that they were not immediately aware that patients were being killed intentionally. Although we shall see that "reliable" nurses who were slated to play central roles in the killing process were told in no uncertain terms what was on the agenda, those with auxiliary roles were left to draw their own conclusions from deviations from normal procedure. Margarete Göbel, for example, was told by the doctor to give an eighty-year-old woman a scopolamine injection once in the morning and then again in the evening—which she considered normal for sedative purposes. The same was ordered on the second day. When she bathed the woman on the third day, she noticed red flecks on the woman's back. The doctor said, "Let us grant her peace." No more medication was given, and the patient died after four or five days.[100]

Göbel's account of her thought process is not entirely clear, but she did come to suspect that *perhaps* the doctor wanted to slowly put the patient to sleep—especially since there were already rumors in Obrawalde that patients were being killed. She did not, however, yet have "concrete grounds" for thinking so; the patient was old and perhaps would have died anyway. On another occasion, Luminal was ordered in several higher-than-normal—but not in themselves lethal—doses over two days. The patient died on the third day. After a third episode, Göbel concluded that patients were being intentionally killed and said to Dr. Mootz, " 'Must we really burden ourselves so?' Dr. M. answered me, 'We have a duty.' "[101]

With other nurses, one incident was apparently sufficient to convince them that a patient's death was intentional. Nurse Lena Estmann was ordered by Dr. Wernicke to administer four to five grams of veronal to a restless patient. Estmann noticed that the patient calmed down after two doses of one-half gram each, so she gave no further doses. After explaining her decision to Dr. Wernicke the next day, "Dr. W. screamed at me that I had to administer what the doctor ordered. She did not take any notice of my objection that the patient had been sedated with the smaller quantity. I did not ask any more questions. In response to the question concerning what I thought about this, I must say that at this moment I realized what Dr. W. intended with the high dose of veronal."[102] This progressive method of killing did sometimes offer gradual insights into the intentions of doctors but also sometimes obscured them. Erna Büchling, for example, once gave veronal—she could not remember how much—to a patient who later died. She insisted, however, that she was not aware that the veronal was intended to kill the patient; after all, the patient had awakened later and had some food. It was only later that the woman was transported to another ward and died.[103]

Rumors—In-House and in Town

Be this as it may, it was inevitable that rumors about the killings would start to circulate. Former nurses reported that the patients themselves were one source of such rumors, even if some nurses like Edith Kloster dismissed them as unreliable: ". . . since it was a question of . . . snippets of conversation of psychiatric patients, I was not absolutely sure whether these rumors that were buzzing around could concern facts."[104] Other nurses accepted patients' statements as further confirmation of what suspicious activity and rumors had already suggested.[105]

In any case, there was no lack of more reliable sources; rumors circulated among nurses as well. Flora Beimer, who worked in the kitchen from late summer 1942 onward, already had her own grounds for suspicion: she kept a food chart and noticed that on some stations food rations went drastically down and deaths went up. "Moreover," she added, "it was whispered in nursing circles that injections were being given, and so it was relatively easy for me to draw some connections."[106] The "insider" Maria Burg confirmed this: "From hearsay, [and] from conversations with colleagues in the cafeteria, I gained certainty in the course of time that killings were being undertaken in various buildings of the institution."[107]

Many nurses reported that the killings were known in town as well.[108] When Elsbet Putzmann went home to Silesia by train sometime in 1944, for example, someone saw the address on her suitcase handle and asked, "Isn't that where people are given lethal injections [*abgespritzt werden*]?" As she continued her testimony, it became clear that this kind of emotional detachment was not shared by relatives who came to Obrawalde for burials and knew that the patient in question had been intentionally killed: "I often heard people cursing and saw how the employee B., who had only to fill out forms in this connection, was reproached."[109]

Neither was it shared by Nurse Mona Lorig, who worked primarily with patients outdoors until her marriage in 1943 and said she learned of the killings only afterward, in Meseritz, when she was working as a Red Cross nurse. Confirmation of these rumors came only vaguely and reluctantly at first, from a colleague she met in town, then clearly and painfully the day she planned to spend a few hours with a boy in the institution to whom she had become attached during her employment. As she headed toward the institution, she met a nurse who told her without explanation that she could spare herself the trip; the boy was dead.[110]

Whatever grounds there may have been for initial doubt about the killings at Meseritz-Obrawalde, nurses eventually carried on their daily professional lives under the "umbrella" of such rumors. How did they think about and adapt to their circumstances once they were confronted with the possibility that they were assisting with murder?

Assistance and the Preservation of Uncertainty: Spaces for Killing and Spaces for Nursing

One of the most revealing testimonies on this question came from Edith Kloster, who was accused of acting as an accessory to murder because she brought patients into the rooms in which they would be killed. One day, she was told by the station nurse's deputy to transport four patients into an examination room. She transported the first two, then fetched the remaining two. Upon her return, she saw the deputy giving one of the patients an unidentified liquid and explaining that it had been prescribed by the chief doctor: "You want to get well again, don't you?" Kloster, in short, was witnessing—and thus had assisted in—murder.[111]

Kloster did already suspect that patients were being killed in the institution: she had heard rumors, from both colleagues and patients, and had noticed larger numbers of bodies being brought to the mortuary. Yet she maintained, in her own defense, that she did not know for *certain* that these four patients were going to be killed: "There could have been many reasons for the transport of the four patients into the examination room. After all, I had to bring patients there from time to time before that. Patients were often transferred from there to other stations. It also happened sometimes that the chief doctor, Dr. W., led a discussion with the patient there. Also, visits from relatives took place on the porch [of the building], and the patients were led there."[112] Rather than *connect* her experience with what was rumored to be an ongoing, covert murder operation, Kloster pointed to the room's various functions as a way of explaining her lack of certainty about the doctor's intentions *in this particular case*. It seems that this argument was not an after-the-fact rationalization but rather a reflection of a very real struggle to preserve the ambivalence of her situation. Even by her own admission, "I . . . always distanced myself on the inside from these things, although they never became conscious to me, unequivocally and absolutely concretely."[113]

We even find similar reasoning in the testimonies of nurses who assisted with the administration of lethal doses of sedatives. Martha Möll, who had been at Meseritz-Obrawalde since 1930, admitted to assisting the accused Nurse Neumann with administering a drink in the bedrooms—that is, raising the headboard of the bed, holding the patient upright, and supporting her so that Neumann could give her the drink. But, like Kloster, Möll insisted that she did not know for sure that the patient was supposed to be killed, although she could "assume" that this was intended. (She had already noticed higher numbers of transports arriving; and earlier, as a transport nurse, she had seen the reckless way patients' belongings were handled at the institution to which they were transported.) The factor that she felt demonstrated her innocence was, again, the *space* in which the liquid was administered: "Since this took place in the bedroom rather than in the isolation room, and I myself did not know the quantity of the dissolved tablets, I was again in a state of considerable doubt since, after all, it was usually in the bedrooms that normal medications were administered to sedate the patients." If this had been done in the special room, she added, she certainly would have known what was going on.[114]

The spaces in which killings took place were also spaces in which perfectly normal procedures not only had been but also *continued to be* carried out; and as long as nurses could preserve in their own minds this ambiguity about the function of particular spaces, they could hold themselves in a state of perpetual uncertainty. These nurses could not shield themselves from rumors that a good many patients in their institution were being killed; but they tried to sustain the possibility in their minds that a *particular* patient, on a particular day, was not being killed.

Thus the fact that killing was carried out amid otherwise normal, routine medical procedures, in medical surroundings, hardly sheltered nurses from information; it seems to have been a factor that they marshaled to preserve uncertainty in particular cases—those cases in which they were involved—and thus to keep the killings on the level of rumor. The "normal," medical side of daily life, combined with the convenient disappearance of the victims, allowed for psychological accommodation. Elfriede Dänemann does not seem to have been the only one who thought that "even if the inhabitants of Obrawalde and Meseritz knew about the goings-on in the institution, most of us did not want to be associated with them."[115]

WE GAIN further insight into how nurses carried on in the midst of rumors when we turn to the testimony of Karin Kremer, who transported patients into a room that nurses referred to among themselves as the "death chamber" (*Sterbezimmer*). It was wellnigh impossible to claim ignorance of the purpose of her activity, and Kremer did not try; rather, she insisted in her testimony that she could offer no details about the killings themselves because she never saw one take place. Moreover, "on account of a certain bad feeling, we nurses never talked about what went on in the so-called little room and how the patients were killed."[116] To be sure, she noticed higher than normal amounts of morphine being delivered to the institution and thus suspected that patients were being killed with injections. She thought there were probably ampoules in the wall cabinet in the "little room." But, she added, "on account of a certain bad feeling, and in the awareness of not wanting to have anything to do with the killings at Obrawalde, I never looked into the wall cabinet and can only express my assumption to that effect."[117] Kremer knew that patients were being killed in this room; yet she, too, seems to have struggled to distance herself from the act by shielding herself as much as possible from knowledge of the details of murder. She was fairly sure of what she would find in that cabinet, which is the reason she chose not to look.[118]

The organization of space and the division of labor aided this kind of self-imposed ignorance: the "death chambers" on several stations, according to nurses, had two entrances, one of which was accessible from the outside.[119] Sometimes patients were transferred into a "death chamber," stayed there several days, and then were moved to another house.[120] Those who brought patients into rooms to be killed were not the same persons who carried their bodies away;[121] thus the failure of a patient to return could mean that the patient was killed, but it could also mean that the patient had been sent to some other ward. If patients simply disappeared, those nurses who were so inclined could consider their fate a matter of permanent speculation.

The Displacement of Responsibility and the Struggle for Innocence

We see then, that the preferable course of action for "helpers" was to avoid the truth about what was going on. Eventually—and the time span may well have been extremely short—they could no longer deny that patients were being killed, and that the nurses themselves were involved. What were the moral implications of their own activity in the eyes of these "helpers"?

Almost without exception, nurses who assisted with killings argued that they did not feel responsible for the killings because they had not been directly involved. Minna Arnold, who "only" transported patients into the "death chamber," reported having had "no guilty conscience whatsoever . . . because I felt in no way directly connected with any killing activities. Moreover, I could not have provided any helping hand or assistance whatsoever with the killings. I was too soft-hearted for that, and I would definitely have had to cry."[122] This argument appears again and again: Edith Kloster insisted that "I could . . . find no connection at all between the required transport of patients into the examination room and any killing that might take place later"[123] despite the fact that she never saw the patients again. Erna Büchling agreed—and added the critical point: "Because I saw no such connection, *it never occurred to me to refuse.*"[124]

Karin Kremer was somewhat more candid, admitting that she naturally had to perceive a connection between her activity and what the station nurse did afterward. Moreover, she believed that killing patients was morally wrong: "I maintained at the time, and had always maintained, that a human being may not kill a living being of his or her own accord. I also considered the psychiatric patients with various degrees of illness in Obrawalde to be human beings. On these grounds I regarded the killing of psychiatric patients as an injustice."[125] Despite her moral *reservations*, however, she maintained that she was not morally *responsible*. She had no intention to kill patients and believed that by limiting her complicity to transport, she had "more or less in an elegant way kept [herself] out of these actions." She continued, "in no way did I have the feeling or even the ability to understand that I had done something wrong or committed an offense." Like Arnold, she added that she would have refused to administer a lethal injection herself; *that*, she would have realized, was punishable (*strafbar*).[126]

This last comment raises a second issue. Nurses who did not feel guilty in their own minds had no reason to feel that their activity was punishable—that is, that they were guilty in the eyes of *others*. Apparently, however, there was a point at which some of them began to worry that they might be *held* responsible even if they did not *feel* responsible. That point seems to have been the one at which they crossed the boundary between helping and direct, single-handed killing. Gisela Feinmann, for example, prepared premeasured quantities of medication to be administered by the senior nurse, and she carried away dead bodies. But in her eyes, "with my constant refusals to assist with the killings directly, I was of the opinion that I had in no way made myself culpable."[127]

Avoiding responsibility did not always convince them that killing patients was a good thing, but it provided them with a kind of psychological "private space" in which they could acknowledge to themselves that the killings were wrong, but remain unassailed by crisis-producing thoughts about whether they could ever be seen as "murderers" in the eyes of others.

THIS willingness to hide one's own moral reservations under a bushel, so to speak, is seen more clearly if we turn to nurses' often-asserted belief in a nonexistent "euthanasia" law. There was usually no basis to their belief other than rumors and a general faith in the goodwill of social institutions. Martha Möll stated that, as far as she remembered, there was talk of a law that permitted the killing of patients. This talk, moreover, made a good deal of sense to her; for if no such law existed, and something was truly amiss, surely the courts would have pursued the matter. What about the medical office, to whom the deaths were reported? Surely it or some other influential authority would have known and, if necessary, intervened in what was going on at Obrawalde.[128]

Möll's position was a perfect reflection of what her professional ethics would have dictated: nurses were neither encouraged nor authorized to question the decisions of superiors in professional life in matters of moral substance. Moreover, even today, people generally rely to some extent on faith in the goodwill of social institutions and for that reason do not demand to see laws in print before they will obey them. The problem with Möll's testimony is that her professional ethics *also* stipulated that it was wrong to grant a "mercy death" or allow suicide, and that there was enough covert, suspicious activity going on to suggest—to those who wanted to know—that something strange and perhaps not quite legal was going on. Indeed, Elsbet Putzmann and her colleagues agreed at the time "that we would not like to be in the place of those who would at some point later be held responsible. With this [comment] we meant those who had organized and ordered these killing operations. . . ."[129]

In short, there is little to suggest that the idea of a law was *completely* convincing. It did not really matter, though; even if it turned out that there was no law, surely *some* other authority *somewhere* higher up was responsible for what was going on. What mattered, in the end, was whether they could believe that responsibility lay someplace else. This, at least, is suggested by the decidedly vague terms in which nurses spoke about it. Erna Büchling testified, "At the time I was always of the opinion that, either from the Ministry of Health or from another high state authority, a corresponding order or a law existed that had the killing of psychiatric patients as its result." As for the orders closer at hand, whereby she transported patients into the "death chamber," "I received an order to do so from a superior. From which [superior], I cannot say anymore."[130]

This is a perfect case of what Zygmunt Bauman calls "free-floating responsibility," where the members of an organization maintain that they have been merely acting on the orders of someone else. Cruelty is far easier to perpetrate under such circumstances because no one feels responsible, yet everyone believes that there is, somewhere, a "proper" authority. "This means," Bauman continues, "that shirking responsibility is not just an after-the-fact stratagem used as a convenient excuse in case charges are made of the immorality, or worse still of illegitimacy, of an action; the free-floating, unanchored responsibility is the very condition of immoral or illegitimate acts taking place with obedient, or even willing participation of people normally incapable of breaking the rules of conventional morality."[131] Free-floating responsibility provided nurses with one more area of uncertainty that could support their feelings of uninvolvement and thus of innocence. That is, not knowing exactly who was responsible offered precisely the same kind of psychological comfort as "not knowing for certain" whether a particular injection on a particular day was lethal.

Reprisals and the Fear of the Unknown

If the assumption of a law and the displacement of responsibility gave nurses a feeling that it was permissible to obey orders in connection with killing, thus giving them a "green light" to participate, the fear of reprisals from Director Grabowski allegedly provided a "red light" for any other course of action. Former nurses and other personnel reported almost without exception that the atmosphere in the institution changed for the worse after his arrival in 1942.[132] As one former nurse remembered, "the relationship among nurses was no longer as it had been before and each was on her guard not to say something rash because one was afraid of being called to Grabowski on account of the most trivial matter."[133] According to another, "the director at the time, Grabowski, was seen by all nurses as a kind of bogeyman. All of us, including me, had a tremendous fear of him. . . ."[134]

It is instructive, and indeed necessary, to examine exactly what it was about Grabowski that inspired this fear. We have already seen in this chapter's introduction, of course, that he was rumored to have a history of murderous activity and established a rather threatening presence for himself in institutional life. According to one former veteran nurse, he often held roll calls and reminded nurses that they were bound from all sides by duties and obligations to everyone but their patients. Should they not accept this obligation voluntarily, there was in any case no chance to quit. The alternative to doing as they were told was a journey to the Warthegau.[135] To supplement this image of an unchallenged and unchallengeable autocrat, Grabowski made it abundantly clear to nurses that he was not someone whom they could hope to influence—even with their female charms. According to one former nurse, he announced in a speech before an assembly of nurses that "his needs, he meant with regard to women, were satisfied and none of us should look at him as, according to his portrayal, a few had permitted themselves to do."[136]

In any case, nurses were not given many opportunities to cultivate a relationship with Grabowski, sexual or otherwise. A number of nurses, including one who at the time had worked at Meseritz-Obrawalde for over a decade, reported that they were not even introduced to Grabowski when he arrived, and learned what they knew about him mainly through conversations with other nurses—unless they landed through some unfortunate circumstance in his office: "When, for example, nurses talked with soldiers from Meseritz during their work outside, he recorded the situation with a photograph and confronted the nurses with it. Under no circumstances did he tolerate nurses' doing anything during their shift other than supervising their patients."[137] As perverse and absurd as this covert surveillance may seem, it is not the kind of activity that in and of itself is likely to inspire the kind of pervasive fear which virtually all nurses reported; while he indeed comes across in these examples as somewhat crude and paranoid, we have not at this point uncovered evidence of the kind of cruelty or violence for which someone like Schmidt was well known.

One could perhaps discover the source of this fear by turning to cases of refusal to participate in killing patients; surely Grabowski would have done more than bare his teeth when confronted by nurses who not only challenged his personal authority but also threatened the legitimacy of the entire enterprise. Such nurses, after all, could inspire others to refuse participation as well or carry their outrage into the extrainstitutional, public sphere.

Let us, then, consider the case of Maria Burg, who was asked by Grabowski in early summer 1942 to take part in the killing of patients. These patients, he explained to her, were "asocial creatures" whose care was not worth the money being spent. Such funds would surely be better spent on soldiers. When Burg refused, Grabowski left her to think about it for a few days and then asked her again. After a second refusal, Grabowski com-

mented that Burg was apparently "not yet imbued with National Socialism . . . and that he would see to it that [she] would
get the opportunity to reconsider the issue in a National Socialist
training camp in Torgau." In the end, Grabowski's solution was
to remove Burg from her position as a nurse and assign her to
messenger duties between the institution and the town of Mes-
eritz(!). After six months, she spent eight weeks in the personnel
office, then was sent to work as a cleaning woman in several
offices. From spring 1943 until the Russian invasion she worked
in a managerial office. Grabowski did not approach her again.[138]

In another case, Edith Bebel defied both the senior nurse and
the personnel manager by refusing to accept a transfer to House
18, which she had heard was a killing station. The next day, she
was transferred to an outdoor work detail. "Outside of the
newly assigned different work, I experienced no detrimental
consequences of my refusal."[139] She learned later that her refusal
had come up at a conference; and Grabowski, of all people, had
maintained that Bebel could not be forced to work in House 18
because she was not an NSDAP member(!).[140] To cite one final
example, one former nurse reported that a colleague of hers who
refused to participate in the killings received no punishment
whatsoever, not even a punitive transfer.[141] Grabowski, in short,
seems to have been a paper tiger.

It is instructive that Grabowski handled violations of a decidedly lesser degree—or, more accurately, of less moral gravity, in
exactly the same way. After working a few years on various stations in the institution, Elsbet Putzmann was assigned in early
1943 to work in the garden and to supervise patient workers
there. Since this was not her idea of nursing, she and a colleague
asked Grabowski for a transfer to a hospital. When he refused,
they took their request to the provincial governor (*Oberpräsident*)
of Pomerania. There too they were unsuccessful, with the added
misfortune that the refusal was channeled back to them through
Grabowski's office. He gave them punitive transfers for this attempt to circumvent his authority; Putzmann ended up with the
cleaning detail.[142]

These examples suggest that Grabowski treated nurses' refusals to kill patients as a purely administrative matter just like any other. It is impossible to know for certain whether this was simply a product of laziness, or whether he had very good reasons for handling refusals in this fashion. Apparently, however, Grabowski did not need to actually send noncompliant nurses to a concentration camp in order to paralyze their colleagues psychologically and thus secure their voluntary participation. A punitive transfer was quite sufficient for handling the handful of refusals: it eliminated the problem at hand by removing the nurse from the source of her conflicts of conscience, and it did so in a way that did not acknowledge, and thus publicize, refusal as a moral gesture. Excessive punishment would undoubtedly have intimidated some; but it also would have created martyrs whose example might have awakened their more reflective colleagues from the state of enforced moral paralysis that they themselves struggled to maintain.

As for those colleagues, maintaining this state of paralysis seems to have entailed fearing consequences that never came. That is, they did not fear Grabowski because of what they knew he would do; they feared him precisely because they *did not know for certain* what he might do. By issuing threats but postponing their fulfillment indefinitely, Grabowski maintained an aura not only of brutality but also of unpredictability. This "not-knowing-for-certain" what might happen seems to have been ultimately highly effective in securing nurses' cooperation. As Kremer explained, "If I had not followed official orders back then, I was certain that I would have been subject to reprisals from Grabowski. *What kind of reprisals these might have been, I could not imagine, but without a doubt I had something to be afraid of.*"[143]

WE HAVE now generated a psychological profile of "helpers" whose most striking characteristic is its groundlessness in matters of fact: nurses testified that they believed that a law or some form of bureaucratic blessing sanctioned the killings, yet they had no proof of it beyond word of mouth and were constantly

confronted with evidence to the contrary, namely, the covert nature of an enterprise involving large shipments of medications
and piles of bodies. They did not feel morally and legally responsible, yet they had only vague ideas about precisely *who*
might be responsible. They felt that they had no other option
than to obey orders, yet it seems that there was absolutely nothing to fear in the way of reprisals.

We have also seen, however, that this state of affairs does not
necessarily imply that these testimonies are after-the-fact rationalizations; rather, buried between the lines of each so-called rationalization is a clue regarding nurses' strategies of psychological accommodation "at the time of the fact." The testimonies
suggest why nurses participated voluntarily as helpers, despite
whatever conflicts of conscience they may have experienced:
they distanced themselves, both physically and psychologically,
from their roles as accomplices.

*Maintaining a Precarious Peace of Mind: The Significance
of Who Does What*

On some level, nurses were painfully conscious of this distance and struggled to remain outside the sphere of direct killing. Elfriede Dänemann, for example, was charged with moving
patients from House 5 to House 3 to be killed. Once the purpose
of such transports became obvious to her and her colleagues—
or, perhaps, once it became impossible to deny the obvious—
"each [of us], if I may put it this way, tried with all her might to
avoid this dreadful task."[144] Dänemann noted that she was unfortunately more robust than the others and thus often ended
up being the executor of this "dreadful task," but this form of
assistance seems to have been psychologically tolerable nevertheless. This cannot be said for the senior nurse's order to give
a patient a (lethal) air injection: "I could not do it and I did not
want to do it and began to cry. Then [the senior nurse] scolded
me and sent me away. . . ."[145]

Interestingly, it seems that low-ranking nurses were not the
only ones struggling in this fashion to remain as far removed as

possible from direct killing. According to Göbel, a senior nurse was placed in charge of administering lethal injections in one particular house and bitterly resented it, once saying that " 'with you I have to come, over there they do it themselves.' She meant that in other houses the nurses would perform killings themselves, whereas in our house she had to do it herself." Göbel continued, "I also remember that she was crying a lot as she said this. In general, I would like to mention that all of us cried a great deal back then."[146]

For this senior nurse, killing patients was an undesirable, perhaps emotionally wrenching, but nevertheless bearable activity. However, Dänemann's loss of composure—her bursting into tears—suggests that a critical line was crossed when she was told to kill patients with her own hands—that the whole psychological apparatus with which she had held her moral qualms at bay came crashing down, and she found herself in a situation where it was impossible to escape the terrible truth, not only about the meaning of what she was asked to do, but also perhaps about the meaning of what she had already done.

Neutralizing Dissent: The Utility of Indirect Participation

Nurses' willingness to remain *involved*, combined with their fervent desire to remain *uninvolved*, did not escape the attention of administrators: it came to their aid when they dealt with nurses who categorically refused to kill patients single-handedly. Such nurses would *not* be required to give an injection of morphine-scopolamine or Luminal dissolved in water; they would be required "only" to transport patients into or out of the "little room" or hold the patient's arm during the injection.

Almost without exception, the testimonies considered for the current study show that this was a highly effective technique for soliciting such nurses' participation. Margarete Göbel, as we have seen above, learned only gradually that the dosages of Luminal being administered on her station were intended to be lethal. Having received adequate confirmation, she told the senior nurse Juwel that she was a faithful Catholic and would not participate any further. Juwel, who reportedly also refused to kill patients,[147] replied, "Things will change," and indeed they did: thereafter the lethal injections in that house were given exclusively by a nurse who only worked at Obrawalde occasionally.[148]

Göbel had occasion to reiterate her position in 1943, when she was moved to a house that was rumored to be a killing station. Upon spotting the "death chamber," she told the attending doctor that under no circumstances did she want to be involved. Dr. Wernicke told her not to worry; Göbel would not be asked to administer any medications, and the doctor would assume responsibility for what went on. The space, she explained, was needed for wounded soldiers. This was evidently tolerable; Göbel and her colleagues carried on, holding patients' hands when Luminal was given.[149]

Beate Holzmann, too, told Dr. Wernicke that she would not single-handedly kill patients, explaining, "We had not given the patients life and therefore could not take it away."[150] This principle did not stop her from assisting with transports of patients and holding them while they were being killed; "before my own conscience," she said, "I have always felt somewhat guilty and tried to get over it and forget it as much as possible."[151]

THE SPATIAL AND DISCURSIVE REINFORCEMENT OF MORAL FLIGHT

With this last example, we are reminded that nurses' strategies for avoiding knowledge, deferring responsibility, and suppressing their own moral reflection were not spun out of thin air but rather were allowed, and at times encouraged, by the institutional environment in which they found themselves. To be sure, Dr. Wernicke's claim that she would assume responsibility for the killings reinforced Göbel's already existing desire to be mercifully left out of the whole affair: she reported having felt "relieved." But at other times, comments by upper-level staff members and administrators went beyond reinforcement and functioned as a tool for "steering" nurses' thoughts in a direction that would render them responsive only to their sense of technical responsibility—that is, their responsibility to facilitate the smooth functioning of institutional life. At the same time, nurses were isolated from competing interpretations of their activity.

Speech as a Tool of Moral Realignment

The nurses of Meseritz-Obrawalde faced no shortage of reminders that their own thoughts and opinions about what was going on in their institution were of absolutely no importance. As we have seen earlier, Grabowski often held roll calls and reminded nurses of their duties and obligations: since the soldiers were protecting them on the front, nurses were obligated to return the favor, so to speak, by carrying on with their own duties in the institution. While reinforcing this sense of responsibility to support a collective effort, he characterized the alternative potential object of responsibility, namely, their patients, as undeserving of any consideration, let alone initiative: *they*, after all, were being spoiled, and this couldn't go on any longer.[152]

The desire of superiors to erase the patient from nurses' moral imagination was manifested in small, but significant, daily encounters. Nurses who characterized their activity as morally questionable were "corrected" by superiors in such way that the same activity could be construed as morally acceptable. We have already encountered one example of this, namely, the exchange involving Nurse Göbel, who asked the doctor whether it was truly necessary that they "burden" themselves with guilt in this way. The doctor's response was "We have a duty."[153] Whatever feelings of responsibility Göbel may have felt for her patients, either spontaneously or as a matter of principle, the doctor's answer reminded her with its icy brevity that those feelings had no place in institutional life.

Another interesting example concerns Gisela Feinmann, who spent most of the war years tending animals for experiments at Meseritz-Obrawalde, but who spent six months of 1944 working on patient wards. One of her duties entailed periodically going into a room where a small bag of premeasured medicine stood on the table. She was to mix the powder with water and prepare syringes, then leave everything on the table in the room. The senior nurse collected these items later and killed patients with them.

Feinmann was aware of the intended use of the medicine and claimed to have told the senior nurse, "Leave me alone, I do not want to have anything to do with it." The senior nurse replied, "You do not have to do anything, but when I don't have time, then prepare that for me."[154] The exchange was short and the language vague, but it was not trivial. Feinmann, of course, was expressing her unwillingness to assist him in murdering *patients*. In response, the senior nurse attempted to redirect her "gaze" and recharacterize the very same activity as a favor to *him*. The moral issue involved was not murder but rather helping one's neighbor.

AN ALTERNATIVE strategy was to tell the nurse that death was nothing more than the deliverance of patients from their suffering, and indeed a number of nurses reported accepting this, at least for a time.[155] Elsbet Putzmann, for example, reported that "at the beginning I was of the opinion that the euthanasia measures introduced in wartime could be a deliverance for absolutely incurable cases." Here, she referred specifically to particularly serious cases, where the patient had already been in the institution for twenty to thirty years.[156]

From a contemporary standpoint, this argument seems nothing more than an act of unconscionable moral presumption thinly disguised as an act of compassion. After all, it seems to have been generally known among the nurses, for those who were willing to admit it, that medical prognosis was hardly the issue. From a historical standpoint, however, we must keep in mind that the nurses of whom we speak were not simply "granting a mercy death" to people who had advanced or severe psychiatric illnesses but otherwise were perfectly healthy; the patients they confronted were often already suffering from hunger and corporeal illnesses. Immediately after the war, one outraged doctor described a scene that nurses would very likely have confronted day after day, week after week: "I walk through a sickroom. It is deathly still. Beds are right next to each other—color-less, emaciated faces with excessively large eyes, which are sleepily closed, lie in the pillows, weak-willed and apathetic."[157] Death rates in institutions were already extremely high without their "help"; nurses were quite literally watching patients starve to death.

The deprivational schemes of the regime, in other words, were not only a demonstration of its refusal to "drag incurable pa-tients through the war"; they produced a state of affairs wherein the idea of "death as deliverance" could be proffered to nurses and, in combination with the variety of factors outlined above, regarded as perhaps not such a bad idea after all. This does not necessarily mean that nurses espoused the kind of death wish often ascribed to psychiatrists, whereby frustration with their persistent lack of therapeutic success generated the desire to kill, quite literally, the source of their humiliation. Rather, it is more likely to have been a gesture of resignation that simultanously afforded emotional comfort. It allowed nurses to maintain the conviction that there was no need to abandon conventional mo-rality entirely under the circumstances; it was indeed possible to synthesize it with the demands being made of them. This was undoubtedly an appealing solution, especially for those who felt helpless and lacked the courage to refuse.

Isolation and the Specter of Shame

Sometimes, however, even the logic of "death as deliverance" could not silence a nurse's conscience, and yet she carried on for other reasons. The testimony of Brunhilde Neumann, who confessed to having participated in the murder of patients, is worth examining in some detail in this connection.[158] Although a Party member, Neumann maintained that this was not the rea-son for her agreement to kill; rather, she felt obligated as a civil servant to follow orders. Besides, at the beginning the killings did not pose a great emotional problem for her: Grabowski told her that death was deliverance for the patients in question, and she believed it. "I can say with a clear conscience that only the most seriously ill on our station were killed." Time and changing circumstances eroded her moral composure: when her father died in 1943, she reported, she "first realized the whole injustice of what was going on at Obrawalde at the time." Unable to reconcile the killings with her Christian beliefs, she cried a great deal and had a deeply guilty conscience.[159] Yet she carried on because, she said, "There always stood over me the compulsion and the duty to execute everything as it was ordered. The environment in which we nurses lived was that of the mentally ill. We hardly got out of the institution, had a lot of work to do, and hardly came into contact with the outside world."[160] In one respect, Neumann was absolutely right: Meseritz-Obrawalde nurses were working as many as fourteen hours per day at the time.[161] It seems, however, that it is not—or not only—the long hours in the institution and the resulting internalization of her duties which explain her complicity. Rather, her isolation from the outside world produced a state of mind wherein she simply did not have any ideas about what form an alternative reaction might take. Even if the idea of refusing occurred to her, she had no mental or procedural precedents that could carry her beyond that impulse. In her mind Neumann the nurse had subsumed Neumann the Christian and thinking individual.

Her feeling of isolation from the outside world was reinforced by the (very likely deliberate) in-house isolation from her colleagues. Having worked from 1926 to 1940 at the Stralsund institution, Neumann was a relative newcomer at Orawalde when the killings began. As a result, "as a former Stralsund nurse I had hardly any contact with the other nurses from Treptow and Obrawalde. We lived together in such a way that only nurses who knew each other from before and had worked together in other institutions came into contact." As a result, from the very beginning of the killings, she "could not bring [herself] to talk about with it with anyone."[162]

Neumann, of course, pointed out that she stood under the duty to remain silent about the killings; and indeed many nurses confirmed that enough mistrust underlay collegial relations that honest, intimate conversation was out of the question. Margarete Göbel, who had a guilty conscience, told her inquisitors, "No one would have helped us nurses if we had refused, and we had no one to whom we could pour out our hearts and whom we could trust."[163] Lena Stein, who was transferred to Meseritz-Obrawalde in 1940, also reported that she did not talk to anyone about the killings for the same reason. "No one knew the political views of the other and thus their views on the killing of psychiatric patients."[164]

However, in Neumann's case—and perhaps in others—there was something more behind this silence than a fear of denunciation. If one reads her testimony further, it is obvious that Neumann hardly needed a rule to silence her: she *reinforced* her isolation by withdrawing from all human contact outside of that which was necessary during her shift. "When I was off duty, I usually went into the woods to find peace. Because of the burdens to which I was subjected as a result of the goings-on in the institution, I did not have the least interest in going into town or otherwise [spending time] among other people."[165] Although she did not say so explicitly, Neumann's desire to avoid other people seems connected with a feeling of acute shame that accompanied her for the rest of her life. After begging her inquisitors to spare her husband the burden of her past, she committed suicide shortly after her interrogation in June 1962.[166]

It seems that even nurses with more psychological stamina shunned personal relationships while they were participating in the killings. Elsa Siemens became friendly with Nurse Erna Einbeck during her six months in the infirmary in 1940. Thereafter, the two women had often met in the evenings; but over time Einbeck was seen less and less frequently and, in 1943, her patients told Siemens that she was involved in the killings. Unable to believe this, Siemens decided to confront Einbeck directly: "First I asked her why she no longer came around. She answered that she had a lot to do and therefore had no more time for visits. Then I asked her if she could accept responsibility for what she was doing in the infirmary, should it someday come to light. [Einbeck] gave me no answer to this. She simply said, 'We have taken an oath and we must do it.' "[167] This connection between involvement in killing and withdrawal from personal relationships manifested itself in other nurses' testimonies as well: Bebel, for example, grounded her refusal to work in House 18 by telling the senior nurse that she was married and would never be able to confront her future children if she obeyed.[168] Gisela Feinmann said that if she had known she would be accused of assisting in murder, she would have refused marriage. "I still do not know today how I should explain everything to my husband and how he will take it."[169] Alone with their thoughts, and unassailed by the questions and potential reproach of colleagues and family, nurses could carry on. Encounters with other human beings would perhaps have stimulated self-criticism and, possibly, shame; such encounters, the testimonies suggest, posed a palpable threat to their emotional equilibrium.[170]

Saving What Can Be Saved

While guilty-minded nurses like Neumann carried on in a state of self-imposed isolation, others carried on but also tried to save what could be saved. One former Eichberg patient, for example, reported that she was subjected to psychological torture by Dr. Schmidt and to physical abuse from Nurse Elsen, eventually receiving a three-week sentence in the bunker with reduced rations and no toilet facilities. Although she quite justifiably could have condemned the entire staff along with the sadistic goings-on at Eichberg, the former patient distinguished between nurses who took a perverse pleasure in patients' suffering and those who were "on their side." The activities of the latter group had a distinctly covert, palliative character and were aimed primarily at sustaining the patient physically and emotionally. This meant not only, for example, bringing food and drink to her when she was in the bunker; it also meant encouraging her to capitulate to the lies and profound injustice of her entire situation. Seidel, in particular, came to her while she was in the bunker and told her to confess to something or else she would never come out. Senior Nurse Seidel was good to her, she remembered, and "definitely would have liked to help me."[171]

Elsbet Putzmann provides an example from Meseritz-Obrawalde. She routinely carried bodies to the mortuary and on at least one occasion transported a patient into the "death chamber." It seems, however, that alongside these activities she tried to save children on her night shifts. Knowing that children who wetted their beds during the night were usually selected to be killed the next day, she said, "I tried everything to keep them dry and to hand them over dry after the night shift."[172]

Such activities, to be sure, were not necessarily grounded in moral outrage over the killings: Seidel said that she indeed suffered unbearable conflicts of conscience, but Putzmann said she did not feel guilty about her assistance in the murder of adults because she was not directly involved. Moreover, it is not clear what, if any, selective criteria these nurses deployed while they were "saving what could be saved," and they may have been simply trying to comfort themselves in the midst of guilt that was compounded daily. It may well be that, as Burleigh suggests, such nurses were trying to cancel out the implications of routine murder through individual acts of charity.[173]

IT MAY also be the case, however, that there is more to be learned from the phenomenon of "saving what can be saved" than this interpretation suggests. While there may have been nurses who coolly calculated strategies of moral compensation in this fashion, the Meseritz-Obrawalde testimonies leave the impression that at least some were responding to a feeling of profound powerlessness. Rather than create a stir that was bound to remain ineffectual in the long run, they seem to have sought to carve out a sphere of activity in which they could, in their own small way, lessen the human costs of the catastrophe by means that had some hope of success.

In other words, it is not necessarily the case that low-level sabotage or general decency toward patients was simply a manifestation of a "moral ego" whose main concern was that good deeds outnumber the evil. In fact, it is precisely in these cases that we finally discover the possibility that some nurses, in spite of the manifold circumstances militating against it, confronted their victims as human beings and manifested those instinctual moral impulses that arise in the presence of others and are the very basis of social life. In the majority of cases that we have considered, moral impulses vis-à-vis patients are difficult to detect. At most, they appear in the form of awkwardly articulated, abstract notions of "death as deliverance" or, in some cases, the assertion that "as Christians" they believed killing was wrong. Individual patients seem to have been reference points for their applying (or not applying) moral principles, not human beings who by their very presence constantly generated a feeling of responsibility anew. Most of the testimonies considered in this chapter confirm Bauman's suggestion that the agents of National Socialism did not have to remove their victims from view in order to destroy individual conscience (although such sequestration undoubtedly helped); moral deliberation and feelings of responsibility for others could be destroyed in their very midst.

There is a final sobering observation to be made in connection with nurses' few, feeble attempts to manifest a remaining spark of moral concern. While they offer a hopeful sign that moral flight may not have been universal, their actual *function* was to make daily life bearable for those nurses; they, too, were thus a strategy of psychological accommodation. They headed off emotional crisis, secured the further participation of such nurses, and thus reinforced the totality of consent that enabled the killings to continue unopposed. Having resigned themselves to a state of powerlessness but still hoping to make some small difference in the lives of a few, those nurses who retained a tiny degree of initiative and courage lighted upon a resolution that ultimately oiled the machinery of death.

Concluding Remarks

I̲t̲ i̲s̲ b̲y̲ n̲o̲w̲ abundantly clear that the architects of the "euthanasia" program did not set out to terrorize nurses openly or otherwise force them to carry out measures that contradicted their most fundamental professional and moral imperatives. They intended, rather, to dampen their sense of alarm, immobilize them through feelings of helplessness, and exploit their desire for emotional equilibrium. Confrontation and crisis were to be avoided; and in those instances where self-conscious awareness of complicity in murder emerged, it was contained with the aid of bureaucratic and discursive pressures, in the realm of the private. In this respect, the National Socialists' psychological insight served them well in maintaining the assistance not only of those who could kill without a guilty conscience but also of those who killed *with* or, more accurately, *in spite of* a guilty conscience.

With this observation, we have come full circle and returned to our point of departure, namely, the relevance of nurses' attitudes toward victims to the explanation of their complicity in murder. Clearly, the regime did not need to obliterate moral feeling to secure nurses' participation in mass murder, nor was it necessary for nurses to subscribe to the idea that patients were "lives unworthy of living." While frustration, a lack of professional satisfaction, and frequent loss of temper may sometimes—and particularly at Eichberg—have triggered violence and eventually evolved into a "death wish,"[1] this is hardly the kind of progression that would have been likely among the majority of nurses encountered in this study. Some nurses were habitual abusers, but others reportedly approached their work

with the patience, fortitude, and tact that the profession required. The Meseritz-Obrawalde testimonies suggest that even
those who were not abusive, and who reported having opposed
the killings, carried out their duties efficiently. This, in the end,
is the most disturbing point: many nurses complied for reasons
that seem to have very little to do with attitudes toward, and
previous relationships with, the victims.

That said, it is indeed the case that patients receded from view
as objects of moral concern in nurses' professional socialization
during the Weimar and National Socialist years, which undoubtedly made them even less likely to be moved by compassion, let
alone to take risks on the victims' behalf. This process had its
roots in the First World War, when the population as a whole—
the "people"—was assigned a moral value to which individuals
ideally subordinated themselves through sacrifice. The idea that
the individual need *not* be the primary object of moral responsibility was thus rendered familiar and respectable through the
experience of war (and, not at all incidentally, through the growing popularity of social Darwinism).

In the immediate postwar years, this process continued
against the background of psychiatrists' battle to overcome
image and financial problems. In a two-pronged attempt to
demonstrate that their professional activity was as socially useful as it was humane, psychiatrists pursued two potentially incompatible goals. The purpose, after all, of casting the individual as an object of humane intent and moral responsibility is to
fortify oneself against the demands of the group, which is interested only in self-preservation through rational means. Morality's function is to reassert the integrity of the individual against
unjust demands of society—to claim that those demands do *not*
justify wholesale sacrifice of the interests and entitlements of the
weak; that the ends do *not* justify the means. In their eagerness
to boost their professional image, psychiatrists obscured this intrinsic logical conflict.

Moreover, they manifested this way of thinking in their conception of nurses' professional responsibilities. Weimar reform-
ism trumpeted the ideal nurse-patient relationship as a funda-

mentally *nonpunitive, noncoercive* one. In place of restraint devices, nurses were to solicit the voluntary cooperation of patients in the framework of occupational therapy and socialize them back to health. Approaching the patient in a spirit of "friendly decisiveness" was not only the most *effective* way to bring patients back into the fold; it was also the most *humane*. Nurses were to resolve the tension between friendliness and authority by placing clear limits on the former: they were to inspire trust but never return that trust; they were to be friendly without becoming friends. What mattered was that patients *believed* in the goodwill of staff members, and that their surroundings *appeared* to be harmonious and orderly. In this sense, nurses were in the business of psychological manipulation, even if at this point such activity seems to have been well-intentioned and harmless. During the Weimar years, their professional activity acquired a theatrical dimension that could easily render them, under changed circumstances, potential agents of insincerity and deception.

At the time, however, this possibility certainly did not appear to be looming on the horizon. To the contrary, publishing nurses and psychiatrists insisted that their humanitarian agenda remained unaffected by the National Socialist takeover. In fact, however, the maintenance of a harmonious, orderly environment—of this "society" in microcosm—was elevated to the supreme goal and supreme moral value. The patient, who was theoretically the "end" for whom this environment was only a "means," suddenly acquired moral status insofar as he or she conformed to the norms of an orderly and harmonious environment. That is, his or her moral value was *derivative* rather than intrinsic. In the midst of these developments, previous techniques for restraining violent patients took on an aggressive, punitive character despite superficial continuities in nursing literature's ethical orientation. In fact, it is the deployment of violence under the pretext of "socializing" the patient that captures the catastrophe of institutional psychiatry in its essence: violence became not only therapeutically legitimate; it became respectable.

A variety of circumstantial factors provided momentum for this development. Nurses were not always supported by supervisory staff and administrators when they had difficulties on their wards, and as a result they may have become more inclined over time to handle uncooperative patients with whatever means they had at their immediate disposal rather than solicit the help of hierarchical superiors. Administrators' toleration of "minor" episodes of abuse that did not cause too much of an uproar and had little potential for public exposure undoubtedly made them braver. Last but not least, it is certainly likely that nurses who witnessed the brutality of cardiazol and insulin shock therapies alongside psychiatrists' crude justifications for them eventually accepted violence as a normal, and morally acceptable, part of a larger endeavor that promised favorable returns down the road. The ends, in short, *could* justify the means.

Parallel to this erosion of patients' moral stature, politics—and the politics of everyday life—militated against self-assertion and courage in nurses' lives, and this too bore fruit during the "euthanasia" programs. Weimar nursing advocates approached their political opponents in a spirit of conciliation, seeking to find common ground for rational, mutually satisfactory solutions rather than confrontation over matters of moral substance. The contradiction between the demand for charity and their entitlements as workers remained imbedded and thus unresolved, leaving psychiatric nurses without discursive and organizational precedents for challenging those in positions of power. In addition, the stresses of institutional life undermined individual initiative and solidarity among Weimar nurses: the betrayal of colleagues and administrators, the unpredictability of patients, disciplinary unevenness, and the tension between rules and collectively tolerated deviance threatened the performance of even the most conscientious nurse. The victory of the National Socialists added administrative opportunism to this brew: nurses suddenly worked under the scrutiny of potential denunciators and administrators who, armed with the BBG, could fire nurses for the flimsiest of reasons. The demand for institutional order, which reigned over and above political considerations, generated a pressure to perform one's duties with discreet and unobtrusive efficiency. This was a profession, in short, that already contained enough instability and insecurity to rock the foundations of even the most emotionally robust person; it was also a profession in which risk taking and self-assertion were likely to backfire, and thus a profession in which taking risks very likely had no appeal. Against the background of these theoretical and practical aspects of nurses' experience, we are reminded that moral impulses, and immoral ones, do not have a life of their own but rather are bound to the contingencies of everyday life.

In this light, we must question the supremacy of attitudes, in this case contempt for "lives unworthy of living," in securing the complicity of "ordinary Germans" in murder. Particularly in the case of nurses, the motivational power of personal convictions was, if anything, undermined: in their professional socialization and the politics of everyday life, they were encouraged to keep personal thoughts—even politically "correct" ones—private. By creating a realm in which the legitimacy of nurses' personal views was implicitly (if cynically) acknowledged, psychiatrists—and the medical profession as a whole—may have generated a kind of moral awareness among nurses that, paradoxically, facilitated their ultimate moral collapse. Tzvetan Todorov describes this best in his own reflections on moral life under totalitarianism: ". . . by deciding to submit 'only' in their outward behavior, in their public words and gestures, [totalitarian subjects] console themselves with the thought that they remain masters of their consciences, faithful to themselves in their private lives." This is not to say that they actually succeed in protecting their innermost selves from the taint of institutionalized barbarism. On the contrary: the provision of a tolerable degree of moral freedom becomes a "weapon in the hands of those in power; it lulls to sleep the conscience of the totalitarian subject, reassures him, and lets him underestimate the seriousness of his public deeds."[2] This turns out to be a boon for those in power because it secures people's uncritical, voluntary participation in pursuing the regime's goals.

This observation has implications for the interpretation of the odd cases of refusal among perpetrators of National Socialist policies of mass murder. In the course of the Goldhagen debate, much has been made of the fact that "ordinary Germans" could refuse to participate without suffering serious consequences, but they participated anyway. This would certainly seem to suggest that they did not have great emotional problems carrying out their assigned tasks; perhaps they even wanted to kill or help killers. In Goldhagen's view, the fact that battalion commanders did not perceive refusals as "a challenge to the moral order" only strengthens the argument that the refusers themselves did not intend them as such.[3]

We have uncovered an alternative possibility here, namely, that the failure of hierarchichal superiors to recognize refusal as a moral gesture was part of a strategy for preserving generalized consent; and this strategy hinged on containing signs of moral reflection in the realm of the private. Grabowski, like the battalion commanders, did not acknowledge refusals as a "challenge to the moral order" but rather handled them as he handled other forms of administrative deviance—even when nurses were explicit about the moral basis of their objection. The conclusion to be drawn from this example, at least, cannot be that these "ordinary Germans" had no conscience. It may very well be the case, on the other hand, that the voice of conscience was not to be acknowledged, legitimated, and thus possibly encouraged in the midst of mass murder.[4]

Thus even explicitly moral opposition could be articulated without threatening the viability of the enterprise as a whole. Meanwhile, the majority of remaining nurses either accepted or tolerated what was going on for a whole constellation of other reasons, availing themselves of the possibilities to adapt that their environment offered. Nurses' thoughts were driven by the urgent psychological need to keep the killings on the level of rumor, in the realm of the uncertain. This attempt to avoid direct knowledge was an attempt to avoid a feeling of responsibility— and perhaps of shame that they were involved without protest. If avoiding knowledge was impossible, they displaced responsibility for their own activity to an unspecified, often unknown, but in any case hierarchically superior bearer. At the most, some nurses seem to have carved out a psychological space in which to "process" their moral reservations privately. Whatever path they chose, those who avoided a critical confrontation with what they were doing participated in their own depersonalization: they gave up their status as moral agents—indeed, cast it away—and took refuge in the status offered to them, namely, that of a follower, an order-taker, and an executioner of official policies, not to mention, in some cases, an executioner in a literal sense.[5]

Although nurses were often conscious agents in this process of moral flight, their behavior was encouraged and reinforced by specific discursive and bureaucratic features of institutional life. That the killings were not openly talked about eliminated uncomfortable external stimuli to confront and articulate precisely what they were doing. Administrators persistently reminded nurses of their responsibilities to uphold the collective effort in the midst of war, thus reviving the rhetorical emphasis on the moral value, and indeed moral priority, of the *Volk*, whose roots we located in the discourse of the previous world war. The victims mercifully disappeared from their sphere of activity, leaving behind only a cloud of possibilities regarding what had actually happened to them. As Hilde Steppe has stated, "The perfection of the bureaucratic execution of the entire extermination program, based on the division of labor, offered each individual the possibility, by virtue of the drastically reduced room for acting and decision making, not to perceive the general picture."[6]

Some nurses attempted to sustain the fiction that bureaucratically organized mass murder could still pass as "humane" by arguing that death was deliverance for the victims. Even this, however, seems to have been less a conviction than it was a way of maneuvering within circumstantial parameters that they lacked the courage to challenge. Humane intent and medical efficiency, which had been uncritically linked in Weimar discourse, could no longer be claimed even by the widest stretch of the imagination. Therapeutic activity had ceased, and patients were being systematically murdered, leaving nothing but the "shell" of their professional world—a series of mechanical procedures, carried out in "normal" medical surroundings. Under such circumstances, it is difficult to believe that nurses complied because they had internalized the ethic of obedience to the point of executing their duties "automatically." It seems plausible, however, that they took refuge in familiar activities—and in the familiar idea that they were essentially benevolent—to head off emotional crisis. They abandoned the moral responsibility that was rooted in their status as medical professionals, and in their proximity to the victims, and took refuge in technical responsibility.[7]

Routine inhumanity, with the aid of "normal" spaces and "normal" language, corrupted nursing from the "inside"—that is, without disturbing the technical and discursive apparatus which had once given the entire psychiatric enterprise its moral and therapeutic legitimacy. In this sense, what links violence and murder in psychiatric nursing is not an *internal* dynamic, but rather the circumstances in which they arose and the subtlety with which they became a legitimate part of daily institutional life. The National Socialist regime's most devastating power lay not in its ability to mobilize people against its victims through propaganda but rather in its ability to deploy propaganda in conjunction with specific physical, discursive, and hierarchical arrangements so that the desire for psychological comfort would prevail over courage.

Notes

Preface

1. For an overview of the political and ideological background of resistance historiography, see the introduction to Theodore Hamerow, *On the Road to the Wolf's Lair: German Resistance to Hitler* (Cambridge, Mass., 1997).

2. Eberhard Zeller writes that *"Moral Motives*, a sense of responsibility for mankind as a whole—something most unusual in political life—played a great role in the uprising . . . they saw beyond Hitler as a person: to them he was an important power, the 'instrument of evil' in our time on earth" (*The Flame of Freedom: The German Struggle against Hitler* [London, 1967], 393). Samuel P. Oliner draws a similar conclusion: "Auschwitz represents the totality of evil and perversion that humanity can stoop to. The Righteous Gentiles stood up to the evil during those years, and said 'no' to tyranny and saved lives" ("The Unsung Heroes of Nazi Occupied Europe: The Antidote for Evil," *Nationalities Papers* 12, no. 1 [Spring 1984], 136).

3. Hannah Arendt, *The Origins of Totalitarianism* (New York, 1951), 452.

4. This is a prominent theme of Robert Gellately's *The Gestapo and German Society: Enforcing Racial Policy, 1933–1945* (Oxford, 1990).

5. Ian Kershaw, *Popular Opinion and Political Dissent in the Third Reich: Bavaria, 1933–1945* (Oxford, 1983), 244.

6. For a discussion of unplanned rescue, see Nechama Tec, *When Light Pierced the Darkness: Christian Rescue of Jews in Nazi Occupied Poland* (Oxford, 1986), 174–176.

7. Zygmunt Bauman, among others, points out that rescuers often simultaneously embraced anti-Jewish legislation (*Modernity and the Holocaust* [Ithaca, N.Y., 1989], 187).

8. See chapter 9 of Richard Rorty's *Contingency, Irony, and Solidarity* (Cambridge, 1989).

9. Bernd-Michael Becker, Sabine Damm, Norbert Emmerich, Ursula Grell, Christina Härtel, Marianne Hühn, and Martina Krüger, "Zu unserer Arbeit," in Arbeitsgruppe zur Erforschung her Geschichte der Karl-Bonhoeffer Nervenklinik, *Totgeschwiegen 1933–1945: Zur Geschichte der Wittenauer Heilstätten, seit 1957 Karl-Bonhoeffer Nervenklinik* (Berlin, 1988), 8.

10. Statistics from Hans-Walter Schmuhl, " 'Euthanasie' im Nationalsozialismus: Ein Überblick," in *Euthanasie in Hadamar: Die nationalsozialistische Vernichtungspolitik in hessischen Anstalten*, ed. Landeswohlfahrtsverband Hessen (Kassel, 1991), 59. Published excerpts of Meseritz-Obrawalde testimonies can be found in Franz Koch, "Die Beteiligung von Kran-

kenschwestern und Krankenpflegern an Massenverbrechen im National-
sozialismus," in *Krankenpflege im Nationalsozialismus,* ed. Hilde Steppe,
Franz Koch, and Herbert Weisbrod-Frey, 3d ed. (Frankfurt, 1986); and
Hilde Steppe, "Mit Tränen in den Augen zogen wir dann die Spritzen auf
... ," in *Krankenpflege im Nationalsozialismus,* ed. Hilde Steppe, 5th ed.
(Frankfurt, 1989).

CHAPTER 1
INTRODUCTION

1. MO, 4:961 (K.K.)

2. Daniel Jonah Goldhagen, *Hitler's Willing Executioners: Ordinary Germans and the Holocaust* (New York, 1996), especially 277–280, 442–443, and
chapter 16; and Christopher R. Browning, *Ordinary Men: Reserve Police Battalion 101 and the Final Solution in Poland* (New York, 1992), especially chapter 18.

3. To cite just one example, Browning pointed out that Ukrainian, Lat-
vian, and Lithuanian "volunteers" (*Hilfswillige,* or Hiwis) and other "spe-
cialists" were recruited to lighten the psychological burden of point-blank
shootings (*Ordinary Men,* 52, 83–85, 162–163).

4. It seems that in the eyes of some men, moral accommodation entailed, for example, allowing women to bring their infants and small children to collection points, despite orders to shoot infants on the spot, or
fulfilling orders to shoot Jews who had worked for them by sparing them
the agony of anticipation and shooting them unawares (ibid., 59 and 154–
155).

5. Götz Aly, "Medizin gegen Unbrauchbare," in *Aussonderung und Tod:
Die klinische Hinrichtung der Unbrauchbaren,* ed. Götz Aly (Berlin, 1985), 29;
and "Der saubere und schmutzige Fortschritt," in *Reform und Gewissen:
"Euthanasie" im Dienst des Fortschritts,* ed. Götz Aly (Berlin, 1985), 9–13, 33.
Hans Stoffels's approach, whereby radicalization was driven by aspira-
tions toward a "health utopia," is a variation on this theme ("Utopie und
Opfer: Sozialanthropologische Überlegungen zu den nationalsoziali-
stischen Krankentötungen," in *Psychiatrie im Abgrund: Spurensuche und
Standortbestimmung nach den NS-Psychiatrie-Verbrechen,* ed. Ralf Seidel and
Wolfgang Franz Werner [Cologne, 1991]).

6. See, for example, Hans-Ludwig Siemen, *Menschen blieben auf der
Strecke . . . : Psychiatrie zwischen Reform und Nationalsozialismus* (Gütersloh,
1987), and Bernd Walter, *Psychiatrie und Gesellschaft in der Moderne: Geisteskrankenfürsorge in der Provinz Westfalen zwischen Kaiserreich und NS-Regime*
(Paderborn, 1996). Both authors attempt to avoid leaving the impression
that psychiatrists' positions were simply reflexive responses to socioeconomic and political developments. Rather, they suggest that against the

background of specific pressures, psychiatrists incorporated certain principles (such as the therapeutic value of work) into their scientific-therapeutic approach and proffered them as scientifically sound in their own right.

7. Michael Burleigh, *Death and Deliverance: "Euthanasia" in Germany, c. 1900–1945* (Cambridge, 1994), especially chapter 8, " 'Medieval' or Modern? 'Euthanasia' Programmes, 1941–1945."

8. This is the approach of Asmus Finzen, "Massenmord und Schuldgefühl: Anmerkungen zur Patho-psychologie des Gewissens," in *Sozialpsychiatrische Informationen* ("Psychiatrie im deutschen Faschismus"), no. 2 (1983).

9. See, for example, Dirk Blasius, *Der verwaltete Wahnsinn: Eine Sozialgeschichte des Irrenhauses* (Frankfurt, 1980), 155–169.

10. Michael Burleigh, *Ethics and Extermination: Reflections on Nazi Genocide* (Cambridge, 1997), 125.

11. See, for example, Henry Friedlander, *The Origins of Nazi Genocide: From Euthanasia to the Final Solution* (Chapel Hill and London, 1995), and Burleigh, *Ethics and Extermination.*

12. Friedlander, *The Origins of Nazi Genocide*, 142–149.

13. Browning, *Ordinary Men*, 163.

14. As a member of Police Battalion 101 explained, "Most of the other comrades drank so much solely because of the many shootings of Jews, for such a life was quite intolerable sober." (Quoted in Browning, *Ordinary Men*, 82.) A stoker at the Hartheim killing center also noted that "because the work [as a stoker] was very strenuous and nerve-shattering, we also received a ¼ liter schnapps every day." (Quoted in Friedlander, *The Origins of Nazi Genocide*, 234.)

15. Friedlander, *The Origins of Nazi Genocide*, xii.

16. Aly, "Medizin gegen Unbrauchbare," 17. Zygmunt Bauman makes this point with reference to the Jews in *Modernity and the Holocaust*, especially 184–200; and Henry Friedlander, with the aid of examples from the "euthanasia" program and the persecution of the Jews, also concludes that "close relations with potential victims, not ideology, thus determined whether a sense of 'moral law' led to opposition" (*The Origins of Nazi Genocide*, 189).

17. The first reaction from some parents was suspicion and so much anxiety that Meltzer was compelled to assure them that the questionnaires were for hypothetical purposes only. In the end, 162 questionnaires were returned, and 73 percent of parents responded that they would agree to a "shortening" of the life of their children if experts ascertained that they were "incurably imbecilic." Of the 27 percent who answered that they would *not* agree to such a "shortening" under these circumstances, half answered that they *might* agree to such a shortening if the parents were no longer alive or if the child were in great pain. Only 20 answered that

in none of these circumstances would they agree to "shortening" the life of their child. In the accompanying comments, one parent wrote, "In principle agreed, only parents may not be asked; it is of course hard for them to uphold a death sentence for their own flesh and blood. However, if it were said that [the child] died of x-sickness, then everyone would be satisfied." (Aly, "Medizin gegen Unbrauchbare," 14–15.) See also Burleigh, *Ethics and Extermination*, 121.

18. Aly, "Medizin gegen Unbrauchbare," 15.

19. Ibid., 49.

20. Ibid.

21. Götz Aly, "Aktion T4: Modell des Massenmordes," in *Aktion T4, 1939–1945: Die "Euthanasie"-Zentrale in der Tiergartenstrasse 4*, ed. Götz Aly (Berlin, 1987), 15–18.

22. Aly, "Der saubere und schmutzige Fortschritt," 25.

23. MO, vol. 4 ("Urteilsbegründing"), 1586.

24. These themes can be found in Koch, "Die Beteiligung," and Antje Wettlaufer, "Die Beteiligung von Schwestern und Pflegern an den Morden in Hadamar," in *Psychiatrie im Faschismus: Die Anstalt Hadamar, 1933–1945*, ed. Dorothee Roer and Dieter Henckel (Bonn, 1986).

Chapter 2
Neither Riffraff nor Saints

1. Höck, "Historische Nachrichten und Bemerkungen über die merkwürdigsten Irrenanstalten (1804)," quoted in Herbert Loos, "Die psychiatrische Versorgung in Berlin im 19. und zum Beginn des 20. Jahrhunderts—Aspekte der sozialen Bewältigung des Irrenproblems in einer dynamischen Großstadtentwicklung," in *Geschichte der Psychiatrie im 19. Jahrhundert*, ed. Achim Thom (Berlin, 1984), 99. After the institution burned down in 1798, the Charité took over the care of Berlin's mentally ill; restraint of patients and violence, however, continued.

2. To be sure, Dirk Blasius notes that nursing staff in Rhein Province institutions tended to remain in service over many years in the late nineteenth century (*Der verwaltete Wahnsinn*, 63). On the other hand, Sabine Damm and Norbert Emmerich observe that at Dalldorf many nurses did indeed quit after only a short time ("Die Irrenanstalt Dalldorf-Wittenau," in Arbeitsgruppe, *Totgeschwiegen*, 19). According to turn-of-the-century surveys, staff turnover was indeed higher in urban areas such as Berlin, where opportunities for other employment were greater, than in rural areas where people were less desultory (Thomas Höll and Paul-Otto Schmidt-Michel, *Irrenpflege im 19. Jahrhundert: Die Wärterfrage in der Diskussion der deutschen Psychiater* [Bonn, 1989], 84). Staff turnover aside, however, maintaining a staff of *competent* nursing personnel remained a con-

cern of administrators both in rural and in urban areas well into the twentieth century.

3. Höll and Schmidt-Michel, *Irrenpflege im 19. Jahrhundert*, 24–29.

4. Ernst Horn, "Beschreibung der in der Irrenanstalt des Königlichen Charitékrankenhauses zu Berlin gebräuchlichen Drehmachinen, ihre Wirkung und Anwendung bei Geisteskranken (1818)," quoted in Loos, "Die psychiatrische Versorgung," 99. For other brief discussions of the (low) quality of nursing candidates in the nineteenth century, see Marianne Elisabeth Hertling, *Die Provinzial- Heil- und Pflegeanstalt Düren: Die Entwicklung einer großen psychiatrischen Antalt der Rheinprovinz von ihrer Gründung, 1878 bis 1934* (Herzogenrath, 1985), 179–180; and Georg Streiter, *Die wirtschaftliche und soziale Lage der beruflichen Krankenpflege in Deutschland*, 2d ed. (Jena, 1924), 21–27.

5. Things had not always been this way, however. Although subjected to strategies of confinement in the context of communal and Church-sponsored care, the insane had a place in the religious and symbolic order of things from the Middle Ages until the seventeenth century. Both a practical and a symbolic liability to absolutist regimes, who put a premium on public order, security, and rational organization, they were interned with the destitute, criminals, and other "asocials" in houses of confinement (Michel Foucault, *Madness and Civilization: A History of Insanity in the Age of Reason*, trans. Richard Howard [New York, 1988], especially chapters 1 and 2. See also Blasius, *Der verwaltete Wahnsinn*, 20–21, and Dieter Jetter, *Grundzüge der Geschichte des Irrenhauses* [Darmstadt, 1981], 2–18).

6. Houses of confinement often doubled as workhouses, in part to stimulate manufacturing: each German house of correction had its own specialty, such as weaving or spinning. An additional—and, some would say, even more important—function was to abolish social uselessness: such houses were "prisons of moral order" whose occupants would be compelled to learn the virtues of hard work. In this sense, the insane, criminals, and paupers were subjected to a great disciplinary experiment in the seventeenth and eighteenth centuries; confinement and administration replaced banishment as the solution to moral deviance (Foucault, *Madness and Civilization*, 51–52, 54–63).

7. Damm and Emmerich, "Die Irrenanstalt Dalldorf-Wittenau," in Arbeitsgruppe, *Totgeschwiegen*, 19–20. The extent to which theory corresponded to practice is a separate issue; the authors point out that in 1980 a few straitjackets were found in old cupboards in the clinic, and that in the first two decades after Wittenau's founding "straitgloves" were used.

8. Blasius, *Der verwaltete Wahnsinn*, 61, and Damm and Emmerich, "Die Irrenanstalt Dalldorf-Wittenau," in Arbeitsgruppe, *Totgeschwiegen*, 21.

9. Siemen, *Menschen blieben auf der Strecke*, 25–29. A reputation for therapeutic success, he argues, would be acquired only through the treatment

of war neuroses during the First World War. In addition, it is worth noting here that psychiatry did not acquire the status of an academic discipline until the founding of the first university chairs in the last quarter of the century. Institutional psychiatrists throughout the century were simply doctors who learned what they knew of psychiatry on the job (Blasius, *Der verwaltete Wahnsinn*, 58).

10. Höll and Schmidt-Michel, *Irrenpflege im 19. Jahrhundert*, 58.

11. Hans Wachsmuth, "Aus alten Akten und Krankengeschichten der nassauischen Irrenanstalt (Eberbach-Eichberg)," part 2, *PNW* 29 (July 9, 1927): 328.

12. Ibid., 330.

13. *Auszug aus der Chronik des Psychiatrischen Krankenhauses Eichberg* (Eltville am Rhein, 1984), 4.

14. Hans Wachsmuth, "Aus alten Akten und Krankengeschichten der nassauischen Irrenanstalt (Eberbach-Eichberg)," part 2, *PNW* 29 (July 9, 1927): 332–333; and part 3, *PNW* 29 (October 29, 1927): 494.

15. R. Snell, "Landesheil- und Pflegeanstalt Eichberg im Rheingau," in *Deutsche Heil- und Pflegeanstalten für psychisch Kranke in Wort und Bild*, ed. Johannes Bresler, vol. 1 (Halle a.S., 1910), 183. Originally administered by the Duchy of Nassau and brought under Prussian state control in 1866, Eichberg's affairs were transferred to the communal administration of the district government of Wiesbaden in 1872, and the institution would remain under its administration throughout the period to be studied (*Auszug aus der Chronik*, 4–5).

16. For a useful case-study analysis of the mutual influence of finances, therapeutic innovation, and demographic pressures in the construction of new institutions, see chapter 2 of Walter, *Psychiatrie und Gesellschaft in der Moderne*.

17. *Auszug aus der Chronik*, 4.

18. Damm and Emmerich, "Die Irrenanstalt Dalldorf-Wittenau," in Arbeitsgruppe, *Totgeschwiegen*, 13–15.

19. Ibid., 18–19.

20. Ibid., 28.

21. For details on types of floor plans and general spatial arrangements, see Wilhelm Weygandt, "Irrenanstalten," in *Das Deutsche Krankenhaus*, ed. J. Grober (Jena, 1922).

22. Koch, "Die Beteiligung," 99.

23. "Tagesordnung für die Anstalten der Stadt Berlin für Geisteskranke, Epileptische und Idioten," January 22, 1905. KBoN.

24. Damm and Emmerich, "Die Irrenanstalt Dalldorf-Wittenau," in Arbeitsgruppe, *Totgeschwiegen*, 21–23. This does not mean that nurses no longer applied restraint devices; rather, these practices were disappearing from official portrayals of their tasks and responsibilities.

25. It is interesting, however, that they were evidently quite successful in enforcing their wishes nevertheless: according to a survey from 1895, marriage was still forbidden in eighteen institutions; it could be undertaken with permission in twenty-five and was allowed without administrative intervention in only six (Höll and Schmidt-Michel, *Irrenpflege im 19. Jahrhundert*, 88).

26. Ibid., 30–31, 37.

27. Ibid., 24, 37–55.

28. Ibid., 46.

29. Ibid., 25 and 45.

30. Claudia Bischoff, *Frauen in der Krankenpflege: Zur Entwicklung von Frauenrolle und Frauenberufstätigkeit im 19. und 20. Jahrhundert* (Frankfurt, 1992), 113. See also Hilde Steppe, "Die historische Entwicklung der Krankenpflege als Beruf: Auswirkungen dieser Entwicklung auf heutige Strukturen," *Deutsche Krankenpflegezeitschrift*, no. 5 (Supplement) (1985), and Heinz Faulstich, *Von der Irrenfürsorge zur "Euthanasie": Geschichte der badischen Psychiatrie bis 1945* (Freiburg, 1993), 53.

31. Because the majority of nurses overall fell under the administrative purview of Church organizations, *all* nurses were excluded as nonemployees from employee protections and benefits (Steppe, "Die historische Entwicklung," 8). For a useful general discussion of working conditions, see Bischoff, *Frauen in der Krankenpflege*, 107–124, and Hilde Steppe, "Pflege bis 1933," in *Krankenpflege im Nationalsozialismus*, ed. Hilde Steppe, 5th ed. (Frankfurt, 1989), 26.

32. Nurse Hermann Peuke, "Der Irrenpfleger und sein Beruf," *DI* 10 (August 1906): 132.

33. Ibid., 131.

34. For a more detailed discussion of the role of charity in the history of nursing, see the dissertation on which this book is based: Bronwyn McFarland-Icke, "Moral Consciousness and the Politics of Exclusion: Nursing in German Psychiatry, 1918–1945" (Ph.D. diss., University of Chicago, 1997).

35. Höll and Schmidt-Michel, *Irrenpflege im 19. Jahrhundert*, 68–69, 71.

36. Ibid., 68–69.

37. Ibid., 46, 51, 57.

38. See, for example, Weygandt, "Irrenanstalten," 417; Hertling, *Die Provinzial Heil- und Pflegeanstalt Düren*, 183; Hugo Schneider, "Die ehemalige Heil- und Pflegeanstalt Illenau: Ihre Geschichte, ihre Bedeutung," *Die Ortenau* 61 (1981): 213; and Faulstich, *Von der Irrenfürsorge zur "Euthanasie"*, 65.

39. Siemen, *Menschen blieben auf der Strecke*, 30–31; and Faulstich, *Von der Irrenfürsorge zur "Euthanasie"*, 75.

40. Siemen, *Menschen blieben auf der Strecke*, 29–30.

41. Faulstich, *Von der Irrenfürsorge zur "Euthanasie"*, 78.

42. Werner Tröster, *Suttrop-Dorpke: Zur Geschichte des Westfälischen Landeskrankenhauses Warstein* (Warstein, 1980), 42.

43. Faulstich, *Von der Irrenfürsorge zur "Euthanasie"*, 82.

44. Dr. Wern. H. Becker, "Unsere Pflichten während des Krieges, *DI* 21 (November 1917): 170.

45. Senior Nurse A. Borsum, "Unsere Pflichten während des Krieges," *DI* 21 (September 1917): 131.

46. Ibid.

47. Dr. Dobrick-Kosten, "Krieg und Volksernährung," *DI* 18 (March 1915): 294.

48. Becker, "Unsere Pflichten," 171.

49. Ibid., 172.

50. "An das Krankenpflege- Massage- und Badepersonal," *Die Sanitätswarte* (December 1918), quoted in Steppe, "Pflege bis 1933," 34.

51. Steppe, "Pflege bis 1933," 38–41.

52. "An das Krankenpflege- Massage- und Badepersonal," *Die Sanitätswarte* (December 1918), quoted in Steppe, "Pflege bis 1933," 34.

53. Steppe, "Pflege bis 1933," 38.

54. Ibid. and Streiter, *Krankenpflege in Deutschland*, 67.

55. For details on the positions of various factions, see Steppe, "Pflege bis 1933." On the history of unionized nursing, see Franz Josef Furtwängler, *ÖTV: Die Geschichte einer Gewerkschaft* (Stuttgart, 1955), 133–139, 213–215, 287, 349, 421–425, 510–511.

56. National labor minister (*Reichsarbeitsminister*) to the provincial governor (*Landeshauptmann*) in Hesse, June 20, 1919, quoted in Streiter, *Krankenpflege in Deutschland*, 73.

57. Dr. Falkenberg reported at the May 1920 meeting of the German Association for Psychiatry that fourteen of fifty-four institutions taken into consideration had implemented the forty-eight-hour week. In five institutions, nurses worked seventy-two hours per week (Streiter, *Krankenpflege in Deutschland*, 71–72). Dalldorf instituted the eight-hour workday in spring 1919, reporting that "during their off-duty time personnel have complete freedom of movement." Whether this would adversely affect nurse-patient relationships, only time would tell ("Mitteilungen," *PNW* 20 [April 12, 1919]: 11).

58. Dr. Gustav Kolb, "Inwieweit sind Änderungen im Betrieb der Anstalten geboten?" *PNW* 22 (July 31, 1920): 136–137. A committee reviewing conditions in the institutions of Baden in 1919 recommended religious instruction of nursing personnel to prevent such "misuse" of free time but realized that even this could not hope to reach the social democratic sympathizers among them who were guilty of "materialism" and "lacking Christianity" (Faulstich, *Von der Irrenfürsorge zur "Euthanasie"*, 85).

59. Kolb, "Änderungen im Betrieb," 136–137.

60. Streiter, *Krankenpflege in Deutschland*, 73.

61. Erwin Brauner, "Geistliche oder weltliche Krankenpflege?" *Die Sanitätswarte*, no. 26 (December 1931): 411. See also Paul Levy, "Freie oder karitative Krankenpflege?" *Die Sanitätswarte*, no. 13 (June 1928): 217–219.

62. The extent of the problem is difficult to assess. Georg Streiter claimed in 1924 that "mental illnesses are not a rare occurrence among nurses in psychiatric institutions. . ." (*Krankenpflege in Deutschland*, 138). Johann Susmann Galant claimed in 1926 that "mental illness occurs still relatively frequently among nurses in psychiatric institutions. . . ." In a footnote, *Die Irrenpflege* editor Dr. Carl Wickel countered, "Coming down with mental illness is not frequent among psychiatric nursing personnel in Germany. In thirty years I have only once seen that a nurse became mentally ill," and his condition was such that he would have become ill regardless of his occupation ("Psychohygiene [Gesunderhaltung des Geistes] und die Irrenpflege," *DI* 30 [March 1926]: 40).

63. Wilhelm Engelter, "Brief aus Goddelau," *Die Sanitätswarte*, no. 5 (March 1928): 90.

64. J. Lerrsen, "Die Wohnung und Verpflegung des Personals," *DI* 36 (November 1932): 176.

65. Joseph Koch, "Rationalisierung im Gesundheitswesen," in *Das Deutsche Pflege- und Anstaltspersonal: Seine berufliche, wirtschaftliche, und rechtliche Lage*, ed. Zentralverband der Arbeitnehmer öffentlicher Betreibe und Verwaltungen (Cologne, 1930), 37, 41, 52.

66. This debate, like the eight-hour workday debate, predated the First World War. The issue was taken up with renewed vigor in the early Weimar Republic as part of a general preoccupation with reconstituting the administrative and legal basis of health care procedures; but it was a particularly urgent matter for public institutions, whose employment contracts applied differently depending on a person's qualifications (Dr. Vocke, "Die Ausbildung des Pflegepersonals in den Irrenanstalten," *PNW* 22 [November 20, 1920]: 263).

67. Georg Streiter, "Ausbildung, Prüfung und Fortbildung in der Krankenpflege (mit besonderer Berücksichtigung der Irrenpflege)," *DI* 29 (August 1925): 115–117.

68. Emil Kandzia, "Die Irrenpflege, ein Spezialgebiet der Krankenpflege," *DI* 23 (November 1919): 132–135.

69. Klaus Uenzen, "Etwas über die Bewertung und Ausbildung des Pflegepersonals," *Geisteskrankenpflege* 34 (October 1930): 150.

70. Emil Kandzia, "Was fordert das Irrenplegepersonal für seine Ausbildung?" *DI* 26 (May 1922): 28.

71. Ibid., 23. Other nurses were somewhat more flexible on this issue. Klaus Uenzen, for example, agreed that psychiatric nurses would be best

off "appended" to a centralized training and certification system, but he was willing to accept a separate set of procedures so long as psychiatric nurses enjoyed the same degree of esteem ("Etwas über die Bewertung," 151–152).

72. Uenzen, "Etwas über die Bewertung," 154.

CHAPTER 3
EDUCATING NURSES IN THE SPIRIT OF THE TIMES

1. This conceptual orientation is borrowed from Siemen, who speaks of a crisis of *Existenzberechtigung*, for example, 23.

2. Siemen, *Menschen blieben auf der Strecke*, 46.

3. See in particular Dr. Spliedt, "Zur gegenwärtigen Lage der Anstalten,"*PNW* 20 (February 1, 1919), and Dr. Quaet-Faslem, "Die Sozialiserung der Heilberufe, speziell des ärztlichen Standes," *PNW* 23 (December 31, 1921). Dr. Quaet-Faslem was also at this time a member of the Prussian state parliament, a fact which cautions us against assuming that the state and psychiatry were separate airtight spheres.

4. For details on the standpoints of individual psychiatrists, see Siegfried Grubitzsch, "Revolutions- und Rätezeit 1918/19 aus der Sicht deutscher Psychiater," *Deutscher Psychiater, Psychologie und Gesellschaftskritik* 33/34 (1985): 23–47.

5. Faulstich, *Von der Irrenfürsorge zur "Euthanasie"*, 76.

6. Director Ilberg, "Die Sterblichkeit der Geisteskranken in den sächsischen Anstalten während des Krieges 1914/1918 und deren Folgen," *Allgemeine Zeitschrift für Psychiatrie* 78 (1922): 58–63, quoted in ibid., 78.

7. Burleigh, *Death and Deliverance*, 26.

8. Faulstich, *Von der Irrenfürsorge zur "Euthanasie"*, 99. He adds that during and after the war, many psychiatrists believed that such men simply wanted an excuse for avoiding their duty to the Fatherland.

9. Hans-Georg Güse and Norbert Schmacke, *Psychiatrie zwischen bürgerlichen Revolution und Faschismus* (Kroneberg, 1976), 417. See also J. E. Meyer, " 'Die Freigabe der Vernichtung lebensunwerten Lebens' von Binding und Hoche im Spiegel der deutschen Psychiatrie vor 1933," *Der Nervenarzt* 59 (1988): 85–91.

10. See, for example, Siemen, *Menschen blieben auf der Strecke*, 32; and Damm and Emmerich, "Die Irrenanstalt Dalldorf-Wittenau," in Arbeitsgruppe, *Totgeschwiegen*, 33.

11. Dr. Adolf Groß, "Zeitgemäße Betrachtungen zum wirtschaftlichen Betrieb der Irrenanstalten," *Allgemeine Zeitschrift für Psychiatrie* 79 (1923): 62–65.

12. For a notable and particularly eloquent exception in this debate, see Dr. Johannes Bresler, "Sparsamkeit in der Irrenanstalt," *PNW* 23 (April 9,

1921); "Noch einmal: Sparsamkeit in der Irrenanstalt," *PNW* 23 (August 13, 1921); and "Zum dritten und nicht letzten Male: Sparsamkeit in Irrenanstalten," *PNW* 23 (November 5, 1921).

13. Bresler, "Zum dritten Male," 189.

14. Dr. R. Carrière, "Sparmaßnahmen und Anstaltsniveau," *PNW* 33 (July 4, 1931): 329. See also Dr. Enge, "Fehlschlüsse und Irrtümer bei Sparmaßnahmen," *PNW* 34 (November 19, 1932): 570.

15. Groß, "Zeitgemäße Betrachtungen," 66.

16. Dr. Erich Friedlaender, "Die wirtchaftlichen Aufgaben der Irrenanstalt," part 2, *DI* 27 (October 1923): 187.

17. Gustav Kolb, director of the Heil- und Pflegeanstalt Erlangen, had found only a handful of supporters for his 1919 proposal to develop forms of outpatient care (Siemen, *Menschen blieben auf der Strecke*, 34–37). But by 1921, Dr. Ast would write that "the most effective measure that may promise to be successful in the foreseeable future is the *expansion of psychiatric care outside the institution* according to the ideas of *Kolb*, which are certainly familiar to all of you" ("Der derzeitige Stand der Krankenpflege in den bayerischen Irrenanstalten," *PNW* 23 [November 19, 1921]: 202; italics in original).

18. Dr. Faltlhauser, "Geisteskrankenfürsorge außerhalb der Anstalten," *DI* 27 (May 1923): 90.

19. Between 1923 and 1929, the number of patients treated in institutions annually rose over 60 percent, from approximately 185,000 to over 300,000 (Siemen, *Menschen blieben auf der Strecke*, 59–60).

20. Ibid., 62–64.

21. Henry Simon's ideas were met with skepticism when he introduced them to his colleagues in 1923, and were not fully embraced until 1927 (ibid., 64, 69–70). Institutional psychiatrists seem to have been much quicker to support work therapy: *Die Irrenpflege* did not start rigorous treatment of the subject until 1925, but the first article from February of that year was based on a continuing education lecture for nurses held at the Wiesloch institution in November 1923 (Dr. Möckel, "Die Arbeitstherapie bei Geisteskranken," *DI* 29 [February 1925]: 17).

22. Hermann Haymann, *Lehrbuch der Irrenheilkunde für Pfleger und Pflegerinnen* (Berlin, 1922), 121.

23. Ibid., 120.

24. Möckel, "Die Arbeitstherapie bei Geisteskranken," 27.

25. Siemen, *Menschen blieben auf der Strecke*, 68–69.

26. Möckel, "Die Arbeitstherapie bei Geisteskranken," 23.

27. Dr. Erich Friedlaender, "Die wirtchaftlichen Aufgaben der Irrenanstalt," part 3, *DI* 28 (January 1924): 5.

28. That is, they preferred to speak of *Beschäftigungsbehandlung* rather than *Arbeitstherapie* (Dr. Buder, "Über die neuen Bestrebungen in der

Beschäftigungsbehandlung der Geisteskranken," *DI* 31 [December 1927]: 190; and Dr. Wickel, "Betätigungsbehandlung," *DI* 31 [May 1927]: 69).

29. There were limits to the irrelevance of economic factors. Patients who wasted expensive materials in the course of their occupation in institutional workshops, for example, were to be transferred to some other kind of activity (Friedlaender, part 3, 6). Also, Groß wrote in 1923 that psychiatrists should combine work therapy with bed treatment during food shortages so that patients would not work up an appetite for quantities of food that were not available. "Above all, those patients who uselessly consume their energy by idly standing or walking around without consciously occupying themselves should systematically be put to bed" (Groß, "Zeitgemäße Betrachtungen," 73).

30. Dr. O. Snell, "Sparsamkeit," *DI* 32 (June 1928): 82. He did not comment further on what kinds of purposeful-but-not-payable work he had in mind. But Dr. Wickel noted that "the activity also extends to looking at pictures, reading, playing, and useful work" ("Betätigungsbehandlung," 66).

31. Möckel, "Die Arbeitstherapie bei Geisteskranken," 23.

32. Ibid., 23–24.

33. For treatment of this question, see Siemen, *Menschen blieben auf der Strecke*, parts 1 and 2.

34. Dr. Paul Reiß, *Im roten Hause: Von der Behandlung des Irren* (Straubing, 1929), 22.

35. Dr. Valentin Faltlhauser was author of *Geisteskrankenpflege: Ein Lehr- und Handbuch für Irrenpfleger*, a widely used text for the instruction of nurses that originally appeared in a series of *Die Irrenpflege* articles in 1922 and 1923. It was later published in several editions as a book. He also edited *Leitfaden für Irrenpflege* (Halle a. S., 1936) and wrote numerous articles in the '20s and '30s in *Die Irrenpflege* and other psychiatric journals such as the *PNW*. This champion of a humanist psychiatry would go on to distinguish himself in the National Socialist years by serving as a planning adviser for the T4 program and, as director of the Kaufbeuren-Irsee institution, head of its children's "euthanasia" ward (Friedlander, *The Origins of Nazi Genocide*, 51, 66).

36. Dr. Faltlhauser, "Geisteskrankenpflege: Zum Unterricht und Selbstunterricht für Irrenpfleger und zur Vorbereitung auf die Pflegerprüfung," *DI* 26 (February 1922): 185–187. Hereafter, the title to Faltlhauser's installments in this series will be shortened simply to "Geisteskrankenpflege."

37. Readers who are familiar with German will recognize that the dual purpose of healing and caring is imbedded in the term for such an institution, the "Heil- und Pflegeanstalt." This term became increasingly fashionable during the Weimar years, while its predecessor, the "Irrenanstalt," was phased out.

38. Faltlhauser, "Geisteskrankenpflege," *DI* 26 (March 1922): 209. This mistrust was fueled, he wrote in the next installment, by allegations of patient mistreatment in institutions—allegations that were sometimes merely symptomatic of an illness but unfortunately sometimes true (*DI* 26 [April 1922]: 10).

39. Reiß, *Im roten Hause*, 18.

40. Faltlhauser, "Geisteskrankenpflege," *DI* 26 (March 1922): 213.

41. See, for example, Weygandt, "Irrenanstalten," 388–425.

42. Faltlhauser, "Geisteskrankenpflege" *DI* 26 (March 1922): 202–207.

43. Prof. Dr. Raeke, "Ursachen der Geisteskrankheiten," part 1, *DI* 23 (August 1919): 77.

44. Ibid., 78–80.

45. Prof. Dr. Raeke, "Ursachen der Geisteskranken," part 2, *DI* 23 (September 1919): 93–94; and Dr. W. Fuchs, "Über Prophylaxe," part 2, *DI* 32 (August 1928): 117–118.

46. Prof. Dr. Raeke, "Über den Umgang mit Psychopathen," *DI* 30 (July 1926): 100.

47. Raeke, "Ursachen der Geisteskrankheiten," part 2, 92.

48. Ibid.

49. Fuchs, "Über Prophylaxe," part 2, 114.

50. Faltlhauser, "Geisteskrankenpflege," *DI* 26 (March 1922): 208.

51. Ibid.

52. Galant, "Psychohygiene," 38.

53. Ibid., 35.

54. It is beyond the scope of the current discussion to explore the possible reasons for this apparent contradiction. Noteworthy, however, is the fact that the few psychiatrists who rejected Binding and Hoche's ideas in *PNW* pointed out that the killing of patients in institutions would constitute a breach of public trust—which, in light of psychiatry's public image problems, would certainly have been an unappealing prospect. Also, the prospect of killing precisely those whom they were supposed to treat may have been less appealing to the institutional psychiatrists writing for *Die Irrenpflege*, who saw those patients every day, than to their more "distant" colleagues at research institutes and universities.

55. Galant, "Psychohygiene," 34–35.

56. Haymann, *Lehrbuch*, 128.

57. See, for example, Faltlhauser, "Geisteskrankenpflege," *DI* 26 (August 1922): 81–89, and *DI* 27 (June 1923): 108.

58. Faltlhauser, "Geisteskrankenpflege," *DI* 26 (September 1922): 112.

59. Faltlhauser, "Geisteskrankenpflege," *DI* 27 (November 1923): 203.

60. Faltlhauser, "Geisteskrankenpflege," *DI* 26 (August 1922): 87.

61. Faltlhauser, "Geisteskrankenpflege," *DI* 26 (July 1922): 73. See also Faltlhauser, "Geisteskrankenpflege," *DI* 26 (May 1922): 34.

62. Faltlhauser, "Geisteskrankenpflege," *DI* 26 (August 1922): 88.

63. Med.-Rat Dr. F. Weisenhorn, "Leibesübungen der Geisteskranken an der Heil- und Pflegeanstalt Illenau im Vergangenheit und Gegenwart," *PNW* 32 (November 15, 1930): 558. See also Haymann, *Lehrbuch*, 122.

64. As with the late nineteenth century, statements concerning the use of force were not always consistent with each other and should be regarded as expressions more of intent than of fact. For example, Faltlhauser wrote in the section "The Transport of a Psychiatric Patient" that although restraint devices were frowned upon (*verpönt*), a straitjacket could be used as an absolute last resort in patient-transport emergencies ("Geisteskrankenpflege," *DI* 27 [October 1923]: 193). Also, while isolation in bare cells had by and large been eliminated in practice, he instructed nurses that a doctor was to be notified when a patient required detention in a "single room" (*Einzelzimmer*) ("Geisteskrankenpflege," *DI* 26 [March 1922]: 213, and *DI* 26 [May 1922]: 33 respectively).

65. E. Menninger v. Lerchenthal, "Über die Eignung zum Irrenpflegeberuf," *DI* 33 (January 1929): 10. An unusually detailed description on how to physically handle patients was provided by Haymann, *Lehrbuch*, 125–128.

66. Dr. Ewald Meltzer, *Leitfaden der Schwachsinnigen- und Blödenpflege*, 2d ed. (Halle a. S., 1930), 10.

67. Haymann, *Lehrbuch*, 112.

68. Faltlhauser, "Geisteskrankenpflege," *DI* 27 (October 1923): 192.

69. Faltlhauser, "Geisteskrankenpflege," *DI* 26 (April 1922): 13. On handling violence, see also Faltlhauser, "Geisteskrankenpflege," *DI* 27 (June 1923): 110–112.

70. Faltlhauser, "Geisteskrankenpflege," *DI* 26 (April 1922): 13.

71. Interestingly, however, one contributing nurse did not dismiss it entirely: "The question of earning a secure and adequate living must in any case be important to us. Every righteous person will be willing to grant us that. However, it must be accompanied by an inner warmth and true enjoyment of the chosen profession. He who thinks otherwise and acts purely materialistically will be disappointed his entire life and seldom become a truly competent nurse" (Nurse Klaus Uenzen, "Älterer Pfleger und Anfänger," *DI* 35 [April 1931]: 50).

72. Senior Nurse Georg Sauer, "Was heißt Pfleger sein?" *DI* 33 (March 1929): 34, 38.

73. To be sure, this principle had nothing to do with "natural" gendered differences, which remained alive and well in nursing instruction. For example, when discussing guidelines for improving the institutional environment, Dr. Friedlaender wrote that "it must be emphasized that, [with regard to] enhancing the appearance of homeyness, female personnel gen-

erally bring more talent and broader interest than the male personnel. This is in no way supposed to be a disparaging criticism, [but] rather simply [the identification of] a fact determined from the outset by the difference between the sexes. But precisely for this reason, the man who works in nursing should also do his best in this respect to take it up [along] with his female colleagues." ("Die wirtschaftlichen Aufgaben in der Irrenanstalt," *DI* 30 [February 1926]: 24).

74. See, for example, Menninger v. Lerchenthal, "Über die Eignung zum Irrenpflegeberuf," 10.

75. Ibid., 3.

76. Ibid.

77. Dr. Walter Fuchs, "Pflegeunterricht," *DI* 33 (July 1929): 107–109.

78. Haymann, *Lehrbuch*, 114.

79. Dr. Wickel, "Lernpfleger und Pfleger," *DI* 31 (June 1927): 93.

80. Faltlhauser, "Geisteskrankenpflege," *DI* 26 (October 1922): 137.

81. Dr. W. Kemper, "Über das Berufsgeheimnis," *Geisteskrankenpflege* 36 (March 1932): 41.

82. Faltlhauser, "Geisteskrankenpflege," *DI* 26 (January 1922): 167. This rule was excepted when one learned, for example, of a person's intention to commit a crime (Kemper, "Über das Berufsgeheimnis," 40).

83. Dr. Erich Friedlaender, "Die wirtchaftlichen Aufgaben der Irrenanstalt," part 1, *DI* 27 (August 1923): 142. See also Walter Morgenthaler, *Die Pflege der Gemuts- und Geisteskranken* (Berlin, 1930), 31.

84. See, for example, Snell, "Sparsamkeit," 85.

85. Faltlhauser, "Geisteskrankenpflege," *DI* 26 (January 1922): 169.

86. Faltlhauser, "Geisteskrankenpflege," *DI* 27 (June 1923): 111.

87. Dr. Bernt Götz, "Die Besuchsstunde," *DI* 32 (May 1928): 66.

88. Faltlhauser, "Geisteskrankenpflege," *DI* 26 (May 1922): 35.

89. As Faltlhauser wrote, "The absolutely necessary requirement, which applies to all such observations, is that they be absolutely reliable. The nurse should not report his own judgment, that is, not what he in any case thinks it could be; he should only closely observe [and] report the naked facts" ("Geisteskrankenpflege," *DI* 26 [June 1922]: 43).

90. Faltlhauser, "Geisteskrankenpflege," *DI* 26 (April 1922): 14.

91. Ibid.

92. Sauer, "Was heißt Pfleger sein?" 37.

93. Morgenthaler, *Die Pflege der Gemuts- und Geisteskranken*, 41.

94. Faltlhauser, "Geisteskrankenpflege," *DI* 26 (January 1922): 168–169.

95. Menninger v. Lerchenthal, "Über die Eignung zum Irrenpflegeberuf," 7–8.

96. This was especially the case on occasions when there was less support than usual, such as during the night shift, and when potentially un-

manageable groups of patients were in question—such as when nurses were supervising patient work out of doors (Faltlhauser, "Geisteskrankenpflege," *DI* 26 [October 1922]: 134, and 26 [August 1922]: 88).

97. Dr. E. Menninger v. Lerchenthal, "Die Bedeutung des Wortes in der Irrenpflege," *DI* 31 (February 1927): 20.

98. Ibid., 20–22.

99. W. Krause, "Einiges über den Irrenpflegeberuf und über Irrenpflege," *DI* 27 (July 1923): 126. See also Georg Schäfer, "Das Benehmen des Pflegers im Dienst," *DI* 34 (January 1930): 10.

100. Faltlhauser, "Geisteskrankenpflege," *DI* 27 (October 1923): 191–193. This instruction appeared in almost identical form in the section "Allgemeines über den Umgang mit Geisteskranken und deren Behandlung," in *Geisteskrankenpflege* 36 (April 1932).

101. Faltlhauser, "Geisteskrankenpflege," *DI* 26 (May 1922): 34. He did not specify which kinds of bad news he had in mind, but the occasional necessity of caution during visits from relatives suggests that the news of a death in the family would be one such example.

102. Menninger v. Lerchenthal, "Die Bedeutung des Wortes in der Irrenpflege," 22–23.

103. Faltlhauser, "Geisteskrankenpflege," *DI* 26 (May 1922): 32.

104. Raeke, "Über den Umgang mit Psychopathen," 99.

105. Faltlhauser, "Geisteskrankenpflege," *DI* 26 (May 1922): 32.

106. Faltlhauser, "Geisteskrankenpflege," *DI* 27 (June 1923): 111.

107. Götz, "Die Besuchsstunde," 67.

108. Gotthold, "Die Pflege der unsauberen, unordentlichen und unsozialen Kranken," *DI* 26 (July 1922): 66.

109. Friedrich Schulhof, *Lehrgang für Irrenpfleger* (Vienna, 1929), 1.

110. Faltlhauser, "Geisteskrankenpflege," *DI* 26 (April 1922): 15.

111. Galant, "Psychohygiene," 39.

112. Faltlhauser, "Geisteskrankenpflege," *DI* 26 (January 1922): 170.

113. Dr. Wickel, "Etwas von der Würde des Menschen," *DI* 33 (February 1929): 26.

114. Ibid., 27. For a strikingly similar portrayal of the connection between animal-like behavior and the loss of dignity, see Meltzer, *Leitfaden*, 16.

115. Meltzer, *Leitfaden*, 15. Italics in original.

116. Faltlhauser, "Geisteskrankenpflege," *DI* 26 (August 1922): 87.

117. Ibid.

118. This is not to say that "uncivilized" or otherwise aberrant behavior always indicated mental illness. Homosexuality was one such example; "very many distinguished men, especially artists and creative types, were homosexual" (Dr. Bernt Götz, "Was der Irrenpfleger von sexuellen Anomalien wissen muß," *DI* 30 [November 1926]: 165). The current discussion

takes already diagnosed patients as its starting point and analyzes criteria of therapeutic "progress."

119. Raeke, "Über den Umgang mit Psychopathen," 102. My italics. The original citation is as follows: ". . . alle Psychopathen durch ihre angeborene Veranlagung minderwertige und darum bedauernswerte Menschen sind, die der Gesunde schonen und stützen soll."

120. Prof. Dr. Julius Raeke, "Psychopathische Kinder," *Geisteskrankenpflege* 34 (July 1930): 105.

121. Hans-Ludwig Siemen, "Reform und Radikalisierung: Veränderungen der Psychiatrie in der Weltwirtschaftskrise," in *Medizin und Gesundheitspolitik in der NS-Zeit*, ed. Norbert Frei (Munich, 1991), 193–194. To be sure, 1929 marked an all-time high for the number of institutionalized patients; but these numbers went sharply down thereafter.

122. Siemen, "Reform und Radikalisierung," 194–195. Wittenau psychiatrists also pioneered in the development of in-house specialization strategies during the 1920s. Their so-called Staffelsystem (also called "Wittenauer System") entailed tailoring specific areas of the institution to the specialized needs of different categories of patients, such as alcoholics, drug addicts, children with better prognoses, and so forth. (Damm and Emmerich, "Die Irrenanstalt Dalldorf-Wittenau," in Arbeitsgruppe, *Totgeschwiegen*, 40–43.)

123. Morgenthaler, *Die Pflege der Gemuts- und Geisteskranken*, 35–36.

124. Ibid., 36. My emphasis.

125. Siemen, "Reform und Radikalisierung, "197.

126. Dr. X.Y., "Heiratet nicht Geisteskranke!" *Die Sanitätswarte*, no. 20 (October 1928): 359–360.

127. Dr. E. Baege, "Über Eugenik, speziell die Sterilisierungsfrage," *Allgemeine Zeitschrift für Psychiatrie* 95 (1931): 440.

128. Dr. B. Kihn,"Die Ausschaltung der Minderwertigen aus der Gesellschaft," *Allgemeine Zeitschrift für Psychiatrie* 98 (1932): 395.

129. Ibid., 403.

130. Ibid., 404.

CHAPTER 4
THE EVASIVENESS OF THE IDEAL

1. "Veranlassung: Störung der Hausordnung und der Ruhe der Kranken durch das Verhalten des Pflegers L. und seines Besuches auf Haus 7, Heil- und Pflegeanstalt Berlin-Buch, 6 März 1924." LA Berlin, A Rep. 003-04-1, no. 17, 87. Berlin-Buch nurses were also not always models of decorum in other areas of conventional respectability. In 1926 a clergyman was given occasion to complain, for example, that nurses who accompanied patients to services had not stood up when requested for the reading of the

Evangelium. "In the future, dissidents should not accompany the patients" ("Auszug aus dem Protokoll der Wirtschaftskonferenz vom 13.7.26, Heil- und Pflegeanstalt Berlin-Buch." LA Berlin, A Rep. 003-04-1, no. 144, 21).

2. Résumé, Managing Station Nurse T.P., 1923. Mecklenburgisches Landeshauptarchiv Schwerin, Ministerium für Unterricht, Kunst, Geist-liche- und Medizinalangelegenheiten, no. 10259, 3.

3. Résumé, Nurse K.D., June 29, 1929. KBoN, PF K.D., 13.

4. Questionnaire for new personnel, June 1929. LWV-Eichberg, PF M.M., 5.

5. Ibid., 5.

6. M.M. to Eichberg administration, May 4, 1929. LWV-Eichberg, PF M.M., 1.

7. Memo, April 1921. KBoN, PF A.R., 24.

8. Winnetal Directorate to the Württemberg Ministry of the Interior, September 8, 1930. Hauptstaatsarchiv Stuttgart, E 151 KVII, 6390, 74b–74d. He did not specify which jobs he had in mind, but women who nursed in psychiatry also often had histories of working as domestic help or shop assistants.

9. Whether and to what extent women were *forced* to leave because of marriage is not clear even in Steppe's work. She writes, "Thus the union reported in 1929 that the last marriage ban for independent nurses had been lifted—which can mean only that up until that time there were still marriage bans" ("Pflege bis 1933," 41).

10. G.R., "Gespräch zwischen Pflegerin und Bäuerin," *DI* 23 (May 1919): 30.

11. File note, May 27, 1931. KBoN, PF E.G., 87.

12. Wittenau Directorate to the Office of the Mayor, May 27, 1931. KBoN, PF E.G., 88.

13. Memo from House 10, November 1930. KBoN, PF E.G., 78.

14. Wittenau Directorate to the Office of the Mayor, May 27, 1931. KBoN, PF E.G., 88.

15. File note, June 15, 1931. KBoN, PF E.G., 87; and head doctor to the Directorate, September 17, 1931. KBoN, PF E.G., 90.

16. Wittenau's involvement in her personal affairs is to be explained by the fact that, as a general rule, institutions constituted part of the adminis-trative network providing outside financial support for employees with children. For example, they partook in arranging child subsidies (*Kinder-beihilfe*); they periodically had to verify how many eligible children a nurse had, whether the children were (still) in school or training programs, and so forth.

17. District Welfare Association (*Bezirksfürsorgeverband*), Ofthavelland, to Wittenau, October 1930; and Nurse R.'s response, November 1930. KBoN, PF A.R., 117 and 118 respectively.

18. Nurse A.R. to the Berlin Municipal Authorities, January 20, 1936. KBoN, PF A.R., 222. See also 165 ff.

19. File note, October 1931. KBoN, PF A.R., 134.

20. P.Z. to the Directorate of the Herzberge Institution, August 1930. KBoN, PF P.Z., 121.

21. P.Z. to the Directorate of the Herzberge Institution, September 10, 1930. KBoN, PF P.Z., 123.

22. Accident report, August 1, 1930. KBoN, PF P.Z., 135.

23. P.Z. to the Directorate of the Herzberge Institution, September 10, 1930. KBoN, PF P.Z., 123.

24. Complaint to the head of the local government (*Landeshauptmann*) in Wiesbaden, November 6, 1922. LWV-Eichberg, PF P.S., 25.

25. Landeshauptmann in Nassau to the Rhein District Shoemakers' Guild, March 28, 1927. LWV-Eichberg, PF H.D., 64.

26. Statement, Nurse K., February 11, 1919. LWV-Eichberg, PF J.M., 41.

27. Statement, Nurse M., February 1919. LWV-Eichberg, PF J.M., 41.

28. Ibid., 42.

29. Statements, Nurses Ku., M., B., and T., February 1919. LWV-Eichberg, PF J.M., 43.

30. Statement, Dr. W., February 1919. LWV-Eichberg, PF J.M., 44.

31. Report, Senior Nurse B., September 3, 1928. KBoN, PF F.B., 27. It appears that the documents of Berlin nurses' employment were kept in a single file that was maintained by the institution in which they worked and accompanied them if they changed institutions. Thus the documentation of Nurse B.'s earlier employment at Berlin-Buch was kept with his Wittenau file, since this is the last place where he worked.

32. Hearing, Nurse K., September 12, 1928. KBoN, PF F.B., 29.

33. Hearing, Nurse B., September 11, 1928. KBoN, PF F.B., 28.

34. Hearing, Nurse B., October 8, 1928. KBoN, PF F.B., 31.

35. Ibid.

36. Hearing, Senior Nurse B., October 8 or 9, 1928. KBoN, PF F.B., 31 and 32.

37. Hearing, Senior Nurse B., September 11, 1928. KBoN, PF F.B., 28.

38. Hearing, Nurse K., September 12, 1928. KBoN, PF F.B., 29.

39. Instruction, October 8, 1928. KBoN, PF F.B., 31.

40. Statement of Nurse S. (minutes of the meeting of the salaried employees committee), November 24, 1926. LA Berlin, A Rep. 003-04-1, no. 77, 4–5.

41. Ibid., 5.

42. Ibid., 5–6.

43. Statement of committee (minutes of the meeting of the salaried employees committee), November 24, 1926. LA Berlin, A Rep. 003-04-1, no. 77, 9.

44. Hearing, salaried employees committee, December 15, 1926. LA Berlin, A Rep. 003-04-1, no. 77, 16–19.

45. Staff council member M. to Berlin-Buch Directorate, December 30, 1926. LA Berlin, A Rep. 003-04-1, no. 77, 28.

46. Dr. S. to staff council member M., December 31, 1926. LA Berlin, A Rep. 003-04-1, no. 77, 28.

47. The records are unfortunately unclear regarding the fate of Siebert and her colleague, although a statement from the Berlin-Buch administration to the Berlin deputation for health care suggests that it accepted the position of the employees committee, which rejected their dismissal on the basis of insufficient proof (Drs. W. and K. to the Deptutation for Health Services, January 10, 1927. LA Berlin, A Rep. 003-04-1, no. 77, 40–42).

48. Minutes of the meeting of the salaried employees committee, May 3, 1930. LA Berlin, A Rep. 003-04-1, no. 77, 90–91.

49. Ibid., 95–96.

50. Minutes of the staff council meeting, June 27, 1930. LA Berlin, A Rep. 003-04-1, no. 77, 164.

51. Ibid., 176.

52. Dr. M.'s response to staff council minutes, July 16, 1930. LA Berlin, A Rep. 003-04-1, no. 77, 133.

53. Chief city medical officer of health Dr. W., response to staff council minutes, December 20, 1930. LA Berlin, A Rep. 003-04-1, no. 77, 191.

54. Dr. V. (Berlin Municipal Authorities) to chairman of the staff council, March 24, 1931. LA Berlin, A Rep. 003-04-1, no. 77, 194.

55. Report of chief doctor, July 1932. KBoN, PF A.W., 72.

56. Congratulatory note, May 1943 and absentee slip, October 22, 1943. KBoN, PF A.W., 109 and 110 respectively.

57. Hearing, District Court, April 16, 1931. LWV-Eichberg, PF G.B., 13.

58. Ibid.

59. District attorney (*Oberstaatsanwalt*) to Eichberg, May 22, 1931. LWV-Eichberg, PF G.B., 11.

60. Landeshauptmann in Nassau to Eichberg, May 23, 1931. LWV-Eichberg, PF G.B., 12.

61. Certificate, Nurse G.B., March 31, 1947. LWV-Eichberg, PF G.B., unnumbered page.

62. Dr. W., August 25, 1921. LWV-Eichberg, PF J.M., 59–60.

63. KBoN, PF H.M., 33, 51–54.

64. A patient accused her of striking her and producing a bruise on her backside. Although the patient without explanation withdrew the accusation, Meyer said that perhaps the patient had hit herself on the iron railing of the bedside as she moved her to change the bed (Reports of Drs. D. and R., October 13, 1925. KBoN, PF H.M., 61).

65. Letter of Patient C. to her parents, undated. KBoN, PF H.M., Subfile "Kündigung der Pflegerin H.M.," 19.

66. Report of Dr. P, April 30, 1931. KBoN, PF H.M., Subfile, 19.

67. Statements of Patients P., Ma., K., C., and Mu., April 30, 1931. KBoN, PF H.M., Subfile, 19–21.

68. Statement of Patient L., May 4, 1931. KBoN, PF H.M., Subfile, 22–23.

69. Proposal of Dr. R., May 21, 1931. KBoN, PF H.M., Subfile, 24.

70. Statement of Nurse H.M., May 2, 1931. KBoN, PF H.M., Subfile, 21–22.

71. Proposal of Dr. R., May 21, 1931. KBoN, PF H.M., Subfile, 24.

72. Statement of salaried employees committee, June 8, 1931, and response of Wittenau (authored by Dr. R.), July 13, 1931. KBoN, PF H.M., 123 and 99 respectively.

73. Hearing report, September 29, 1931, and instruction of senior civil servant D., October 3, 1931. KBoN, PF H.M., 134 and 135 respectively.

74. H.M. to the mayor of Berlin, October 11, 1931. KBoN, PF H.M., 136.

75. Explanation of decision, labor court, November 4, 1931. KBoN, PF H.M., 140.

76. Lawyer Dr. B. to the district labor court, December 31, 1931. KBoN, PF H.M., 149.

77. Record of proceedings, district labor court, January 4, 1932, and note on reverse side by the wage contract office. KBoN, PF H.M., 154.

78. H.M. to the Wittenau Directorate, June 3, 1932. KBoN, PF H.M., 155–156.

79. File note, Dr. P., June 6, 1932, and Wittenau Directorate to H.M., June 8, 1932. KBoN, PF H.M., 157 and 158 respectively.

80. H.M. to the Wittenau Directorate, June 14, 1932. KBoN, PF H.M., 159.

81. Director to H.M., June 17, 1932. KBoN, PF H.M., 161.

CHAPTER 5
CLEANING HOUSE IN WITTENAU

1. Founded in the late 1920s, the NSBO evolved into what Martin Broszat calls a "party formation with certain trade union characteristics." Before 1933, it functioned as an organ for anti-Marxist, anticapitalist propaganda and for the organization of Nazi workers (Martin Broszat, *Hitler and the Collapse of Weimar Germany*, trans. V. R. Berghahn [New York, 1987], 66). He writes that the NSBO was founded in 1928, while Karl-Dietrich Bracher states that it was 1929 (*Die deutsche Diktatur* [Cologne, 1969], 236).

2. Gordon Craig, *Germany, 1866–1945* (New York, 1978), 579. For a useful summary in English of the scope and implementation of the law, see

Jane Caplan, *Government without Administration: State and Civil Service in Weimar and Nazi Germany* (Oxford, 1988), 41–49.

3. Hans Mommsen, *Beamtentum im Dritten Reich* (Stuttgart, 1966), 39. The decree stated in §15 that "the regulations for civil servants are to be applied correspondingly to salaried employees and workers" ("Gesetz zur Wiederherstellung des Berufsbeamtentums," *Reichsgesetzblatt*, part 1, no. 34 [April 7, 1933]: 177). Paragraph 1 of the Second Implementation Ordinance defined eligible salaried employees and workers as "persons who are or have been in public service to the Reich, states, communities, and communal associations" ("Zweite Verordnung zur Durchführung des Gesetzes zur Wiederherrstellung des Berufsbeamtentums," *Reichsgesetzblatt*, no. 46 [May 4, 1933]: 233).

4. For example, the decree affected so many employees of the rail and postal services that, despite high unemployment, their continued function would be threatened by rigorous enforcement (Mommsen, *Beamtentum im Dritten Reich*, 53).

5. Ibid., 21–22, 46, 52–53, 58–59. See also "Dritte Verordnung zur Durchführung des Gesetzes zur Wiederherrstellung des Berufsbeamtentums. Vom 6. Mai 1933," *Reichsgesetzblatt*, no. 48 (May 6, 1933): 248.

6. Karl-Dietrich Bracher, Wolfgang Sauer, and Gerhard Schulz, *Die nationalsozialistische Machtergreifung: Studien zur Errichtung des totalitären Herrschaftssystems in Deutschland, 1933/34* (Cologne and Opladen, 1960), 508.

7. There are no reliable statistics on the number of nurses employed at Wittenau for any year other than 1937, when the figure was 447 nurses for 1,783 patients (not including those in family care). Four years earlier, there were only 1,600 patients but presumably more funding for personnel; thus it is not necessarily the case that the number of nurses was correspondingly lower. I have provided a broad estimate here simply to give the reader an idea of the proportions in question. (Statistics from Norbert Emmerich, "Die Wittenauer Heilstätten, 1933–1945," in Arbeitsgruppe, *Totgeschwiegen*, 77 and 90. See also Marianne Hühn, "Psychiatrie im Nationalsozialismus am Beispiel der Wittenauer Heilstätten," in *Aktion T4, 1939–1945: Die "Euthanasie"-Zentrale in der Tiergartenstraße 4*, ed. Götz Aly [Berlin, 1989], 186.)

8. Seventy-six nurses were dismissed out of a total of 643 male and non-civil-servant female nurses. Owing to the absence of civil-servant female nurses in the latter figure, the dismissal rate must be considered approximate (LA Berlin, A Rep. 003-04-1, no. 23 [Verwaltungsberichte], 129 and 151).

9. Faulstich, *Von der Irrenfürsorge zur "Euthanasie"*, 146. He reports that in 1933, the institution had 578 patients, and that same year a ministerial decree reduced the nurse-patient ratio to 1:5.5 patients. (In 1930 the ratio

had been 1:3.8.) Since approximately 60 nurses total would have been the *end* result of the decree's implementation, the figure must be considered a minimum (*Von der Irrenfürsorge zur "Euthanasie"*, 160 [table 4], 165, and 156).

10. Sonja Schröter, "Psychiatrie in Waldheim/Sachsen von ihren Anfängen bis zum Ende des zweiten Weltkrieges (1716–1946): Ein Beitrag zur Geschichte der forensischen Psychiatrie in Deutschland" (Med. diss., University of Leipzig, 1993), 104.

11. Indeed, the case of Wittenau, combined with a systematic analysis of nurse dismissals in the rest of Prussia, would perhaps corroborate Mommsen's observation that BBG dismissal rates were higher in Prussia (*Beamtentum im Dritten Reich*, 56).

12. Emmerich, "Die Wittenauer Heilstätten,"in Arbeitsgruppe, *Totgeschwiegen*, 87.

13. Personnel files H.T. and A.J. (KBoN) provide examples.

14. See, for example, KBoN, PF H.T.

15. The form was printed in the *Reichsgesetzblatt*, no. 48 (May 6, 1933): 253–256.

16. "Fragebogen gemäß Anordnung des Staatskommissars in der Hauptstadt Berlin vom 8. August 1933." See, for example, KBoN, PF F.B.

17. Ibid.

18. See Mommsen, *Beamtentum im Dritten Reich*, 53, and the "Drittes Gesetz zur Änderung des Gesetzes zur Wiederherstellung des Berufsbeamtentums," *Reichsgesetzblatt*, no. 104 (September 23, 1933): 655.

19. "Gesetz zur Wiederherstellung des Berufsbeamtentums," *Reichsgesetzblatt*, no. 34 (April 7, 1933): 175.

20. Mommsen, *Beamtentum im Dritten Reich*, 47.

21. "Erste Verordnung zur Durchführung des Gesetzes zur Wiederherstellung des Berufsbeamtentums," *Reichsgesetzblatt*, no. 37 (April 11, 1933): 195.

22. "Zweite Verordnung zur Durchführung des Gesetzes zur Wiederherstellung des Berufsbeamtentums," *Reichsgesetzblatt*, no. 46 (May 4, 1933): 233.

23. "Zweite Verordnung zur Änderung und Ergänzung der zweiten Verordung zur Durchführung des Gesetzes zur Wiederherrstellung des Berufsbeamtentums," *Reichsgesetzblatt*, no. 107 (September 28, 1933): 678. That Braasch was aware of this is indicated by his letter to the Main Health Office (HGA), July 28, 1933. KBoN, PF F.B., 105.

24. Appended page, BBG questionnaire, July 8, 1933. KBoN, PF F.B., 110.

25. Ibid., 110.

26. Braasch to the HGA, October 14, 1933. KBoN, PF F.B., 123.

27. BBG supplemental questionnaire, August 1933. KBoN, PF R.W., 105.

28. R.W. to the Wittenauer Heilstätten, September 1933. KBON, PF R.W., 109.

29. File note of mayor, September 1933. KBoN, PF R.W., 114.

30. BBG dismissal proposal, September 7, 1933. KBoN, PF R.W., 113.

31. File note of mayor, September 1933. KBoN, PF R.W., 114.

32. Office of the Prussian chief minister to R.W., April 1934. KBoN, PF R.W., 124a. Also, Braasch to the HGA, January 1934, and mayor to the provincial governor (*Oberpräsident*), January 26, 1934.

33. BBG questionnaire, July 17, 1933. KBoN, PF P.W., 78.

34. File note, January 5, 1934. KBoN, PF P.W., 92.

35. Employee questionnaire and statement, February 25, 1922. KBoN, PF A.J., 1 and 8 respectively.

36. Mayor to Nurse A.J., April 15, 1933. KBoN, PF A.J., 60.

37. Statement from the Wittenau NSBO, May 12, 1933. KBoN, PF A.J., 63.

38. Hearing, Herr S. August 2, 1933. KBoN, PF A.J., 67.

39. "Zweite Verordnung zur Durchführung des Gesetzes zur Wiederherstellung des Berufsbeamtentums," *Reichsgesetzblatt*, no. 46 (May 4, 1933): 234.

40. Employee questionnaire, January 2, 1929. KBoN, PF E.M., née J., 2.

41. File note, February 10, 1932. KBoN, PF E.M., née J., 36.

42. E.M. to Wittenau administration, March 24, 1932. KBoN, PF E.M., née J., 40.

43. Wittenau to E.M., April 15, 1933. KBoN, PF E.M., née J., 49.

44. Memos to E.M. from the mayor on March 25, 1933 and May 2, 1933, and a file note, April 24, 1933. KBoN, PF E.M., née J., 48, 52, and 51 respectively.

45. Supplemental questionnaire, August 17, 1933. KBoN, PF E.M., née J., 57.

46. Protocol, cleaning woman S., September 6, 1933. KBoN, PF E.M., née J., 61. My italics. It is tempting to speculate that the administration, already having its "suspicion" but no proof of Macher's hostility toward National Socialism, had engaged S. in a bit of detective work and instructed her to keep her ear cocked for precisely this kind of exchange. L. would later report in her account of the course of events that she had been alone with Macher until S. entered the room and joined the conversation (Hearing, September 9, 1933. KBoN, PF E.M., née J., 63).

47. Hearing, September 8, 1933. KBoN, PF E.M., née J., 62.

48. Hearing, September 9, 1933, and September 12, 1933. KBoN, PF E.M., née J., 63 and 64 respectively.

49. BBG §4 dismissal form, September 15, 1933. KBoN, PF E.M., née J., 65.

50. Instruction, autumn 1933. KBoN, PF E.M., née J., 73.

51. Office of the Mayor to H.T., April 15, 1933. See also Office of the Mayor to H.T., March 25, 1933. KBoN, PF H.T., 131 and 132 respectively.

52. H.T. to senior civil servant P., with the request to forward to State Commissioner E., April 23, 1933. KBoN, PF H.T., 135.

53. Supplemental questionnaire, August 21, 1933. KBoN, PF H.T., 141. There is no evidence in the file concerning whether these references were checked.

54. Braasch to the HGA, September 5, 1933. KBoN, PF H.T.

55. Hearing, September 23, 1933. KBoN, PF H.T., 146.

56. Certificate, October 20, 1933. KBoN, PF H.T., 153.

57. Office of the Mayor, January 1934. KBoN, PF H.T., 177.

58. Hearing, January 25, 1934. KBoN, PF H.T., 169.

59. Ibid. This is very likely a reference to the Reichstag fire of February 27.

60. See Robert Gellately, "Denunciations in Twentieth-Century Germany: Aspects of Self-Policing in the Third Reich and the German Democratic Republic," and John Connelly, "The Uses of *Volksgemeinschaft*: Letters to the NSDAP Kreisleitung Eisenach, 1939–1940," both in *Accusatory Practices: Denunciation in Modern European History, 1789–1989*, ed. Sheila Fitzpatrick and Robert Gellately (Chicago and London, 1997); and Gisela Diewald-Kerkmann, *Politische Denunziation im NS-Regime oder Die kleine Macht der "Volksgenossen"* (Bonn, 1995).

61. Although it is difficult to determine how widespread this kind of administrative mercy was, an example from the Rheinland supports the argument at hand. A senior doctor and the NSBO representative defended two former SPD members with the following explanation: "As both of them explained to me, they looked after the economic interests of the SPD but were not active in a Marxist sense. It is of course true that they were signed up as members of the SPD until March, but then they signed off because they were convinced that the workers had been lied to and deceived" (Heinrich Graf, "Die Situation der Patienten und des Pflegepersonales der rheinischen Heil- und Pflegeanstalten in der Zeit des Nationalsozialismus," in *Verlegt nach unbekannt: Sterilisation und Euthanasie in Galkausen, 1933–1945*, ed. Matthias Leipert, Rudolf Styrnal, and Winfried Schwarzer [Cologne, 1987], 42–43).

62. Declaration, BBG questionnaire of Nurse J.L., August 19, 1933. KBoN, PF J.L., 172.

63. Declaration under oath, February 14, 1933. KBoN, PF J.L., 174.

64. Report, senior nurse, and instruction, Braasch, September 14, 1933. KBoN, PF J.L., 170.

65. Head doctor to Braasch, October 27, 1933. KBoN, PF J.L., 170.

66. "Zweite Verordnung zur Durchführung des Gesetzes zur Wieder-herrstellung des Berufsbeamtentums," *Reichsgesetzblatt*, no. 46 (May 4, 1933): 234. My Italics. According to Mommsen, "The proviso that such positions could not filled again was in a number of cases circumvented" (*Beamtentum im Dritten Reich*, 50).

67. BBG questionnaires. KBoN, PF M.W., 72 and 77.

68. BBG dismissal, September 13, 1933. KBoN, PF M.W., 75.

69. File note, September 20, 1933. KBoN, PF M.W., 77.

70. Ibid., 77.

71. Ibid., 78. Although the mayoral official voiced the intention in his protest to uphold his earlier decision to have her dismissed on the basis of contractual terms rather than the BBG, Wittenau wrote to the Labor Office in December 1935 about Weinz's financial difficulties and asserted therein that she had been dismissed on the basis of §6.

72. Statement, NSBO representative, August 1933. KBoN, PF I.R., 131.

73. File note, Office of the Mayor, September 20, 1933. KBoN, PF I.R., 140.

74. Statement, Dr. Lippert, September 28, 1933. KBoN, PF I.R., 140.

75. Notice (*Kündigung*), October 5, 1933, and certificate, March 31, 1934. KBoN, PF I.R., 141 and 163 respectively.

76. Employee questionnaire, undated (but format indicates it predates 1933). KBoN, PF E.M., née T., unnumbered first document at front of file.

77. File note, April 10, 1931. KBoN, PF E.M., née T., 101.

78. BBG questionnaire. KBoN, PF E.M., née T., 126.

79. Report, Senior Nurse B., September 14, 1933. KBoN, PF E.M., née T., 128.

80. BBG §6 dismissal form, September 14, 1933. KBoN, PF E.M., née T., 129.

81. File note, November 1933. KBoN, PF E.M., née T., 138.

82. Supplemental questionnaire, September 5, 1933. KBoN, PF A.R., 172.

83. BBG dismissal, September 14, 1933. KBoN, PF A.R., 174.

84. Memo, August 1920. KBoN, PF A.R., 9.

85. Report, June 1933. KBoN, PF A.R., 161.

86. A.R. to Wittenau Directorate, June 19, 1934. KBoN, PF A.R., 187–188.

87. File notes of city inspector and head doctor, June 25, 1934. Instruction, Braasch, July 6, 1934. KBoN, PF A.R., 188 and 189 respectively.

88. Police report, July 19, 1934. KBoN, PF A.R., 196.

89. File note, July 24, 1935. KBoN, PF A.R., 189.

90. A.R. to the Berlin Municipal Authorities, January 20, 1936. KBoN, PF A.R., 222.

91. Ibid., 222.

92. Office of the Mayor to A.R., March 6, 1936; A.R. to the Berlin Municipal Authorities, July 6, 1938; and Braasch to A.R., July 25, 1938. KBoN, PF A.R., unnumbered documents.

93. Report of Herzberge Directorate, February 13, 1936. KBoN, PF A.R., 226.

94. Bracher, *Die deutsche Diktatur*, 234.

95. Minister of the interior to E.M., April 1, 1935. KBoN, PF E.M., née J., 74.

CHAPTER 6
REEDUCATING NURSES IN THE SPIRIT OF THE TIMES

1. Excerpt from Hermann Groß, *Die Irrenanstalten zugleich als Heilanstalten betrachtet* (Kassel, 1832), quoted in *Geisteskrankenpflege* 37 (November 1933): 175.

2. Gaupp, "Das Gesetz zur Verhütung erbkranken Nachwuchses und die Psychiatrie," *Klinische Wochenschrift* 13 (1934): 1, quoted in Gisela Bock, *Zwangssterilisation im Nationalsozialismus: Studien zur Rassenpolitik und Frauenpolitik* (Opladen, 1986), 192.

3. Bruno Steinwallner, "Geplante Zulassung der Sterbehilfe in England," *PNW* 38 (November 14, 1936): 583–584.

4. For a more detailed description, see Burleigh, *Death and Deliverance*, 43–46.

5. *Die Rheinprovinz* 12 (1936): 409 ff., quoted in Graf, "Die Situation der Patienten und des Pflegepersonales," 45.

6. Burleigh, *Death and Deliverance*, 43, and Bock, *Zwangssterilisation im Nationalsozialismus*, 195.

7. Dr. Grimme, "Ein Fehler in der Ausbildung für die allgemeine Krankenpflege," *PNW* 38 (August 8, 1936): 392–393.

8. Party Member Götzinger, "Stätten des Grauens: Besuch in fränkischen Pflegeanstalten für Erbkranke—Die Bedeutung der Erbgesundheitsgesetze in Bild und Wort," *Fränkische Zeitung* (Nuremberg), no. 269 (November 17, 1935). Archiv des Diakonischen Werkes der evangelischen Kirche Deutschlands (Berlin), CA, G-S 48. Emphasis in original.

9. Ibid.

10. Ibid.

11. *Neues Volk*, no. 2, 1934, reprinted in *Krankenpflege im Nationalsozialismus*, ed. Hilde Steppe, 5th ed. (Frankfurt, 1989), 66.

12. Grimme, "Ein Fehler in der Ausbildung," 393.

13. Liselotte Katscher, *Krankenpflege und "Drittes Reich": Der Weg der Schwesternschaft des Evangelischen Diakonievereins, 1933–1939* (Stuttgart, 1990), 166, and Graf, "Die Situation der Patienten und des Pflegepersonales," 47.

14. Siemen, *Menschen blieben auf der Strecke*, 143.

15. See ibid.; Burleigh, *Death and Deliverance*, 61, and Bock, *Zwangssterilisation im Nationalsozialismus*, 260.

16. Bock, *Zwangssterilisation im Nationalsozialismus*, 259 and 262.

17. Siemen, *Menschen blieben auf der Strecke*, 143.

18. Archiv des Landschaftsverbands Rheinland, Pulheim-Brauweiler, Graf Collection, interview with former patient J., quoted in Graf, "Die Situation der Patienten und des Pflegepersonales," 44.

19. Bock, *Zwangssterilisation im Nationalsozialismus*, 269–271.

20. "Bericht über die Durchführung des Gesetzes zur Verhütung erbkranken Nachwuchses (Württemberg)," September 30, 1934. Hauptstaatsarchiv Stuttgart, E151K VII 1020 II, Doc. 34.

21. Bock, *Zwangssterilisation im Nationalsozialismus*, 272.

22. Ibid., 271–272. Obviously, this kind of opportunism did not always prevail. To cite just one example, a chief medical official reported in late 1934 that one institutional director had refused to report a case of mental deficiency for reasons of conscience ("Bericht über die Durchführung des Gesetzes zur Verhütung erbkranken Nachwuchses [Württemberg]," October 10, 1934. Hauptstaatsarchiv Stuttgart, E151K VII 1020 II, Doc. 34C). Moral reservations of psychiatrists were dismissed by Party propaganda as "uncalled-for mawkishness (sentimentality), sentimental humanitarianism [*Humanitätsduselei*], or feminine instincts" (Bock, *Zwangssterilisation im Nationalsozialismus*, 293).

23. Burleigh, *Death and Deliverance*, 56–61.

24. Bock, *Zwangssterilisation im Nationalsozialismus*, 260.

25. Ibid., 274.

26. Burleigh, *Death and Deliverance*, 56.

27. Joachim E. Meyer, "Psychiatrie im Nationalsozialismus," in *Dienstbare Medizin: Ärzte betrachten ihr Fach im Nationalsozialismus*, ed. H. Friedrich and W. Matzow (Göttingen, 1992), 45.

28. Bock, *Zwangssterilisation im Nationalsozialismus*, 284.

29. Ibid., 282–283.

30. Ibid., 284.

31. Dr. Enge, "Das Gesetz zur Verhütung erbkranken Nachwuchses in Laienbetrachtung und ärztliche Erfahrungen als Gutachter im Erbgesundheitsverfahren," *PNW* 39 (January 2, 1937): 8.

32. Siemen, *Menschen blieben auf der Strecke*, 144–146.

33. Hans-Walter Schmuhl, "Kontinuität oder Diskontinuität? Zum epochalen Charakter der Psychiatrie im Nationalsozialismus," in *Nach Hadamar: Zum Verhältnis von Psychiatrie und Gesellschaft im 20. Jahrhundert*, ed. Franz-Werner Kersting, Karl Teppe, and Bernd Walter (Paderborn, 1993), 119. For statistical information on the Reich as a whole and the Erlangen institution in particular, see Siemen, *Menschen blieben auf der Strecke*, 146 ff.

On Hesse, see Burleigh, *Death and Deliverance*, 49–50; on the Rheinland, see Graf, "Die Situation der Patienten und des Pflegepersonales," 46.

34. Heinz Faulstich has pointed out that at the institute near Konstanz, this state of affairs correlated with higher death rates from tuberculosis in the 1930s: only one patient died of tuberculosis in 1931, the last year before major reductions. Nine died in 1934; and in each of the years 1937 and 1938, ten died (*Von der Irrenfürsorge zur "Euthanasie"*, 171).

35. Horst Dickel, "Alltag in einer Landesheilanstalt im Nationalsozialismus: Das Beispiel Eichberg," in *Euthanasie in Hadamar: Die nationalsozialistische Vernichtungspolitik in hessischen Anstalten*, ed. Landeswohlfahrtsverband Hessen (Kassel, 1991), 106.

36. Administrator Sack, "Die Heil- und Pflegeanstalten, ihre wirtschaftlichen, finanziellen und sonstigen Verhältnisse," part 1, *PNW* 40 (May 27, 1938): 247–248.

37. Archiv des Landschaftsverbandes Rheinland, Graf Collection, interview with the witness J., quoted in Graf, "Die Situation der Patienten und des Pflegepersonales," 48.

38. Monika Daum, "Arbeit und Zwang, das Leben der Hadamarer Patienten im Schatten des Todes," in *Psychiatrie im Faschismus: Die Anstalt Hadamar, 1933–1945*, ed. Dorothee Roer and Dieter Henkel (Bonn, 1986), 187.

39. Siemen reports that German psychiatrists remained skeptical until 1935 (*Menschen blieben auf der Strecke*, 154).

40. Burleigh, *Death and Deliverance*, 85–88.

41. Emmerich, "Die Wittenauer Heilstätten," in Arbeitsgruppe, *Totgeschwiegen*, 84.

42. Siemen, *Menschen blieben auf der Strecke*, 156.

43. Burleigh, *Death and Deliverance*, 84.

44. Siemen, *Menschen blieben auf der Strecke*, 156, and Emmerich, "Die Wittenauer Heilstätten," in Arbeitsgruppe, *Totgeschwiegen*, 84.

45. Siemen, *Menschen blieben auf der Strecke*, 159 and 184.

46. Ibid., 158.

47. Ibid., 159.

48. Burleigh, *Death and Deliverance*, 89, and Siemen, *Menschen blieben auf der Strecke*, 156–157, 160–161.

49. Administrator Sack, "Die Heil- und Pflegeanstalten, ihre wirtschaftlichen, finanziellen und sonstigen Verhältnisse," part 2, *PNW* 40 (June 4, 1938): 257.

50. Peter Stolz, "Die Rolle der Irrenanstalten im Faschisierungsprozeß der deutschen Psychiatrie," *Recht und Psychiatrie*, no. 2 (1983): 66.

51. Dr. Enge, "Welchen Irrtümern und Mißverständnissen begegnet man bei Laien über die Erbpflegegesetze?" *Geisteskrankenpflege* 42 (March 1938): 34. For a similar position, see Sack, part 2, 258.

52. Enge, "Irrtümern und Mißverständnissen," 34.

53. Dr. Wittneben, "Erziehung, Behandlung und Pflege Geistes-schwacher," *Geisteskrankenpflege* 38 (October 1934): 146.

54. Dr. med. Hans Hoffmann, "Die Sterilisierung (Unfruchtbarma-chung) Minderwertiger aus eugenischen Gründen," *Geisteskrankenpflege* 37 (October 1933): 157.

55. Nurse Georg Roos, "Aus der Praxis eines Pflegers für Geistes-kranke," *Geisteskrankenpflege* 41 (July 1937): 110.

56. Nurse Georg Roos, "Beziehung des Krankenpflegers zum Arzt," *Geisteskrankenpflege* 41 (December 1937): 180–181.

57. Ibid., 181.

58. Chief medical officer of health Dr. Reimann, "Einige Ausführungen über den Beruf eines Geisteskrankenpflegers," *Geisteskrankenpflege* 41 (August 1937): 123.

59. Nurse W. Philippi, "Ein Pfleger für Geisteskranke schildert seinen Beruf," *Geisteskrankenpflege* 40 (May 1936): 78.

60. Reimann, "Einige Ausführungen," 121.

61. Senior Nurse Muth, "Einige Hinweise für den Dienst," *Geisteskran-kenpflege* 39 (August 1935): 118. The motto "Put yourself in his place!" was a common one in nursing textbooks. See Ludwig Scholz, *Leitfaden für Irren-pfleger*, 23d ed. (Halle a. S., 1935), 5, and Nurse Karin Neuman-Rahn, *Der seelisch kranke Mensch und seine Pflege* (Jena, 1939), 140.

62. Nurse Lutz Wilms, "Die Pflege des Geistes in der Geisteskranken-pflege," *Geisteskrankenpflege* 43 (August 1939): 121.

63. Deacon W. Thielmann, "Der Pfleger und der Kranke," *Geisteskran-kenpflege* 41 (January 1937): 11.

64. Dr. med. Bruckner, "Als Patient in einer Heil- und Pflegeanstalt," *Geisteskrankenpflege* 39 (May 1935): 76.

65. Wittneben, "Erziehung, Behandlung und Pflege Geistesschwacher," 153, and Dr. med. Gustav Donalies, "Die Verhütung des Selbstmordes in der Anstalt," *Geisteskrankenpflege* 38 (June 1934): 86.

66. The following discussion is based on the journal *Geisteskrankenpflege*, but Dr. Valentin Faltlhauser's *Geisteskrankenpflege: Ein Lehr- und Handbuch für Irrenpfleger* (Halle a. S., 1939) contains the same points.

67. Dr. Wickel, "Der Umgang mit Geisteskranken, ihre Beobachtung und Pflege," *Geisteskrankenpflege* 39 (October 1935): 151.

68. Dr. Ferdinand Hürten, "Das Bewahrhaus unter besonderer Berück-sichtigung der Diestaufgaben des Pflegepersonals," *Geisteskrankenpflege* 40 (March 1936): 42.

69. Nurse Clemens Köhler, "Die Pflege der geisteskranken Rechts-brecher," *Geisteskrankenpflege* 41 (September 1937): 130.

70. Nurse Albert Erbe, "Schwachsinnige, ihr Leiden und ihre Behand-lung durch den Pfleger," *Geisteskrankenpflege* 42 (July 1938): 106.

71. Roos, "Aus der Praxis," 109.

72. Wickel, "Der Umgang mit Geisteskranken," 151.

73. Arms should be kept at the patient's back so that they could not get caught on the edge of the bed and break. The nurse holding the patient's head was not to exert pressure on the ears for fear of injury. If, when deposited in isolation, the patient attempted to escape as the nurse left, the latter was to take care to avoid slamming the patient's fingers in the door (ibid., 152).

74. Ibid. Lest it be thought that this was an unusual argument during the 1930s, it should be pointed out that Dr. Schulze-Bünte of Berlin's Herzberge institution entertained similar notions, emphasizing the importance of prevention and nipping disputes in the bud with calm, verbal methods of distraction. "Also here, the use of force is to be avoided as much as possible." He also regarded isolation as a last resort and understood its purpose as one of allowing a patient time "to think about himself and to calm down again" ("Über die Gestaltung der Freizeit in den Heilanstalten," *Geisteskrankenpflege* 43 [September 1939]: 131–132).

75. Dr. M. Kesselring, "Die Bedeutung und Pflege des geistigen Lebens in der Anstalt," *Geisteskrankenpflege* 39 (December 1935): 185.

76. Dr. med. Erwin Bücken, "Die gerichtliche Unterbringung von Geisteskranken in Heilanstalten," *Geisteskrankenpflege* 44 (February 1940): 12.

77. Nurse Heinrich Becker, "Einiges zur Pflege unserer Kranken," *Geisteskrankenpflege* 41 (June 1937): 92.

78. Dr. Enge, "Beobachtungsberichte des Pflegepersonals," *Geisteskrankenpflege* 37 (August 1933): 113.

79. Erbe, "Schwachsinnige," 106.

80. Dr. R. Spaar, "Das Gesetz zur Verhütung erbkranken Nachwuchses vom 14. Juli 1933," *Geisteskrankenpflege* 38 (April 1934): 55–56.

81. Roos, "Aus der Praxis," 108.

82. Reimann, "Einige Ausführungen," 122.

83. Wickel, "Der Umgang mit Geisteskranken," 146.

84. Thielmann,"Der Pfleger und der Kranke," 11.

85. Wickel, "Der Umgang mit Geisteskranken," 147.

86. Roos, "Aus der Praxis," 108.

87. Wickel, "Der Umgang mit Geisteskranken," 145–146.

88. Philippi, "Ein Pfleger für Geisteskranke," 78–79.

89. Kesselring, "Bedeutung und Pflege des geistigen Lebens," 182.

90. Schulze-Bünte, "Über die Gestaltung der Freizeit," 131.

91. Ibid., 130–131.

92. Ibid., 135.

93. Becker, "Einiges zur Pflege unserer Kranken," 92. This nurse published an almost identical passage in an article written three years later, when it would certainly have offered any nurses involved in the T4 pro-

gram confirmation of the idea that they had a role to play in upholding life as well as in "facilitating" death ("Die Geisteskrankenpflege," *Geisteskrankenpflege* 44 [May 1940]: 51–52).

94. Wettlaufer, "Die Beteiligung von Schwestern und Pflegern an den Morden in Hadamar," 310. See also Angelika Ebbinghaus, "Kostensenkung, 'Aktive Therapie' und Vernichtung: Konsequenzen für das Anstaltswesen," in *Heilen und Vernichten im Mustergau Hamburg*, ed. Angelika Ebbinghaus, Heidrun Kaupen-Haas, and Karl-Heinz Roth (Hamburg, 1984), 140.

95. Nurse Clemens Köhler, "Der Kolonnenpfleger," *Geisteskrankenpflege* 42 (October 1938): 149.

96. Nurse Albert Erbe, "Auf was wird der Pfleger achten, wenn er einen Patienten zum Besucher bringt?" *Geisteskrankenpflege* 41 (June 1937): 90.

97. Siemen, *Menschen blieben auf der Strecke*, 162; Cornelia Hoser and Birgit Weber-Dickmann, "Zwangssterilisationen an Hadamarer Anstaltsinsassen," in *Psychiatrie im Faschismus: Die Anstalt Hadamar, 1933–1945*, ed. Dorothee Roer and Dieter Henkel (Bonn, 1986), 140.

98. Spaar, "Das Gesetz zur Verhütung erbkranken Nachwuchses," 45. For an almost identical formulation five years later, see Enge, ""Irrtümern und Mißverständnissen," 33.

99. Hoffmann, "Die Sterilisierung Minderwertiger," 148.

100. Medical Officer Dr. Snell, "Die Notwendigkeit der Steriliseriung der Erbkranken," *Geisteskrankenpflege* 43 (September 1939): 140.

101. Hoffmann, "Die Sterilisierung Minderwertiger," 149 and 158.

102. Ibid., 152–153.

103. Ibid., 155.

104. Ibid.

105. Ibid. See also Spaar, "Das Gesetz zur Verhütung erbkranken Nachwuchses," 51, and Enge, "Irrtümern und Mißverständnissen," 35.

106. Burleigh, *Death and Deliverance*, 57–58. Approximately five thousand people died in the aftermath of the procedure (0.1 percent of men and 0.5 percent of women sterilized) (Meyer, "Psychiatrie im Nationalsozialismus," 46). That the accompanying psychological trauma was very real and debilitating has been documented by Gisela Bock in *Zwangssterilisation im Nationalsozialismus*.

107. Hoffmann, "Die Sterilisierung Minderwertiger," 150.

108. City councilman H. Drechsler, *Aktenstaub*, quoted in Hoffmann, "Die Sterilisierung Minderwertiger," 151.

109. Hoffmann, "Die Sterilisierung Minderwertiger," 150–151. Nurses were not only treated to vivid portrayals of female decadence in their journal; they were also explicitly advised to regard their female patients as irresponsible and sexually promiscuous: "We know, for example, that

feebleminded girls in particular become pregnant outside the institution, and they require special supervision inside the institution as well" (Dr. R. Herrmann, "Geisteskrankenpfleger und Erbkunde," *Geisteskrankenpflege* 38 [February 1934]: 22).

110. Enge, "Irrtümern und Mißverständnissen," 35.

111. Ibid. For excerpts of similar propaganda directed at the public at large, see Bock, *Zwangssterilisation im Nationalsozialismus*, 282–283.

112. Wittneben, "Erziehung, Behandlung und Pflege Geistesschwacher," 153.

113. He recalled an episode in 1922, when a "feebleminded," mute woman lay dying of tuberculosis. On the day she died, Wittneben had entered her room to hear her clearly singing, "Where does the soul find its home, peace. . . . peace, peace, heavenly peace. . . ." She smiled briefly, and then "the soul vanished from the fetters of the body" (ibid.).

114. Ibid., 154.

115. Donalies, "Die Verhütung des Selbstmordes," 86.

116. Ibid.

117. Spaar, "Das Gesetz zur Verhütung erbkranken Nachwuchses," 50.

118. Herrmann, "Geisteskrankenpfleger und Erbkunde," 20.

119. Ibid., 21.

120. Spaar, "Das Gesetz zur Verhütung erbkranken Nachwuchses," 51.

121. Enge, "Beobachtungsberichte des Pflegepersonals," 114.

122. In addition, when nurses were accused of abuse during the doctor's visit, "one should remain completely calm and speak only at the request of the doctor" (Wickel, "Der Umgang mit Geisteskranken," 145).

123. Reimann, "Einige Ausführungen," 122. My italics.

124. Muth, "Einige Hinweise," 118–119.

125. Erbe, "Schwachsinnige," 106.

126. Wittneben, "Erziehung, Behandlung und Pflege Geistesschwacher," 150.

127. Ibid., 149.

128. Ibid., 150.

129. Erbe, "Schwachsinninge," 105. See also Roos, "Aus der Praxis," 110.

130. Erbe, "Schwachsinninge," 104.

131. Köhler, "Die Pflege der geisteskranken Rechtsbrecher," 131.

132. Wilms, "Die Pflege des Geistes," 121. See also Neumann-Rahn, *Der seelisch kranke Mensch und seine Pflege*, 144.

133. Köhler, "Der Kolonnenpfleger," 149.

134. Becker, "Die Geisteskrankenpflege," 50.

135. Kesselring, "Bedeutung und Pflege des geistigen Lebens," 180.

136. Ibid., 182.

137. Dr. Hürten, "Das Bewahrhaus," 43.

138. This idea that mental illness was not a sufficient "excuse" for deviant behavior was not limited to nursing texts. According to an administrator writing for the *PNW*, "it is generally acknowledged today that the mentally ill must learn to incorporate themselves into the working community *in spite of their mental disorder....*" Work was not a treatment aimed at the elimination of a particular illness but rather something to which patients were obligated regardless of that condition (Sack, "Die Heil- und Pflegeanstalten," part 1, 246; my italics).

139. Kesselring, "Bedeutung und Pflege des geistigen Lebens," 180.

140. Ibid., 184.

141. Ibid., 182.

142. Siemen has made a similar observation: "The Active Therapy of Simon ... became exclusively a means to unfold an almost terrorist therapy-dictatorship in the institutions.... The institution itself, which was also the place where the mentally ill person—indeed, in miserable conditions—could still be a little crazy, turned into a system that allowed the norms of society to become the guiding principle of daily life (*Menschen blieben auf der Strecke*, 152).

143. Kesselring, "Bedeutung und Pflege des geistigen Lebens," 182.

144. Hürten, "Das Bewahrhaus," 42. My italics.

145. Ibid.

146. Ibid., 43.

147. Ibid., 44.

148. Ibid., 44–45.

149. Bücken, "Die gerichtliche Unterbringung," 9.

150. Bücken pointed out that patients were not simply deposited in institutions by the courts; rather, every two to three years the court would review the patient's progress and consider release (ibid., 12).

151. See, for example, Senior Nurse W. Krause, "Der Pfleger bei der Außenarbeit," *Geisteskrankenpflege* 37 (July 1933): 100; Philippi, "Ein Pfleger für Geisteskranke," 79; and Reimann, "Einige Ausführungen," 122–123.

152. Prof. Dr. med. Jahrmärker, "Zu Fragen der Verantwortlichkeit in der psychiatrischen Praxis," *Geisteskrankenpflege* 47 (March 1943): 28. Italics in original.

153. Ibid., 29.

154. Senior civil servant Kühne, "Die wirtschaftlichen Aufgaben des Pflegepersonals im Kriege," *Geisteskrankenpflege* 47 (August 1943): 64.

155. Ibid., 66.

156. Administrative Chief Inspector Sieben, "Betriebswirtschaftliche Mitarbeit des Pflegeaufsichtspersonals," *Geisteskrankenpflege* 42 (May 1938): 77–78.

157. See, for example, Dr. med. Möckel, "Die wirtschaftliche Seite der Anstalten," *Geisteskrankenpflege* 46 (October 1942).

158. Nurse Georg Roos, "Forderungen der Krankenpflege," *Geisteskrankenpflege* 44 (October 1940): 120.

159. Ibid.

160. Ibid., 121.

CHAPTER 7
POLITICS AND PROFESSIONAL LIFE UNDER NATIONAL SOCIALISM

1. These lines describe the beauty and sense of renewal that each spring brings—a sense of renewal which, in the author's view, is akin to the experience of Germans under National Socialist rule. The first year, he writes, "exterminated what was already lost, indeed born more of what is good and new." Hitler, he declares, "has brought us the springtime of humanity." (Poem by Otto L. [signature illegible], for the "Kamaradschaftsabend des Personals der Heil- und Pflegeanstalt Buch am 3. Februar 1934." LA Berlin, A Rep. 003-04-1, no. 258, unnumbered document.)

2. Other items on the evening's program strengthen this impression, such as the "Song of Work" (*Das Lied der Arbeit*) and, on the same occasion in 1935, the song "Work Is Happiness" (*Arbeit ist Glück*) ("Kamaradschaftsabend des Personals der Heil- und Pflegeanstalt Buch am 3. Februar 1934" and February 1935. LA Berlin, A Rep. 003-04-1, no. 258, unnumbered documents).

3. Burleigh, *Death and Deliverance*, 51. The provincial governor of the Rheinland suggested that the refusal to observe the Hitler Salute be punished with dismissal: "Otherwise the authority of the state, which absolutely must push for the most exact compliance with its orders, would be greatly diminished" (Archiv der RLK Bedburg—Hau, no. 23, quoted in Graf, "Die Situation der Patienten und des Pflegepersonales," 42).

4. In 1937 Berlin-Buch nurse (and active Party member) Hans Kopp was presented with a copy of *Mein Kampf* in honor of twenty-five years of service (city of Berlin to the HGA, October 20, 1937. LA Berlin, A Rep. 003-04-1, no. 262, PF H.K.).

5. *Sturmführer* to the staff council of the Wittenauer Heilstätten, March 25, 1934. KBoN, PF A.H., 2.

6. Braasch to the HGA, April 23, 1934. KBoN, PF A.H., 6.

7. See, for example, LWV-Eichberg, PF N.G., 2 and 8.

8. Although there are references to his wish for reemployment as early as 1935, he formally requested reemployment at Wittenau in a letter dated November 13, 1936 (KBoN, PF P.W., 103).

9. NS personnel office manager to the Office of the State Commissioner, October 1936. KBoN, PF P.W., 98.

10. Letter of reference from the German Labor Front, November 14, 1936. KBoN, PF P.W., 104.

11. Braasch to the HGA, January 15, 1937. KBoN, PF P.W., 103.

12. Hearing, Nurse K., March 15, 1939. KBoN, PF R.E., 72.

13. Instruction, Braasch, March 23, 1939. KBoN, PF R.E., 73.

14. Instruction, Braasch, March 26, 1938. KBoN, PF F.L., 261.

15. Directorate of the Heilanstalt Winnetal to the Württemberg Ministry of the Interior, August 8, 1936. Hauptstaatsarchiv Stuttgart, E151K VII 6386, doc. 6.

16. Directorate of the Heilanstalt Weinsberg to the Württemberg Ministry of the Interior, September 2, 1936. Hauptstaatsarchiv Stuttgart, E151K VII 6386, doc. 6, enclosure 2.

17. Director Bender to the HGA, March 19, 1940. LA Berlin, A Rep. 003-04-1, no. 100, 34.

18. Instruction, Dr. Bender, June 27, 1940. LA Berlin, A Rep. 003-04-1, no. 100, 35. "Methodical economization" was the regime's euphemistic reference to the T4 program.

19. Bender was handpicked to attend a July 1939 meeting of "reliable" doctors who were to help plan the "euthanasia" program (Ernst Klee, "*Euthanasie*" *im NS-Staat: Die "Vernichtung lebensunwerten Lebens"* [Frankfurt, 1983], 83; see also Friedlander, *The Origins of Nazi Genocide*, 66). In light of this, it seems almost superfluous to add that the East German Communist Party's *Betriebsparteiorganisation* at the Berlin-Buch Clinic thus wholly misrepresented Bender's views on the subject of "euthanasia" when it suggested that he regarded these "economization" measures as anything other than a relief: "When the Nazi leadership intended to spread their infamous murder operation T4, the killing of the chronically ill, to the Berlin-Buch institution, Dr. Bender refused coresponsibility and reported to the Front" (Betriebsparteiorganisation der SED des Klinikums Berlin-Buch, Kommission Betriebsgeschichte, ed., *Klinikum Berlin-Buch: Beiträge zur Betriebsgeschichte* [Berlin, 1987], 1:14).

20. "Bericht über die Zustände in den Irrenanstalten des Regierungs Wiesbaden seit 1932," November 26, 1946. HHSAW, Abt. 461, no. 32442 (Eichberg Trial, Volume 3, Roll 20910, 16).

21. HHSAW, Abt. 461, no. 32442 (Eichberg Trial),4:2 (Hinsen testimony), quoted and translated by Burleigh, *Death and Deliverance*, 47.

22. Quoted and translated by Burleigh, *Death and Deliverance*, 50 and 90.

23. Memo, Director Hinsen, November 25, 1937. LWV-Eichberg, PF N.G.

24. Decision, Landesarbeitsgericht, July 15, 1936 (Nurse E.F. vs. the city of Berlin), and instruction, March 18, 1937. LA Berlin, A Rep. 003-04-1, nos. 137, 114, and 123 respectively.

25. Archiv der RLK Bedburg—Hau, no. 20, quoted in Graf, "Die Situation der Patienten und des Pflegepersonales," 48.

26. Report, Senior Nurse H., April 20, 1941. LWV-Eichberg, PF A.G., 37.

27. File note, Mennecke, April 26, 1941. LWV-Eichberg, PF A.G., 37.

28. Certificate, sent by Mennecke to the Labor Front, April 30, 1941. LWV-Eichberg, PF A.G.

29. Questionnaire, 1929. KBoN, PF L.H., 1.

30. Request, L.H., August 1927. KBoN, PF L.H., 34.

31. L.H. to *Der Schwarze Korps*, forwarded by the latter to State Commissioner Dr. Lippert, April 4, 1936. KBoN, PF L.H., unnumbered document.

32. Excerpt from the personnel file of Nurse K.T., August 1928; statement of the HGA, September 1928; and L.H. to Director W., September 1928. KBoN, PF L.H., 54, 55, and 56 respectively.

33. "Bericht an die Direktion der Wittenauer Heilstätten," by L.H., December 15, 1935. KBoN, PF L.H., 173.

34. Instruction, Office of the Mayor, April 2, 1936 (summary of pages 76–81, 104–107, and 127–128 of KBoN, PF L.H.), and HGA to Wuhlgarten, June 10, 1932. KBoN, PF L.H., 217 and 141 respectively.

35. File notes, October, 1933. KBoN, PF L.H., 148.

36. Report, Senior Nurse E., March 9, 1936; and certificate, March 31, 1936. KBoN, PF L.H., 192 and 227 respectively.

37. Statement, Patient D., March 6, 1936; and Braasch to the HGA, March 14, 1936. KBoN, PF L.H., 193 and 191 respectively.

38. To cite one example among many—at the time of her transfer to Wittenau, Holstein explained, Senior Nurse B. had been informed of the conditions of Holstein's further employment: in the event of the slightest complaint, she would be dismissed. Senior Nurse B. had proceeded to exploit Holstein's precarious situation by holding her in a state of terror: " 'If I report you, you will land on the street!' . . . One must try to imagine," Holstein reminded administrators, "with what fear and trembling I reported to work, always afraid that she could find something today or tomorrow" ("Bericht an die Direktion der Wittenauer Heilstätten," by L.H., December 15, 1935. KBoN, PF L.H., 173).

39. L.H. to *Der Schwarze Korps*, forwarded by the latter to state commissioner Dr. Lippert, April 4, 1936. KBoN, PF L.H., unnumbered document.

40. File note, Braasch, January 1936. KBoN, PF L.H., 175.

41. Ibid.

42. L.H. to the Charlottenburg labor court, March 27, 1936. KBoN, PF L.H., 207.

43. File note, Office of the Mayor, April 25, 1936. KBoN, PF L.H., 227.

44. F.L. to the HGA, October 1934. KBoN, PF F.L., 133.

45. Statement, Dr. Bender, November 1934. KBoN, PF F.L.

46. F.L. to the HGA, January 8, 1935. KBoN, PF F.L.

47. F.L. to the Betriebsverfahrensamt, RVK, November 19, 1935. KBoN, PF F.L., 182.

48. File comment of administrative officer H., January 3, 1936. KBoN, PF F.L.

49. Hufeland administrative director to the HGA, March 10, 1936. KBoN, PF F.L., 197.

50. Reports of Senior Nurse S., February 2, 1937, March 18, 1937, and March 19, 1937; Senior Nurse E., April 1937; and Senior Nurse D., July 14, 1937. KBoN, PF F.L., 216, 224, 225, 226, and 228–233.

51. Senior Doctor K. to the Rudolf Virchow Hospital Directorate, February 2, 1927. KBoN, PF F.L., 216.

52. Hearing, February 12, 1937. KBoN, PF F.L., 217.

53. Statement, F.L., September 20, 1937. KBoN, PF F.L., 248.

54. Instruction, administrative director (signature unreadable), March 26, 1938. KBoN, PF F.L., 260.

55. Ibid., 262.

56. Ibid.

57. File note, Directorate, May 1939, and certificate, May 1943. KBoN, PF F.L., 279–280 and 302 respectively.

58. Instruction, administrative director, March 26, 1938. KBoN, PF F.L., 261.

59. A.H. to the Wittenau Directorate, March 18, 1936. KBoN, PF A.H., 76.

60. NSV's report to the district welfare and youth office (*Bezirkswohlfahrt- und Jugendamt*), Wedding, March 19, 1936. KBoN, PF A.H., 78.

61. Ibid. It appears that the NSV's participation in disciplining deviant Party members was not an isolated phenomenon. In his research on practices of denunciation and self-policing in Eisenach, John Connelly has found similar examples (Connelly, "The Uses of *Volksgemeinschaft*," 912).

62. The family welfare (*Familienfürsorge*) representative visited Harz's new apartment on March 21 and, finding no sign of dereliction, returned the infant to the parents. However, Harz and his wife still refused to acknowledge their own responsibility for their financial problems, blaming those problems instead on their unfavorable environment (Wedding welfare and youth office to the personnel department of Wittenau, March 30, 1936. KBoN, PF A.H., 92).

63. Braasch to the HGA, April 18, 1936. KBoN, PF A.H., 95.

64. Office of the Mayor to the labor court in Berlin, May 22, 1936. KBoN, PF A.H., unnumbered document.

65. File note, Braasch, July 1934. KBoN, PF R.W., 131.

66. File note, Braasch, July 1935. KBoN, PF R.W., 137.

67. Letter of R.W., forwarded to the Labor Front from the Gestapo, August 1936. KBoN, PF R.W., 1 of subfile.

68. Braasch to the HGA, July 1935, and again on October 9, 1936. KBoN, PF R.W., 137 and 7 of subfile.

69. HGA to the main personnel administration (*Hauptpersonalverwaltung*), October 13, 1936; Office of the State Commissioner to the Office of the Mayor, October 1936; and Office of the Mayor to the Office of the State Commissioner, October 19, 1936. KBoN, PF R.W., subfiles 5–8.

70. NSDAP, Berlin *Gauleitung*, to the Office of the Mayor, September 1937. KBoN, PF R.W., subfile.

71. The *Gauleitung* noted that it was responding to correspondence from the Office of the Mayor dated June 15, 1937, and this same June correspondence was referred to again in 1939 when Wittenau considered and then rejected yet another application for employment from Wendel (KBoN, PF R.W., subfile 22).

72. Stamp of the NSDAP, August 17, 1940. KBoN, PF P.Z., 154.

73. P.Z. to the personnel office of the Wittenauer Heilstätten, August 12, 1941. KBoN, PF P.Z., 165.

74. File note to the letter sent by P.Z. on August 12, 1941, Braasch. KBoN, PF P.Z., 165.

75. P.Z. to the Directorate, September 23, 1941. KBoN, PF P.Z., 167.

76. File note to the letter sent by P.Z. on September 23, 1941, Braasch. KBoN, PF P.Z., 167.

77. File note, Dr. F., September 26, 1941. KBoN, PF P.Z., 168. Although the Citizenship Law of November 14, 1935, divided non-Aryans into Jews and *Mischlinge*, and the latter group was more or less unaffected by later measures against the Jews, *Mischlinge* remained non-Aryans in terms of the enforcement of earlier laws and ordinances (Raul Hilberg, *The Destruction of the European Jews*, student edition [New York, 1985], 32).

78. Instruction, Braasch, September 26, 1941, and certificate, P.Z., September 24, 1941. KBoN, PF P.Z., 168 and 169 respectively.

79. NSDAP to Wittenau, September 2, 1937; NSDAP to E.H., December 4, 1937; E.H. to the Wittenau Directorate, October 18, 1937; and file note, October 12, 1937. KBoN, PF E.H., 357, 360, 361, and 363.

80. Report, April 1, 1938 and district manager of the NSV to the Wittenau Directorate, April 29, 1938. KBoN, PF E.H., 369 and 367 respectively.

81. Wittenau Directorate to the district mayor of Reinickendorf, May 16, 1938. KBoN, PF E.H., 368.

82. District manager to Wittenau, June 16, 1937 and district manager to the district mayor of Reinickendorf, June 20, 1938. KBoN, PF E.H., 370 and 371 respectively.

83. Instruction, Braasch, July 13, 1938. KBoN, PF E.H., 371.

84. Instruction, Braasch, September 14, 1938; Conti to the district mayor of Reinickendorf, November 10, 1938; E.H. to the Wittenau Directorate and file note, Braasch, November 12, 1938; and E.H. to the Wittenau Directorate, March 1, 1939. KBoN, PF E.H., unnumbered documents.

85. ". . . it seems credible to me when a woman with no connection to politics claims not to have known about the Communist orientation of the RGO" (Ministry of the Interior to the State Commissioner of Berlin, March 5, 1935. KBoN, PF A.J., 80). "Nurse A.J. in my opinion found her way unknowingly into the RGO and probably was not aware of [its] political character" (NSBO representative, April 3, 1935. KBoN, PF A.J., 85).

86. File note, Braasch, April 1, 1935. KBoN, PF A.J., 103.

87. Nurse Jost was more than willing to withdraw the appeal provided that accrued benefits in the form of pay, vacation, health insurance, and pension were preserved; otherwise she would have to pursue the appeal as planned. The Office of the Mayor rejected this demand, insisting that her dismissal had been perfectly legal and that her reemployment was being considered solely as a gesture of goodwill (*aus Billigkeitsgründen*). Unwilling to be bullied (and, in the event of reemployment, exploited) in this fashion, Nurse Jost reaffirmed that she would accept another position at Wittenau only with the guarantee that she would enjoy her accrued benefits. This was the final word heard from her (Office of the Mayor, April 12, 1935 and Braasch to the HGA, July 6, 1935. KBoN, PF A.J., 86 and 94 respectively).

88. Wittenau nurse Käthe Hackbarth was also fired for RGO membership in 1933 and rehired in 1935. If rehiring an alleged former Communist was considered a gamble, it paid off for the architects of mass murder: Hackbarth was selected along with Flora Lenz and two other Wittenau nurses to "serve" in the T4 program five years later (testimony of Hackbarth, 1948, Kriminalamt Dessau, quoted in Hühn, who uses the nurse's real name, "Psychiatrie im Nationalsozialismus am Beispiel der Wittenauer Heilstätten," 193). Further details on the reasons for her reemployment could not be included in this study because her personnel file could no longer be found at the Karl-Bonhoeffer-Nervenklinik.

89. Unfortunately, research for this study turned up only one document that sheds light on how female nurses may have felt about this kind of condescension—and even more unfortunately, it was penned by the hysterical and paranoid Holstein. At any rate, she seems to have regarded political consciousness as a burden: she came to Berlin with the political innocence shared by all Bavarian women, who had been saddled with the right to vote without being told much more about "left-wing elements" than that they were great murderous criminals. "We didn't want it [the right to vote] and are still today willing, with heart and soul, to put it back into the hands of men, where this duty belongs" (L.H. to *Der Schwarze Korps*, forwarded by the latter to state commissioner Dr. Lippert, April 4, 1936. KBoN, PF L.H., unnumbered document).

90. Fuller had joined the NSDAP in May 1933 (personal data, KBoN, PF E.F., 126).

91. Report, July 1936. KBoN, PF E.F., 159.

92. C.G. to Director Braasch, August 15, 1936. KBoN, PF E.F.

93. HGA to Wittenau, October 16, 1936. KBoN, PF E.F., 199.

94. In February 1938 a friend of G. informed the Wittenau administration that the affair continued and was threatening G.'s marriage. G. was frequently spending time at her apartment, and the landlord was in the process of having him legally banned from the building. A few days later Fuller's landlord complained to the Directorate himself, noting that she was two months behind in her rent. Although Braasch asked the HGA either to dismiss or to transfer her, the HGA refused once more to comply (hearing, February 10, 1938; building administrator A. to Braasch, February 14, 1938; Braasch to the HGA, March 25, 1938; HGA to Braasch; and notice (*Kündigung*), August 11, 1938. KBoN, PF E.F., 238, 239, 249, 270).

95. Deutscher Gemeindetag to the provincial governor, Stettin, August 24, 1936. Bundesarchiv Koblenz, R36, no. 1848.

96. Ibid., and the provincial governor, Stettin, to the Deutscher Gemeindetag, July 8, 1936. Bundesarchiv Koblenz, R36, no. 1848.

97. Wilma Lutz, for example, worked as a nurse in Berlin for six years before her first marriage in 1910 and resumed work after her divorce in 1926. She married again in 1938 and left her position at Wittenau even though, at the age of fifty-seven, having children was presumably no longer an issue (Résumé, 1927, and W.L. to the Wittenauer Directorate, February 1938. KBoN, PF W.L., 14 and unnumbered document).

98. "Stellenverzeichnis für Versorgungsanwärter (Angestellten)," January 1, 1937. LA Berlin, A Rep. 003-04-1, no. 27, 103.

99. "Vortrag, Schaffung einer Schwesternschule, Heilbu Direktion," January 18, 1937. LA Berlin, A Rep. 003-04-1, no. 27, 176–177. Nothing came of this idea in the short term, and it was eventually shelved to allow administrators to devote their full attention to mass murder: "The attempt to build a nursing school in our institution is for the time being not being further pursued in light of the serious measures in connection with the scheduled economization of the psychiatric institutions and the conversion of the Berlin-Buch institution into a hospital" (instruction of administrative director, June 1940. LA Berlin, A Rep. 003-04-1, no. 42, 1849).

100. HGA to the Berlin-Buch institution, October 7, 1935. LA Berlin, A Rep. 003-04-1, no. 42, 185. Italics in original.

101. Instruction, Berlin-Buch administration, September 16, 1937. LA Berlin, A Rep. 003-04-1, no. 42, 193.

102. 1938 Report on Nurses of House 8. LA Berlin, A Rep. 003-04-1, no. 25, 246.

103. Ibid.

104. Minutes, Examination Committee, September 2, 1928. HHStA Wiesbaden, 430/1–12435.

105. Landesrat Bernotat to the Deutscher Gemeindetag, November 17, 1938. Other respondents also considered the second measure highly impractical and added their own reservations: one pointed out that institutions which accommodated their Jews on separate wards would gain a bad reputation, and another deemed such measures unnecessary; Aryan patients generally were not in a condition to feel offended by the presence of Jews in the first place (the Oberpräsident of Lower Silesia, to the Deutscher Gemeindetag, October 10, 1938, and the Oberpräsident of East Prussia to the Deutscher Gemeindetag, November 29, 1938). All of the above from Bundesarchiv Koblenz, R 36, Nr. 1842.

106. File note, Hinsen, January 15, 1938. LWV-Eichberg, PF K.J.

107. Instruction, draft to Herr. K. of the Labor Front, November 2, 1936. KBoN, PF E.H., 343–344.

108. K.K. to the Oberpräsident via the Directorate of Eichberg, October 13, 1939. LWV-Eichberg, PF K.K., 29.

109. Head regional superintendant (*Landesoberinspektor*) W. to the Oberpräsident, October 19, 1939. LWV-Eichberg, PF K.K., 29.

110. K. to K.K., October 31, 1939, and November 14, 1939. LWV-Eichberg, PF K.K., 31.

111. E.M. to the Office of the Mayor, wage contract office (*Tarifvertragsamt*), November 8, 1935, and exchange between the general administration (*Allgemeine Hauptverwaltung*) and the main personnel administration (*Hauptpersonalverwaltung*), December 12, 1935. KBoN, PF E.M., 113 and 119.

112. Office of the Mayor to E.M., December 18, 1935. KBoN, PF E.M., 119.

113. Gau-Hauptstellenleiter of the NSDAP to the Office of the Mayor, September 1, 1936. LA Berlin, A Rep. 003-04-1, no. 261 (PF G.E.), 84.

114. Office of the Mayor to G.E., September 12, 1936. LA Berlin, A Rep. 003-04-1, no. 261 (PF G.E.), 85.

115. NSDAP to the Office of the Mayor, August 25, 1937. LA Berlin, A Rep. 003-04-1, no. 261 (PF G.E.), 89.

116. Office of the Mayor to G.E. LA Berlin, A Rep. 003-04-1, no. 261 (PF G.E.), 90.

117. W.S. to Hitler, sent by the Labor Front to the wage contract office, December 11, 1936. KBoN, PF W.S., 128. Memos between offices of the employment bureacracy over the following years suggest that Sommer would indeed have been transferred if a suitable position had been available, but he remained a psychiatric nurse until 1941, when a doctor's confirmation of his physical unsuitability for the job sufficed to secure his release.

118. Gellately, "Denunciations in Twentieth-Century Germany," 950.

119. Detlev Peukert, *Inside Nazi Germany: Conformity, Opposition, and Racism in Everyday Life*, trans. Richard Deveson (New Haven, Conn., 1987), 72.

120. A.J. to the Wittenau Directorate, March 29 and May 15, 1934; file note, Braasch, May 31, 1934; instruction, Braasch, October 4, 1934, and April 20, 1935; and Braasch to A.J., October 4, 1934. KBoN, PF A.J., 188, 192, 196, and 203 respectively.

121. "Bericht über die praktische Tätigkeit," May 16, 1936. KBoN, PF L.B., 167.

122. Career description. KBoN, PF L.B. Unfortunately, further documents offering details on her career after spring 1937 are no longer in the file.

123. Graf, "Die Situation der Patienten und des Pflegepersonales," 43.

124. Report of Dr. Klein, sent by the Prussian state commissioner of the Central Health Administration (*Zentrale Gesundheitsverwaltung*) to the Zentralverwalteten Krankenhäuser, Hospitäler und Heil- und Pflegeanstalten, March 20, 1933. LA Berlin, A Rep. 003-04-1, no. 264, 128.

125. Dr. K. to the Zentralverwalteten Krankenhäuser, Hospitäler und Heil- und Pflegeanstalten. LA Berlin, A Rep. 003-04-1, no. 264, 128.

126. Archiv des Landschaftsverbands Rheinland, Pulheim-Brauweiler, Graf Collection, Interview with former patient J., quoted in Graf, "Die Situation der Patienten und des Pflegepersonales," 44.

127. Here, the author concludes the poem cited at the outset of this chapter by celebrating the camaraderie of the Berlin-Buch ("Heilbu") staff. Not surprisingly, his understanding of the term includes not only goodwill but also the idea that the staff members are all of "one mind." (Poem by Otto L. [signature illegible], for the "Kamaradschaftsabend des Personals der Heil- und Pflegeanstalt Buch am 3. Februar 1934." LA Berlin, A Rep. 003-04-1, no. 258, unnumbered document.)

CHAPTER 8
WAR, MASS MURDER, AND MORAL FLIGHT

1. MO, 4:927 (M.A.).

2. According to Hans-Walter Schmuhl, the figure lies somewhere between 100,000 and 200,000 (" 'Euthanasie' im Nationalsozialismus," 59). More recently, Henry Friedlander has narrowed the scope by stating that more victims died in the second phase of "euthanasia" than in the first, which claimed over 70,000 victims (*The Origins of Nazi Genocide*, 151).

3. Quoted in Faulstich, *Von der Irrenfürsorge zur "Euthanasie"*, 206–207.

4. Quoted in Graf, "Die Situation der Patienten und des Pflegepersonales," 50.

5. Klee, *"Euthanasie" im NS-Staat*, 430, and Faulstich, *Von der Irrenfürsorge zur "Euthanasie"*, 320.

6. Christina Härtel, Marianne Hühn, and Norbert Emmerich, "Krankenmorde in den Wittenauer Heilstätten," in Arbeitsgruppe, *Totgeschwiegen*, 185–188.

7. Norbert Emmerich, "Die Wittenauer Heilstätten, 1933–1945," in Arbeitsgruppe, *Totgeschwiegen* , 78–79, 85–87. The Berlin-Buch institution was closed in October 1940, and by the beginning of 1943 the Herzberge and Wuhlgarten institutions had been converted into hospitals.

8. Siemen, *Menschen blieben auf der Strecke*, 180 ff.

9. Deutscher Gemeindetag to the Württemberg Ministry of the Interior, February 22, 1940. Bundesarchiv Koblenz, R 36, no. 1820.

10. Schröter, "Psychiatrie in Waldheim/Sachsen," 112.

11. MO, 4:964 (F.E.).

12. Koch, "Die Beteiligung," 99, and Heike Bernhardt, "Die Anstaltspsychiatrie in Pommern 1939–1945: Ein Beitrag zur Aufhellung nationalsozialistischer Tötungsaktionen unter besonderer Berücksichtigung der Landesheilanstalt Ueckermünde" (Med. diss., University of Leipzig, 1992), 27. See also Christina Härtel, "Transporte in den Tod: Die Verlegungen von den Wittenauer Heilstätten nach Obrawalde bei Meseritz," in Arbeitsgruppe, *Totgeschwiegen*, 191–193.

13. Koch, "Die Beteiligung," 100.

14. Fritz Niemand, "Ich war in der Tötungsanstalt Meseritz-Obrawalde: Erinnerungen, Erfahrungen, Dokumente (zusammengestellt von Stefan Romey)," in *Krankenpflege im Nationalsozialismus*, ed. Hilde Steppe, 5th ed. (Frankfurt, 1989), 170–171.

15. Ibid., 171–172.

16. Klee, *"Euthanasie" im NS-Staat*, 405, and Koch, "Die Beteiligung," 105.

17. Statistics from postwar testimonies and a Russian investigative report, quoted in Klee, *"Euthanasie" im NS-Staat*, 403. One nurse who carried out killings and was executed in 1945 estimated that as many as 18,000 people were killed there. See also Friedlander, *The Origins of Nazi Genocide*, 161.

18. For example, testimony of A.G., quoted in Steppe, "Mit Tränen in den Augen," 152.

19. Klee, *"Euthanasie" im NS-Staat*, 409–410.

20. Koch, "Die Beteiligung," 101.

21. Christina Härtel, "Transporte in den Tod," in Arbeitsgruppe, *Totgeschwiegen*, 192–193.

22. MO, 4:1051 (E.P.), and MO, 4:1011 (Dr. J.L.).

23. Horst Dickel, "Anstaltsalltag in einer Landesheilanstalt im Nationalsozialismus," in *Euthanasie in Hadamar: Die nationalsozialistische Vernichtungspolitik in hessischen Anstalten*, ed. Landeswohlfahrtsverband Hessen (Kassel, 1991), 105, and Friedlander, *The Origins of Nazi Genocide*, 159.

24. Burleigh, *Death and Deliverance*, 245. This, as pointed out above, was no mere by-product of wartime scarcity but rather the will of Bernotat, Schmidt, and Mennecke. Only on the children's station, established in

April 1941, were hygienic standards and food rations better; the reason seems to have been a desire to formulate more reliable prognoses during an initial observation period. This, however, did not stop Schmidt and his close assistants from killing approximately 430 of their charges before war's end, and sending their brains to the University of Heidelberg for research (Dickel, "Anstaltsalltag in einer Landesheilanstalt," in Landeswohlfahrtsverband Hessen, *Euthanasie in Hadamar*, 105 and 110).

25. Burleigh, *Death and Deliverance*, 48.

26. Dickel, "Anstaltsalltag in einer Landesheilanstalt," in Landeswohlfahrtsverband Hessen, *Euthanasie in Hadamar*, 112.

27. Burleigh, *Death and Deliverance*, 73. For various firsthand details, see the following Eichberg testimonies (here, and henceforth, listed by *microfilm* page number): HHSAW Abt. 461, no. 32442(1), 2039 (J.H.); HHSAW Abt. 461, no. 32442(1), 1949 (J.S.); HHSAW Abt. 461, no. 32442(3), 2484–2485 (former patient). According to a former doctor, nurses were not allowed to put patients in the bunker without doctor's orders but did so anyway (HHSAW Abt. 461, no. 32442[1], 1909 [Dr. V.]).

28. HHSAW Abt. 461, no. 32442(1), 1949 (J.S.), and HHSAW Abt. 461, no. 32442(1), 1951 (former nurse E.V.).

29. HHSAW Abt. 461, no. 32442(2), 2219 (I.H.)

30. HHSAW Abt. 461, no. 32442(2), 2220 (K.P.)

31. HHSAW Abt. 461, no. 32442(3), 2486.

32. HHSAW Abt. 461, no. 32442(1), 1921 (Nurse J.M.); HHSAW Abt. 461, no. 32442(1), 2041–2042 (H.D.); HHSAW Abt. 461, no. 32442(1), 1937 (Dr. L.); HHSAW Abt. 461, no. 32442(1), 1929 (A.T.)

33. HHSAW Abt. 461, no. 32442(1), 1937 (Dr. L.)

34. HHSAW Abt. 461, no. 32442(1), 1921 (J.M.)

35. HHSAW Abt. 461, no. 32442(2), 2261 (K.S.). Schmidt wound up bringing the patient to the bunker himself and issuing the nurse a punitive transfer to the Weilmünster institution on account of this "insubordination." He then changed his mind and had the nurse returned to Eichberg after all, remarking during their brief meeting, "There are some people for whom religion is more important than the final victory."

36. HHSAW Abt. 461, no. 32442(1), 2067–2068 (H.S.). See also HHSAW Abt. 461, no. 32442(3), 2319 (D.W.). Seidel could have saved herself the trouble, since according to Dr. Hinsen, Traupel himself had been longing for a "euthanasia" law since at least the mid-1930s (Burleigh, *Death and Deliverance*, 47).

37. HHSAW Abt. 461, no. 32442(1), 1929 (A.T.). Seidel seems to have considered Schmidt a kind of partner of conscience: she reportedly told a doctor once that "Schmidt did not have a clear conscience and at night saw the children coming up to him." HHSAW, Abt. 461, no. 32442(1), 1937 (Dr. L.). On Klein and Huber, see Burleigh, *Death and Deliverance*, 252.

38. HHSAW Abt. 461, no. 32442(1), 1921 (J.M.).

39. HHSAW Abt. 461, no. 32442(1), 1949 (J.S.); HHSAW Abt. 461, no. 32442(1), 1921 (J.M.); HHSAW Abt. 461, no. 32442(1), 2033 (A.S.).

40. Burleigh, *Death and Deliverance*, 251.

41. HHSAW Abt. 461, no. 32442(1), 2025–2026. (M.F.).

42. HHSAW Abt. 461, no. 32442(2), 2219 (I.H.).

43. HHSAW Abt. 461, no. 32442(2), 2218 (L.H.).

44. HHSAW Abt. 461, no. 32442(1), 2010 (E.N.), 2087 (W.S.), and 2089 (C.S). See also 2010 (Nurse D.R. and former patient A.R.) and 2088 (Dr. M.).

45. Meyer, "Psychiatrie im Nationalsozialismus," 51.

46. The nature of the so-called review process is demonstrated by the example of "expert" Dr. Hermann Pfannmüller, director of the Eglfing-Haar psychiatric institution, who allegedly reviewed over two thousand cases in addition to his other duties during three weeks at the end of 1940 (Friedlander, *The Origins of Nazi Genocide*, 80). On the absence of overarching logic in the selection process, see Gerhard Schmidt, *Selektion in der Heilanstalt, 1939–1945* (Stuttgart, 1965), and Friedlander, *The Origins of Nazi Genocide*, chapter 4.

47. T4 killing centers were established in the institutions at Brandenburg/Havel, Brandenburg/Saale, Sonnenstein/Pirna, Hadamar/Limburg, Grafeneck (Württemberg), and Hartheim/Linz. Layovers were intended to help camouflage the ultimate destination—and fate—of deported patients (Landeswohlfahrtsverband Hessen, *Euthanasie in Hadamar*, 32).

48. Until recently, the reasons that the T4 program was halted on August 21, 1941, were a source of debate among historians. Possible explanations included the following: the spread of knowledge about the killings and resulting disquiet in the German public; Bishop von Galen's August 3 sermon in which he condemned the killings in dangerously explicit terms; reports of the killings that were being spread abroad; the German invasion of the Soviet Union's opening up a vast frontier on which exterminatory policies might be implemented out of the public's view; and the fact that the original target of 70,000 dead had been reached. (Schmuhl, " 'Euthanasie' im Nationalsozialismus," 63; Michael Burleigh and Wolfgang Wippermann, *The Racial State: Germany, 1933–1945* [Cambridge, 1991], 153). Most recently, Henry Friedlander has argued persuasively that public disquiet was in fact the main reason (*The Origins of Nazi Genocide*, 107 and 111 ff.).

49. Former nurse B., quoted in Horst Brombacher, "Das Euthanasieprogramm für 'unheilbar Kranke' (1939–1941) und seine Durchführung in den Anstalten Mittebadens," *Die Ortenau* 65 (1987): 454.

50. Ernst T. Mader, *Das erzwungene Sterben von Patienten der Heil- und Pflegeanstalt Kaufbeuren-Irsee zwischen 1940 und 1945 nach Dokumenten und*

Berichten von Augenzeugen (Blöcktach, 1982), 20, quoted in Graf, "Die Situation der Patienten und des Pflegepersonales," 49–50.

51. Statement, 1945, quoted in Karl Morlok, *"Wo bringt ihr uns hin?"*— *Geheime Reichssache Grafeneck* (Stuttgart, 1985), 48.

52. Faulstich, *Von der Irrenfürsorge zur "Euthanasie"*, 271. For other examples, see Tröster, *Suttrop-Dorpke*, 125, and HHSAW Abt. 461, no. 32442(2), 2154–2155 (Nurse E.C.). One depressed nurse from the Wiesloch institution (Baden), however, went beyond resignation and decided to inquire for herself as to what had become of her charges. When she attempted to enter the grounds of Grafeneck, however, she was accosted by SS personnel. In response to her inquiry, they laughed, "They like it so much at Grafeneck that they never want to leave again!" (Faulstich, *Von der Irrenfürsorge zur "Euthanasie"*, 273).

53. Morlok, *"Wo bringt ihr uns hin?"*, 48.

54. Friedlander, *The Origins of Nazi Genocide*, 136 ff.

55. MO, 4:1193 (A.S.).

56. MO, 4:1193, 1194 (A.S.).

57. MO, 4:1198 (A.S.).

58. MO, 4:1195–1196 (A.S.).

59. MO, 4:1191 (A.S.).

60. MO, 4:1209 (E.D.).

61. MO, 4:1060 (M.M.).

62. HHSAW Abt. 461, no. 32442(2), 2260 (K.S.).

63. HHSAW Abt. 461, no. 32442(2), 2257 (K.S.) See also testimonies of Nurses E.C. (HHSAW Abt. 461, no. 32442[2], 2254) and F.P. (HHSAW Abt. 461, no. 32442[2], 2057).

64. HHSAW Abt. 461, no. 32442(2), 2257 (K.S.).

65. HHSAW Abt. 461, no. 32442(2), 2057 (F.P.).

66. HHSAW Abt. 461, no. 32442(2), 2153 (J.H.). His deputy, A.S., also maintained that Hadamar was not specified as a destination and there was no talk of killing patients (HHSAW Abt. 461, no. 32442[2], 2153).

67. HHSAW Abt. 461, no. 32442(1), 2017 (J.H.).

68. HHSAW Abt. 461, no. 32442(2), 2262 (K.E.). See also the testimony of A.S., HHSAW Abt. 461, no. 32442(1), 2033. Sending patients off with a stamped postcard may have been a common tactic used by suspicious and concerned nurses to covertly investigate the purpose of the transports; it was also attempted, with the same unsettling results, by personnel of the Lauenburg institution in Pomerania (Bernhardt, "Die Anstaltspsychiatrie in Pommern," 29).

69. HHSAW Abt. 461, no. 32442(1), 1949 (J.S.).

70. HHSAW Abt. 461, no. 32442(1), 1952 (J.M.).

71. HHSAW Abt. 461, no. 32442(1), 1950 (K.B.).

72. One notable exception at Eichberg was Nurse E.C. (HHSAW Abt. 461, no. 32442[2], 2154–2155).

73. Nurse Elfriede Conrad, for example, said she and her colleagues originally assumed that the T4 questionnaires were intended to help with evacuation and selection of workers. After she heard a rumor from a priest and patient relative in late 1940 about killings in other institutions, she sought to leave her position and, failing that, tried to save some patients from transport in January 1941 by urging relatives pick them up. Tragically, she was successful in only a few cases because many relatives were not in a position to do so on short notice, and she was unable to tell them the true reason for her request. Even so, her activities put her on a bad footing with Mennecke, who accused her of trying to sabotage the transports. By the end of February 1941, she had fallen ill and succeeded in getting a transfer from Eichberg (HHSAW Abt. 461, no. 32442[2], 2154–2155). Senior Nurse Heidrun Seidel apparently also had this difficulty when she attempted to save the sister of a friend of hers, who was also a nurse. When the friend responded that she would prefer to have her sister visit during the summer, Seidel sent a personal messenger to explain, in no uncertain terms, the true grounds and urgency of her request (HHSAW Abt. 461, no. 32442[3], 2319 [Nurse D.W.]).

74. HHSAW Abt. 461, no. 32442(1), 1949 (J.S.).

75. HHSAW Abt. 461, no. 32442(2), 2257 (K.S.).

76. Reported by Nurse E.C., HHSAW Abt. 461, no. 32442(2), 2154–2155.

77. Meyer, "Psychiatrie im Nationalsozialismus," 53. From spring 1942 onward patient transports were carried out under the auspices of "Action Brandt," whereby such patients were allegedly being protected from air raids.

78. Meseritz-Obrawalde testimony of M.T., quoted in Steppe, "Mit Tränen in den Augen," 156.

79. MO, 4:1023–1024 (E.S.).

80. MO, 4:990 (L.S.), and MO, 4:1006 (E.B.) respectively.

81. HHSAW Abt. 461, no. 32442(1), 1921 (J.M.).

82. HHSAW Abt. 461, no. 32442(2), 2153 (A.S.).

83. MO, 3:752 (M.G.).

84. HHSAW Abt. 461, no. 32442(1), 2067–2068 (H.S.).

85. MO, 3:752 (M.G.); MO, 4:1079 (H.G.) and 1066 (M.M.) respectively.

86. MO, 4:1009 (F.B.).

87. MO, 4:1062 (M.M.).

88. MO, 4:1018–1019 (I.W.).

89. HHSAW Abt. 461, no. 32442(1), 2041–2042 (H.D.).

90. HHSAW Abt. 461, no. 32442(2), 2153 (A.S.). For similar arguments, see HHSAW Abt. 461, no. 32442(1), 2058 (A.S.), and HHSAW Abt. 461, no. 32442(1), 1921 (J.M.).

91. Steppe, "Mit Tränen in den Augen," 138.

92. HHSAW Abt. 461, no. 32442(1), 1928 (A.T.).

93. HHSAW Abt. 461, no. 32442(1), 1933 (K.E.).

94. For example, testimonies of Nurse K.E. and former nurse J.S., HHSAW Abt. 461, no. 32442(2), 2262, and HHSAW Abt. 461, no. 32442(1), 1949 respectively.

95. HHSAW Abt. 461, no. 32442(1), 1920 (J.M.). Nurse A.S. also testified that Schmidt was known among the nursing staff as a "mass murderer." HHSAW Abt. 461, no. 32442(1), 2056–2057.

96. HHSAW Abt. 461, no. 32442(1), 1921 (J.M.).

97. HHSAW Abt. 461, no. 32442(1), 2019 (G.B.).

98. HHSAW Abt. 461, no. 32442(1), 2056–2057 (A.S.). For an almost identical description of this sequence of events, see the testimony of Nurse K.S., HHSAW Abt. 461, no. 32442(2), 2260–2261.

99. HHSAW Abt. 461, no. 32442(1), 2022 (S.H.).

100. MO, 3:746 (M.G.).

101. MO, 3:746–747 (M.G.). Göbel reported that she was not certain whether she administered all of the dosages herself.

102. Meseritz-Obrawalde testimony of L.E., quoted in Steppe, "Mit Tränen in den Augen," 148–149.

103. MO, 4:1002–1003 (E.B.).

104. MO, 4:1046 (E.K.).

105. MO, 4:1052 (E.P.).

106. MO, 4:1008 (F.B.).

107. MO, 4:864 (M.B.).

108. See MO 4:1090 (M.B.) and 1081 (H.K.); the latter reported that her mother learned about the killings at her local bakery.

109. MO, 4:1052 (E.P.). See also MO, 4:1090 (M.B.).

110. MO, 4:943–944 (M.L.).

111. MO, 4:1043–1045 (E.K.).

112. MO, 4:1045–1046 (E.K.). She was not the only nurse to defend her uncertainty on these grounds. Erna Büchling, who also participated in in-house transports, maintained that patients were sometimes sent to House 10, a killing ward, without having veronal first and even walked there themselves (4:1003).

113. MO, 4:1047 (E.K.).

114. MO, 4:1065–1066 (M.M.).

115. MO, 4:990 (E.D.).

116. MO, 4:956 (K.K.).

117. MO, 4:957 (K.K.).

118. It is instructive that a similar comment was made by a veteran Eichberg male nurse, who said that nurses lived in fear of reprisals if they even talked about what was going on at Eichberg. "Therefore one did not

want to see what was going on up there" (HHSAW, Abt. 461, no. 32442[1], 1953 [P.S.]).

119. See testimonies MO, 4:1063 (M.M.) (children's station) and MO, 4:957 (K.K.) (women's killing station).

120. MO, 4:912 (G.F.).

121. Martha Möll said that although she sometimes brought bodies to the mortuary, at one point a graveyard work detail of male nurses was established for this purpose and nurses no longer had access to the mortuary (MO, 4:1060–1061 (M.M.).

122. MO, 4:928 (M.A.).

123. MO, 4:1046 (E.K.).

124. MO, 4:1005 (E.B.). My italics.

125. MO, 4:961 (K.K.).

126. MO, 4:960–961 (K.K.).

127. MO, 4:915 (G.F.).

128. MO, 4:1066–1067 (M.M). For a similar example, see MO, 4:1046 (E.K.).

129. MO, 4:1055 (E.P.).

130. MO, 4:1004–1005 (E.B.).

131. Bauman, *Modernity and the Holocaust*, 163.

132. See, for example, MO, 4:875 (E.H.).

133. MO, 4:1067 (M.M).

134. MO, 4:960 (K.K.).

135. MO, 3:744 (M.G.).

136. MO, 4:1047 (E.K.).

137. MO, 4:1024 (E.S.).

138. MO, 4:865 (M.B.).

139. MO, 4:886–887 (E.B.).

140. MO, 4:887 (E.B.).

141. MO, 4:987 (L.S.).

142. MO, 4:1051 (E.P.).

143. MO, 4:961 (K.K). My italics.

144. MO, 4:1211 (E.D.).

145. MO, 4:1212 (E.D.).

146. MO, 3:751 (M.G.).

147. Juwel is said to have told Martha Möll that she refused on religious grounds to take the oath Grabowski tried to impose on her. Juwel apparently did not specify the reasons she was asked to take oath to begin with, but Möll noticed that on days when Juwel was on duty, killings did *not* take place on her station (MO, 4:1059 and 1063 [M.M.]).

148. MO, 3:748 (M.G.).

149. MO, 3:749–750 (M.G.).

150. MO, 3:697 (B.H.).

151. MO, 3:703 (B.H.).

152. MO, 3:744 (M.G.).

153. MO, 3:746–747 (M.G.).

154. MO, 4:915 (G.F.).

155. See, for example, MO, 4:916 (G.F.) and 902 (B.N.).

156. MO, 4:1054 (E.P.).

157. Quoted by Klee, *"Euthanasie" im NS-Staat,* 432.

158. A large segment of testimony has been published in Koch, "Die Beteiligung," 117–122.

159. MO, 4:903–904 (B.N.).

160. MO, 4:904 (B.N.).

161. MO, "Urteilsbegründung," 1554.

162. MO, 4:891, 897 (B.N.). Although at Meseritz-Obrawalde for only four months, Maxine Lang confirmed that nurses arriving from other institutions (in her case Treptow) were isolated from other nurses (MO, 4:859–860 [M.L.]).

163. MO, 3:752–753 (M.G.).

164. MO, 4:990 (L.S.). See also 4:1079 (H.K.).

165. MO, 4:905 (B.N)

166. MO, 4:906, 890 (B.N.).

167. MO, 4:1023 (E.S.).

168. MO, 4:886 (E.B.).

169. MO, 4:917 (G.F.).

170. This is not, of course, to say that the killings were a taboo subject of conversation at Meseritz-Obrawalde; they were not. Nurses whispered among themselves and spoke indirectly about the killings, which were by many accounts an "open secret." It seems, however, that these conversations took place among nurses who considered themselves safely at a distance from the whole horrifying business; those who experienced conflicts of conscience, such as Neumann and Kremer, do not seem to have been so eager to chatter about what was going on. On conversations about the killings, see MO, 4:876 (E.H.) and 1055 (E.P.).

171. HHSAW, Abt. 461, no. 32442(3), 2484–2485.

172. MO, 4:1055 (E.P.).

173. Burleigh, *Death and Deliverance,* 252.

CHAPTER 9
CONCLUDING REMARKS

1. Koch, "Die Beteiligung," 128.

2. Tzvetan Todorov, *Facing the Extreme: Moral Life in the Concentration Camps,* trans. Arthur Denner and Abigail Pollak (New York, 1996), 129.

3. Goldhagen, *Hitler's Willing Executioners,* 252.

4. Goldhagen unfortunately obscures this possibility beyond recognition in his own example by emphasizing that when police battalion members had problems shooting innocent people, this was only an expression of visceral opposition, *not* moral opposition (ibid.). He unwittingly reproduces precisely the conceptual dichotomy that the men themselves may have been encouraged to adopt. Visceral opposition, if treated as something quite different from moral feeling, made an ideal safety valve, so to speak, for the system as a whole: allowing men to opt out because they were too "weak" for such a task settled the problem on the spot and obviated their expressing or thinking about their refusal in any other way, let alone confronting the moral magnitude of what they were doing. Opting out on those grounds, as Browning pointed out, "did not challenge basic police discipline or the authority of the regime in general" (Browning, *Ordinary Men*, 74). Therein lay its utility.

5. Todorov makes this same point with reference to concentration camp guards (*Facing the Extreme*, 165 ff.).

6. Steppe, "Mit Tränen in den Augen," 164.

7. The importance of this substitution of technical for moral responsibility is, according to Bauman, a defining feature of silencing moral concern (*Modernity and the Holocaust*, 192–198).

Bibliography

Unpublished Sources

Archiv der Karl-Bonhoeffer-Nervenklinik, Berlin (personnel files, job descriptions).

Archiv des Diakonischen Werkes der evangelischen Kirche Deutschlands (Berlin), CA, G-S 48.

Archiv des Landeswohlfahrtsverbandes Hessen, Eichberg branch (personnel files).

Bundesarchiv Koblenz, R36 (Deutscher Gemeindetag), R96 (Reichsarbeitsgemeinschaft Heil- und Pflegeanstalten).

Dokumentationsstelle Pflege, Frankfurt (copies of Meseritz-Obrawalde trial records).

Hauptstaatsarchiv Stuttgart, E151K VI, VII (Ministerium des Innern, Gesundheitswesen).

Hessisches Hauptstaatsarchiv, Wiesbaden, Abt. 430 (administrative records, Eichberg) and 461 (Eichberg trial records).

Landesarchiv Berlin, A Rep. 003-04-1 (Städtische Heil- und Pflegeanstalt Buch).

Mecklenburgisches Landeshauptarchiv (Schwerin), Ministerium für Kunst, Geistliche- und Medizinalangelegenheiten (administrative records and personnel files, Landesheil- und Pflegeanstalt Schwerin-Sachsenberg).

Printed Primary Sources

Official Publications

Reichsgesetzblatt. No. 34, April 7, 1933.
———. No. 37, April 11, 1933.
———. No. 46, May 4, 1933.
———. No. 48, May 6, 1933.
———. No. 104, September 23, 1933.
———. No. 107, September 28, 1933.

Books, Textbooks, Dissertations

Abendroth, Erna von. "Der Beruf der Krankenpflegerin mit besonderer Berücksichtigung der sächsischen Verhältnisse." PhD. diss., University of Leipzig, 1921. Quoted in Hilde Steppe, "Das Selbstverständnis der Krankenpflege," *Deutsche Krankenpflegezeitschrift*, no. 5 (1990): 4–5.

Bresler, Johannes. *Deutsche Heil- und Pflegeanstalten für psychisch Kranke in Wort und Bild*. 2 vols. Halle a. S., 1910–1912.

Catel, Werner, ed. *Die Pflege des Gesunden und Kranken Kindes*. Leipzig, 1939.

Enge, Johannes. *Soziale Psychiatrie*. Berlin, 1919.

———. *Ratgeber für Angehörige von Geisteskranken*. 2d ed. Halle a. S., 1924.

Faltlhauser, Valentin. *Geisteskrankenpflege: Ein Lehr- und Handbuch für Irrenpfleger*. Halle a. S., 1939.

———, ed. *Leitfaden für Irrenpflege*. Halle a. S., 1936.

Groß, Hermann. *Die Irrenanstalten zugleich als Heilanstalten betrachtet*. Kassel, 1832. Quoted in *Geisteskrankenpflege* 37 (November 1933): 175.

Gütt, Alfred, et al., eds. *Der Amtsarzt: Ein Nachschlagewerk für Medizinal- und Verwaltungsbeamte*. Jena, 1936.

Haymann, Hermann. *Lehrbuch der Irrenheilkunde für Pfleger und Pflegerinnen*. Berlin, 1922.

Jahreis, Christian, ed. *Schwestern Erzählen: Ein Buch von irdischer Not und helfender Liebe*. Nuremberg, 1936.

Maes, Ullinca. *Die Schwestern in den Krankenanstalten Deutschlands*. Berlin, 1922. Quoted in Hilde Steppe, "Das Selbstverständnis der Krankenpflege," *Deutsche Krankenpflegezeitschrift*, no. 5 (1990): 4.

May, Franz. "Von den wesentlichen Eigenschaften eines rechtschaffenden Krankenwärters." In *Unterricht für Krankenwärter*. Mannheim, 1782. Quoted in Eduard Seidler, *Geschichte der Pflege des kranken Menschen*, 156. 2d ed. Stuttgart, 1966.

Meltzer, Ewald. *Leitfaden der Schwachsinnigen und Blödenpflege*. 2d ed. Halle a. S., 1930.

Morgenthaler, Walter. *Die Pflege der Gemuts- und Geisteskranken*. Berlin, 1930.

Neuman-Rahn, Karin. *Der seelisch kranke Mensch und seine Pflege*. Jena, 1939.

Reiß, Paul. *Im roten Hause: Von der Behandlung des Irren*. Straubing, 1929.

Rittershaus, Ernst. *Die Irrengesetzgebung in Deutschland nebst einer vergleichenden Darstellung des Irrenwesens in Europa (für Ärzte, Juristen u. gebildete Laiaen)*. Berlin and Leipzig, 1927.

Schlöß, Heinrich. *Leitfaden für Irrenpfleger*. Vienna, 1909.

Scholz, Ludwig. *Leitfaden für Irrenpfleger*. 23d ed. Halle, 1935.

Schulhof, Friedrich. *Lehrgang für Irrenpfleger*. Vienna, 1929.

Die Schwester vom Roten Kreuz. Berlin, 1919. Quoted in Hilde Steppe, "Pflege bis 1933," in *Krankenpflege im Nationalsozialismus*, edited by Hilde Steppe, 33. 5th ed. Frankfurt, 1989.

, Johannes. "Sparsamkeit in der Irrenanstalt." *PNW* 23 (April 9, 1921).

———. "Noch einmal: Sparsamkeit in der Irrenanstalt." *PNW* 23 (August 13, 1921).

———. "Zum dritten—und nicht letzten Male: Sparsamkeit in Irrenanstalten." *PNW* 23 (November 5, 1921).

———. "Sparsamkeit in der Irrenanstalt." *DI* 25 (December 1921).

———. "Bermerkungen zu den 'Vorschlägen zu einem Fürsorgegesetz für Geistes- und Gemütskranke' von Dr. Beyer, Oberregierungsrat im Ministerium für Volkswohlfahrt." *PNW* 26 (November 15, 1924).

Bruckner. "Als Patient in einer Heil- und Pflegeanstalt." *Geisteskrankenpflege* 39 (May 1935).

Bücken, Erwin. "Die gerichtliche Unterbringung von Geisteskranken in Heilanstalten." *Geisteskrankenpflege* 44 (February 1940).

Buder. "Über die neuen Bestrebungen in der Beschäftigungsbehandlung der Geisteskranken." *DI* 31 (December 1927).

Carrière, R. "Sparmaßnahmen und Anstaltsniveau." *PNW* 33 (July 4, 1931).

Dickhoven, J. "Ein Besuch in der Prov.-Heilanstalt Gütersloh i. W." *DI* 30 (April 1926).

Dobrick-Kosten. "Krieg und Volksernährung." *DI* 18 (March 1915).

Donalies, Gustav. "Die Verhütung des Selbstmordes in der Anstalt." *Geisteskrankenpflege* 38 (June 1934).

Enge, Johannes. "Der Schutz der persönlichen Rechte der Geisteskranken und die Schaffung eines Reichsirrengesetzes." *DI* 23 (January 1919).

———. "Fehlschlüsse und Irrtümer bei Sparmaßnahmen." *PNW* 34 (November 19, 1932).

———. "Beobachtungsberichte des Pflegepersonals." *Geisteskrankenpflege* 37 (August 1933).

———. "Das Gesetz zur Verhütung erbkranken Nachwuchses in Laienbetrachtung und ärztliche Erfahrungen als Gutachter im Erbgesundheitsverfahren." *PNW* 39 (January 2, 1937).

———. "Welchen Irrtümern und Mißverständnissen begegnet man bei Laien über die Erbpflegegesetze?" *Geisteskrankenpflege* 42 (March 1938).

———. "Berufs- und Dienstgeheimnis des Krankenpflegepersonals." *Geisteskrankenpflege* 44 (September 1940).

Engelter, Wilhelm. "Brief aus Goddelau." *Die Sanitätswarte*, no. 5 (March 1928).

Erbe, Albert. "Auf was wird der Pfleger achten, wenn er einen Patienten zum Besucher bringt?" *Geisteskrankenpflege* 41 (June 1937).

———. "Schwachsinnige, ihr Leiden und ihre Behandlung durch den Pfleger." *Geisteskrankenpflege* 42 (July 1938).

Simon, Hermann. *Aktivere Krankenb.* [
1929.

Stangenberger, J. *Unter dem Deckmantel*
Quoted in Hilde Steppe, "Die histori.
pflege als Beruf: Auswirkungen die:
Strukturen," supplement to *Deutsche N*
(1985): 8.

Storchen, J. "Die wohlunterrichtete Krancken-W.
Hilde Steppe, "Das Dilemma der pflegerische
trische Informationen 2 (1988): 17.

Streiter, Georg. *Die wirtschaftliche und soziale Lage der*
pflege in Deutschland. 2d ed. Jena, 1924.

Weygandt, Willhelm. "Irrenanstalten." In *Das Deutsche Kr.*
by J. Grober. Jena, 1922.

Zentralverband der Arbeitnehmer öffentlicher Betriebe
tungen, ed. *Das deutsche Pflege- und Anstaltspersonal: Sei.*
wirtschaftliche, und rechtliche Lage. Cologne, 1930.

Periodical Literature

"An das Krankenpflege- Massage- und Badepersonal." *Die Sanitätsw.*
(December 1918). Quoted in Hilde Steppe, "Pflege bis 1933," in *Kra.*
kenpflege im Nationalsozialismus, edited by Hilde Steppe, 34. 5th ed.
Frankfurt, 1993.

Ast, Fritz. "Der derzeitige Stand der Krankenpflege in den bayerischen
Irrenanstalten." *PNW* 23 (November 19, 1921).

Baege, E. "Über Eugenik, speziell die Sterilisierungsfrage." *Allgemeine*
Zeitschrift für Psychiatrie 95 (1931).

Becker, Heinrich. "Einiges zur Pflege unserer Kranken." *Geisteskranken-*
pflege 41 (June 1937).

———. "Kleinigkeiten, die wichtig sind." *Geisteskrankenpflege* 43 (November 1939).

———. "Die Geisteskrankenpflege." *Geisteskrankenpflege* 44 (May 1940).

Becker, Wern. H. "Unsere Pflichten während des Krieges." *DI* 21 (November 1917).

Bonhoeffer, Karl. "Jahresversammlung des Deutschen Vereins für Psychiatrie in Hamburg am 27. und 28. Mai 1920." *Allgemeine Zeitschrift für Psychiatrie* 76 (1920).

Borsum, A. "Unsere Pflichten während des Krieges." *DI* 21 (September 1917).

Brauner, Erwin. "Geistiche oder weltliche Krankenpflege?" *Die Sanitäts-*
warte, no. 26 (December 1931).

Faltlhauser, Valentin. "Geisteskrankenpflege: Zum Unterricht und Selbstunterricht für Irrenpfleger und zur Vorbereitung auf die Pflegerprüfung" (hereafter simply "Geisteskrankenpflege"). *DI* 26 (January 1922).

———. "Geisteskrankenpflege." *DI* 26 (February 1922).

———. "Geisteskrankenpflege." *DI* 26 (March 1922).

———. "Geisteskrankenpflege." *DI* 26 (April 1922).

———. "Geisteskrankenpflege." *DI* 26 (May 1922).

———. "Geisteskrankenpflege." *DI* 26 (June 1922).

———. "Geisteskrankenpflege." *DI* 26 (July 1922).

———. "Geisteskrankenpflege." *DI* 26 (August 1922).

———. "Geisteskrankenpflege." *DI* 26 (September 1922).

———. "Geisteskrankenpflege." *DI* 26 (October 1922).

———. "Geisteskrankenfürsorge außerhalb der Anstalten." *DI* 27 (May 1923).

———. "Geisteskrankenpflege." *DI* 27 (June 1923).

———. "Geisteskrankenpflege." *DI* 27 (October 1923)

———. "Geisteskrankenpflege." *DI* 27 (November 1923).

Friedlaender, Erich. "Die wirtschaftlichen Aufgaben der Irrenanstalt," part 1. *DI* 27 (August 1923).

———. "Die wirtschaftlichen Aufgaben der Irrenanstalt," part 2. *DI* 27 (October 1923).

———. "Die wirtschaftlichen Aufgaben der Irrenanstalt," part 3. *DI* 28 (January 1924).

———. "Die wirtschaftlichen Aufgaben in der Irrenanstalt." *DI* 30 (February 1926).

Fuchs, W. "Über Prophylaxe," part 1. *DI* 32 (July 1928).

———. "Über Prophylaxe," part 2. *DI* (August 1928).

———. "Pflegeunterricht." *DI* 33 (July 1929).

Galant, Johann Susmann. "Psychohygiene (Gesunderhaltung des Geistes) und die Irrenpflege." *DI* 30 (March 1926).

Gaupp, "Das Gesetz zur Verhütung erbkranken Nachwuchses und die Psychiatrie." *Klinische Wochenschrift* 13 (1934): 1. Quoted in Gisela Bock, *Zwangssterilisation im Nationalsozialismus: Studien zur Rassenpolitik und Frauenpolitik*, 192. Opladen, 1986.

Gebhardt. "Zu den Artikeln 'Drohende Rückschritte im Irrenwesen Deutschlands' in den Nummern 23–24 und 29–30 der Psych.-Neurolog. Wochenschrift." *PNW* 26 (December 13, 1924).

Gotthold. "Die Pflege der unsauberen, unordentlichen und unsozialen Kranken." *DI* 26 (July 1922).

Götz, Bernt. "Was der Irrenpfleger von sexuellen Anomalien wissen muß." *DI* 30 (November 1926).

———. "Die Besuchsstunde." *DI* 32 (May 1928).

Grimm, Auguste. "Der Dienst im Wachsaal." *DI* 23 (November 1919).

Grimme. "Ein Fehler in der Ausbildung für die allgemeine Kranken-pflege." *PNW* 38 (August 8, 1936).

Groß, Adolf. "Zeitgemäße Betrachtungen zum wirtschaftlichen Betrieb der Irrenanstalten." *Allgemeine Zeitschrift für Psychiatrie* 79 (1923).

Herrmann, R. "Geisteskrankenpfleger und Erbkunde." *Geisteskrankenpflege* 38 (February 1934).

Hoffmann, Hans. "Die Sterilisierung (Unfruchtbarmachung) Minderwer-tiger aus eugenischen Gründen." *Geisteskrankenpflege* 37 (October 1933).

Hürten, Ferdinand. "Das Bewahrhaus unter besonderer Berücksichtigung der Diestaufgaben des Pflegepersonals." *Geisteskrankenpflege* 40 (March 1936).

Ilberg. "Die Sterblichkeit der Geisteskranken in den sächsischen Anstalten während des Krieges 1914/1918 und deren Folgen." *Allgemeine Zeitschrift für Psychiatrie* 78 (1922): 58–63. Quoted in Heinz Faulstich, *Von der Irrenfürsorge zur "Euthanasie": Geschichte der badischen Psychia-trie bis 1945*, 78. Freiburg, 1993.

Jahrmärker. "Zu Fragen der Verantwortlichkeit in der psychiatrischen Praxis." *Geisteskrankenpflege* 47 (March 1943).

Julie. "Gebildete Mädchen in der Irrenpflege." *DI* 13 (September 1909).

K., S. "Der Acht-Stunden-Tag in der Krankenpflege." *Unterm Lazaruskreuz* (Berlin), 1920. Quoted in Hilde Steppe, "Pflege bis 1933," in *Kranken-pflege im Nationalsozialismus*, edited by Hilde Steppe, 33. 5th ed. Frank-furt, 1989.

Kandzia, Emil. "Die Irrenpflege, ein Spezialgebiet der Krankenpflege." *DI* 23 (November 1919).

———. "Die Ausbildung des Pflegepersonals." *DI* 24 (November 1920).

———. "Was fordert das Irrenpflegepersonal für seine Ausbildung?" *DI* 26 (May 1922).

Karll, Agnes. "Zeitenwende." *Unterm Lazaruskreuz* (Berlin), 1919. Quoted in Hilde Steppe, "Pflege bis 1933," in *Krankenpflege im Nationalsozialis-mus*, edited by Hilde Steppe, 33. 5th ed. Frankfurt, 1989.

Kemper, W. "Über das Berufsgeheimnis." *Geisteskrankenpflege* 36 (March 1932).

Kesselring, M. "Die Bedeutung und Pflege des geistigen Lebens in der An-stalt." *Geisteskrankenpflege* 39 (December 1935).

Kihn, B. "Die Ausschaltung der Minderwertigen aus der Gesellschaft." *Allgemeine Zeitschrift für Psychiatrie* 98 (1932).

Koch, Josef. "Rationalisierung im Gesundheitswesen." In *Das Deutsche Pflege- und Anstaltspersonal: Seine berufliche, wirtschaftliche, und recht-liche Lage*, edited by the Zentralverband der Arbeitnehmer öffentlicher Betriebe und Verwaltungen. Cologne, 1930.

Köhler, Clemens. "Die Pflege der geisteskranken Rechtsbrecher." *Geisteskrankenpflege* 41 (September 1937).

————. "Der Kolonnenpfleger." *Geisteskrankenpflege* 42 (October 1938).

Kolb, Gustav. "Inwieweit sind Änderungen im Betrieb der Anstalten geboten?" *PNW* 22 (July 31, 1920).

Krause, W. "Einiges über den Irrenpflegeberuf und über Irrenpflege." *DI* 27 (July 1923).

————. "Der Pfleger bei der Außenarbeit." *Geisteskrankenpflege* 37 (July 1933).

Kühne. "Die wirtschaftlichen Aufgaben des Pflegepersonals im Kriege." *Geisteskrankenpflege* 47 (August 1943).

Lerrsen, J. "Die Wohnung und Verpflegung des Personals." *DI* 36 (November 1932).

Levy, Paul. "Freie oder karitative Krankenpflege?" *Die Sanitätswarte*, no. 13 (June 1928).

Menninger v. Lerchenthal, E. "Die Bedeutung des Wortes in der Irrenpflege." *DI* 31 (February 1927).

————. "Über die Eignung zum Irrenpflegeberuf." *DI* 33 (January 1929).

Möckel. "Die Arbeitstherapie bei Geisteskranken." *DI* 29 (February 1925).

————. "Die wirtschaftliche Seite der Anstalten." *Geisteskrankenpflege* 46 (October 1942).

Müller, Marie. "Erziehung der Geisteskranken." *DI* 30 (October 1926).

Muth. "Einige Hinweise für den Dienst." *Geisteskrankenpflege* 39 (August 1935).

Peuke, Hermann. "Der Irrenpfleger und sein Beruf." *DI* 10 (August 1906).

Philippi, W. "Ein Pfleger für Geisteskranke schildert seinen Beruf." *Geisteskrankenpflege* 40 (May 1936).

Piontek, Hermann. "Einiges über den Umgang mit Geisteskranken." *DI* 30 (January 1926).

Quaet-Faslem. "Die Sozialiserung der Heilberufe, speziell des ärztlichen Standes." *PNW* 23 (December 31, 1921).

R. "Erwiderung an Schwester Julie!" *DI* 13 (December 1909).

R., G. "Gespräch zwischen Pflegerin und Bäuerin." *DI* 23 (May 1919).

Raeke, Julius. "Ursachen der Geisteskrankheiten," part 1. *DI* 23 (August 1919).

————. "Ursachen der Geisteskranken," part 2. *DI* 23 (September 1919).

————. "Über den Umgang mit Psychopathen." *DI* 30 (July 1926).

————. "Psychopathische Kinder." *Geisteskrankenpflege* 34 (July 1930).

Ranker, J. "Wie können einfache Pflegepersonen Bildung erhalten?" *DI* 13 (February 1910).

Ranker, J. C. "Wer hat das Recht, zum Beruf der Irrenpflege zu greifen?" *DI* 24 (April 1920).

Reimann. "Einige Ausführungen über den Beruf eines Geisteskrankenpflegers." *Geisteskrankenpflege* 41 (August 1937).

Rhein. "Staatliche Anerkennung für das Pflegepersonal der Heil- und Pflegeanstalten für Geisteskranke." *PNW* 33 (January 10, 1931).

Roos, Georg. "Aus der Praxis eines Pflegers für Geisteskranke." *Geisteskrankenpflege* 41 (July 1937).

———. "Beziehung des Krankenpflegers zum Arzt." *Geisteskrankenpflege* 41 (December 1937).

———. "Forderungen der Krankenpflege." *Geisteskrankenpflege* 44 (October 1940).

Sack. "Die Heil- und Pflegeanstalten, ihre wirtschaftlichen, finanziellen und sonstigen Verhältnisse," part 1. *PNW* 40 (May 27, 1938).

———. "Die Heil- und Pflegeanstalten, ihre wirtschaftlichen, finanziellen und sonstigen Verhältnisse," part 2. *PNW* 40 (June 4, 1938).

Sauer, Georg. "Was heißt Pfleger sein?" *DI* 33 (March 1929).

Schäfer, Georg. "Das Benehmen des Pflegers im Dienst." *DI* 34 (January 1930).

Schmid, Therese. "Einfache Mädchen in der Irrenpflege." *DI* 13 (December 1909).

Schneider, O. "Die Frau als Krankenpflegerin." *Die Krankenpflege*, 1903. Quoted in Hilde Steppe, "Die historische Entwicklung der Krankenpflege als Beruf: Auswirkungen dieser Entwicklung auf heutige Strukturen," supplement to *Deutsche Krankenpflegezeitschrift*, no. 5 (1985): 5.

Schulze-Bünte. "Über die Gestaltung der Freizeit in den Heilanstalten." *Geisteskrankenpflege* 43 (September 1939).

Sieben. "Betriebswirtschaftliche Mitarbeit des Pflegeaufsichtspersonals." *Geisteskrenkenpflege* 42 (May 1938).

Snell. "Die Notwendigkeit der Sterilisierung der Erbkranken." *Geisteskrankenpflege* 43 (September 1939).

Snell, O. "Sparsamkeit." *DI* 32 (June 1928).

Snell, R. "Landesheil- und Pflegeanstalt Eichberg im Rheingau." In *Deutsche Heil- und Pflegeanstalen für psychisch Kranke in Wort und Bild*, vol. 1, edited by Johannes Bresler. Halle a. S., 1910.

Spaar, R. "Das Gesetz zur Verhütung erbkranken Nachwuchses vom 14. Juli 1933." *Geisteskrankenpflege* 38 (April 1934).

Spliedt. "Zur gegenwärtigen Lage der Anstalten." *PNW* 20 (February 1, 1919).

Steinwallner, Bruno. "Geplante Zulassung der Sterbehilfe in England." *PNW* 38 (November 14, 1936).

Streiter, Georg. "Ausbildung, Prüfung und Fortbildung in der Krankenpflege (mit besonderer Berücksichtigung der Irrenpflege)." *DI* 29 (August 1925).

Thielmann, W. "Der Pfleger und der Kranke." *Geisteskrankenpflege* 41 (January 1937).

Uenzen, Klaus. "Etwas über die Bewertung und Ausbildung des Pflegepersonals." *Geisteskrankenpflege* 34 (October 1930).

―――. "Älterer Pfleger und Anfänger." *DI* 35 (April 1931).

Vocke. "Die Ausbildung des Pflegepersonals in den Irrenanstalten." *PNW* 22 (November 20, 1920).

Wachsmuth, Hans. "Aus alten Akten und Krankengeschichten der nassauischen Irrenanstalt (Eberbach-Eichberg)," part 2. *PNW* 29 (July 9, 1927).

―――. "Aus alten Akten und Krankengeschichten der nassauischen Irrenanstalt (Eberbach-Eichberg)," part 3. *PNW* 29 (October 29, 1927).

―――. "Aus alten Akten und Krankengeschichten der nassauischen Irrenanstalt Eberbach-Eichberg," part 6, *PNW* 32 (March 8, 1930).

―――. "Aus alten Akten und Krankengeschichten der nassauischen Irrenanstalt Eberbach-Eichberg," part 6, *PNW* 32 (March 15, 1930).

Weisenhorn, F. "Leibesübungen der Geisteskranken an der Heil- und Pflegeanstalt Illenau im Vergangenheit und Gegenwart." *PNW* 32 (November 15, 1930).

Wickel, Carl. "Psychohygiene [Gesunderhaltung des Geistes] und Irrenpflege." *DI* 30 (March 1926).

―――. "Betätigungsbehandlung." *DI* 31 (May 1927).

―――. "Lernpfleger und Pfleger." *DI* 31 (June 1927).

―――. "Die Ausbildung des Pflegepersonals und ihre Erfordernisse in den Anstalten." *DI* 31 (July 1927).

―――. "Etwas von der Würde des Menschen." *DI* 33 (February 1929).

―――. "Der Umgang mit Geisteskranken, ihre Beobachtung und Pflege." *Geisteskrankenpflege* 39 (October 1935).

Wilms, Lutz. "Die Pflege des Geistes in der Geisteskrankenpflege." *Geisteskrankenpflege* 43 (August 1939).

Wittneben. "Erziehung, Behandlung und Pflege Geistesschwacher." *Geisteskrankenpflege* 38 (October 1934).

Y., X. "Heiratet nicht Geisteskranke!" *Die Sanitätswarte*, no. 20 (October 1928).

Selected Secondary Works

Aly, Götz. "Medizin gegen Unbrauchbare." In *Aussonderung und Tod: Die klinische Hinrichtung der Unbrauchbaren*, edited by Götz Aly. Beiträge zur nationalsozialistischen Gesundheits- und Sozialpolitik, vol. 1. Berlin, 1985.

―――. "Der saubere und schmutzige Fortschritt." In *Reform und Gewissen: "Euthanasie" im Dienst des Fortschritts*, edited by Götz Aly. Beiträge zur nationalsozialistischen Gesundheits- und Sozialpolitik, vol. 2. Berlin, 1985.

———, ed. *Aussonderung und Tod: Die klinische Hinrichtung der Unbrauchbaren.* Beiträge zur nationalsozialistischen Gesundheits- und Sozialpolitik, vol. 1. Berlin, 1985.

———, ed. *Reform und Gewissen: "Euthanasie" im Dienst des Fortschritts.* Beiträge zur nationalsozialistischen Gesundheits- und Sozialpolitik, vol. 2. Berlin, 1985.

———, ed. *Aktion T4, 1939–1945: Die "Euthanasie"-Zentrale in der Tiergartenstrasse 4.* Berlin, 1989.

Aly, Götz, and Karl-Heinz Roth. *Die restlose Erfassung: Volkszählen, Identifizieren, Aussondern im Nationalsozialismus.* Berlin, 1984.

Aly, Götz, and Christian Pross, eds. *Der Wert des Menschen: Medizin in Deutschland, 1918–1945.* Berlin, 1989.

Arbeitsgruppe zur Erforschung der Geschichte der Karl-Bonhoeffer Nervenklinik. *Totgeschwiegen 1933–1945: Zur Geschichte der Wittenauer Heilstätten, seit 1957 Karl-Bonhoeffer Nervenklinik.* Berlin, 1988.

Arendt, Hannah. *The Origins of Totalitarianism.* New York, 1951.

Auszug aus der Chronik des Psychiatrischen Krankenhauses Eichberg. Eltville am Rhein, 1984.

Bastian, Till. *Von der Eugenik zur Euthanasie.* Bad Wörishofen, 1981.

Bauer, Franz. *Geschichte der Krankenpflege: Handbuch der Entstehung und Entwicklung der Krankenpflege von der Frühzeit bis zur Gegenwart.* Kulmbach, 1965.

Bauer, Fritz, ed. *Justiz und NS-Verbrechen: Sammlung der Strafurteile wegen nationalsozialistischer Tötungsverbrechen, 1945–1966.* Amsterdam: University Press, 1968–1981.

Bauman, Zygmunt. *Modernity and the Holocaust.* Ithaca, N.Y., 1989.

Bernhardt, Heike. "Die Anstaltspsychiatrie in Pommern, 1939–1945: Ein Beitrag zur Aufhellung nationalsozialistischer Tötungsaktionen unter besonderer Berücksichtigung der Landesheilanstalt Ueckermünde." Med. diss., University of Leipzig, 1992.

Betriebsparteiorganisation der SED des Klinikums Berlin-Buch, Kommission Betriebsgeschichte, ed. *Klinikum Berlin-Buch: Beiträge zur Betriebsgeschichte.* Vol. 1. Berlin, 1987.

Bischoff, Claudia. *Frauen in der Krankenpflege: Zur Entwicklung von Frauenrolle und Frauenberufstätigkeit im 19. und 20. Jahrhundert.* Frankfurt, 1992.

Blasius, Dirk. *Der verwaltete Wahnsinn: Eine Sozialgeschichte des Irrenhauses.* Frankfurt, 1980.

———. "Psychiatrischer Alltag im Nationalsozialismus." In *Die Reihen fast geschlossen: Beiträge zur Geschichte des Alltags unterm Nationalsozialismus,* edited by Detlev Peukert and Jürgen Reulecke. Wuppertal, 1981.

———. *Umgang mit Unheilbaren: Studien zur Sozialgeschichte der Psychiatrie.* Bonn, 1986.

———. "Der Historikerstreit und die historische Erforschung des 'Euthanasie'-Geschehens." *Sozialpsychiatrische Informationen* 17 (1988).

———. "Die 'Maskerade des Bösen'? Psychiatrische Forschung in der NS-Zeit." In *Medizin und Gesundheitspolitik in der NS-Zeit,* edited by Norbert Frei. Schriftenreihe der Vierteljahreshefte für Zeitgeschichte. Munich, 1991.

———. "Psychiatrie und Krankenmord in der NS-Zeit: Probleme der historischen Urteilsbildung." In *Psychiatrie im Abgrund: Spurensuche und Standortbestimmung nach den NS-Psychiatrie Verbrechen,* edited by Ralf Seidel and Wolfgang Franz Werner. Dokumente und Darstellungen zur Geschichte der Rheinischen Provinzialverwaltung und des Landschaftsverbandes Rheinland, vol. 6. Cologne, 1991.

Bleker, Johanna, and Norbert Jachertz, eds. *Medizin im Dritten Reich.* Cologne, 1989.

Bock, Gisela. *Zwangssterilisation im Nationalsozialismus: Studien zur Rassenpolitik und Frauenpolitik.* Opladen, 1986.

Bracher, Karl-Dietrich. *Die deutsche Diktatur.* Cologne, 1969.

Bracher, Karl-Dietrich, Wolfgang Sauer, and Gerhard Schulz. *Die nationalsozialistische Machtergreifung: Studien zur Errichtung des totalitären Herrschaftssystems in Deutschland, 1933/34.* Schriften des Instituts für Politische Wissenschaft, vol. 14. Cologne and Opladen, 1960.

Brombacher, Horst. "Das Euthanasieprogram für 'unheilbar Kranke' (1939–1941) und seine Durchführung in den Anstalten Mittelbadens." *Die Ortnau* 65 (1987).

Broszat, Martin. *Hitler and the Collapse of Weimar Germany.* Translated by V. R. Berghahn. New York, 1987.

Browning, Christopher R. *Ordinary Men: Reserve Police Battalion 101 and the Final Solution in Poland.* New York, 1992.

Burleigh, Michael. *Death and Deliverance: "Euthanasia" in Germany, c. 1900–1945.* Cambridge, 1994.

———. *Ethics and Extermination: Reflections on Nazi Genocide.* Cambridge, 1997.

Burleigh, Michael, and Wolfgang Wippermann. *The Racial State: Germany, 1933–1945.* Cambridge, 1991.

Caplan, Jane. *Government without Administration: State and Civil Service in Weimar and Nazi Germany.* Oxford, 1988.

Connelly, John. "The Uses of *Volksgemeinschaft*: Letters to the NSDAP Kreisleitung Eisenach, 1939–1940." In *Accusatory Practices: Denunciation in Modern European History, 1789–1989,* edited by Sheila Fitzpatrick and Robert Gellately. Chicago and London, 1997.

Craig, Gordon. *Germany, 1866–1945.* New York, 1978.

Daum, Monika. "Arbeit und Zwang, das Leben der Hadamarer Patienten im Schatten des Todes." In *Psychiatrie im Faschismus: Die Anstalt Hadamar, 1933–1945*, edited by Dorothee Roer and Dieter Henkel. Bonn, 1986.

Delius, Peter. *Das Ende von Strecknitz: Die Lübecker Heilanstalt und ihre Auflösung, 1941*. Kiel, 1988.

Dickel, Horst. "Alltag in einer Landesheilanstalt im Nationalsozialismus: Das Beispiel Eichberg." In *Euthanasie in Hadamar: Die nationalsozialistische Vernichtungspolitik in hessischen Anstalten*, edited by Landeswohlfahrtsverband Hessen. Kassel, 1991.

Diewald-Kerkmann, Gisela. *Politische Denunziation im NS-Regime oder Die kleine Macht der "Volksgenossen."* Bonn, 1995.

Dörner, Klaus. "Nationalsozialismus und Lebensvernichtung." *Vierteljahreshefte für Zeitgeschichte* 15 (1967).

———. *Bürger und Irre: Zur Sozialgeschichte und Wissenschaftssoziologie der Psychiatrie*. Frankfurt, 1975.

———. "Anstaltsalltag in der Psychiatrie und NS-Euthanasie." In *Medizin im Dritten Reich*, edited by Johanna Bleker and Norbert Jachertz. Cologne, 1989.

Dörner, Klaus, et al., eds. *Der Krieg gegen die psychisch Kranken*. Rehburg-Loccum, 1980.

Ebbinghaus, Angelika. "Kostensenkung, 'Aktive Therapie' und Vernichtung: Konsequenzen für das Anstaltswesen." In *Heilen und Vernichten im Mustergau Hamburg*, edited by Angelika Ebbinghaus, Heidrun Kaupen-Haas, and Karl-Heinz Roth. Hamburg, 1984.

Ebbinghaus, Angelika, Heidrun Kaupen-Haas, and Karl-Heinz Roth, eds. *Heilen und Vernichten im Mustergau Hamburg*. Hamburg, 1984.

Evangelische Bildungs- und Pflegeanstalt "Hephata," ed. *Der Eichberg: Opfer und Täter*. Gersenheim, 1983.

Faulstich, Heinz. *Von der Irrenfürsorge zur "Euthanasie": Geschichte der badischen Psychiatrie bis 1945*. Freiburg, 1993.

Finzen, Asmus. *Auf dem Dienstweg: Die Verstrickung einer Anstalt in die Tötung psychisch Kranker*. Rehburg-Loccum, 1983.

———. "Massenmord und Schuldgefühl: Anmerkungen zur Patho-psychologie des Gewissens." *Sozialpsychiatrische Informationen*, no. 2 (1983).

Fitzpatrick, Sheila, and Robert Gellately, eds. *Accusatory Practices: Denunciation in Modern European History, 1789–1989*. Chicago and London, 1997.

Foucault, Michel. *Madness and Civilization: A History of Insanity in the Age of Reason*. Translated by Richard Howard. New York, 1988.

Frei, Norbert, ed. *Medizin- und Gesundheitspolitik in der NS-Zeit*. Schriften-reihe der Vierteljahreshefte für Zeitgeschichte, edited by Institut für Zeitgeschichte. Munich, 1991.

Freudenberger, Klaus, and Walter Murr. "Wo bringt ihr uns hin? Zur Deportation und Ermordung behinderten Menschen aus der Anstalt Kork im Jahre 1940." *Die Ortenau* 70 (1990).

Friedlander, Henry. *The Origins of Nazi Genocide: From Euthanasia to the Final Solution*. Chapel Hill and London, 1995.

Friedländer, Saul. *Nazi Germany and the Jews: The Years of Persecution, 1933–1939*. London, 1997.

Furtwängler, Franz Josef. *ÖTV: Die Geschichte einer Gewerkschaft*. Stuttgart, 1955.

Ganssmüller, Christian: *Die Erbgesundheitspolitik des Dritten Reichs: Planung, Durchführung, und Durchsetzung*. Cologne, 1987.

Gellately, Robert. *The Gestapo and German Society: Enforcing Racial Policy, 1933–1945*. Oxford, 1990.

———. "Denunciations in Twentieth-Century Germany: Aspects of Self-Policing in the Third Reich and the German Democratic Republic." In *Accusatory Practices: Denunciation in Modern European History, 1789–1989*, edited by Sheila Fitzpatrick and Robert Gellately. Chicago and London, 1997.

Goldhagen, Daniel Jonah. *Hitler's Willing Executioners: Ordinary Germans and the Holocaust*. New York, 1996.

Graf, Hendrik. " 'Betrifft: Überführung von Kranken': Kranken- und Irren-pflege im Nationalsozialismus." *Deutsche Krankenpflegezeitschrift* (Stuttgart), no. 5 (1983).

———. "Die Situation der Patienten und des Pflegepersonales der rhei-nischen Heil- und Pflegeanstalten in der Zeit des Nationalsozialis-mus." In *Verlegt nach unbekannt: Sterlilisation und Euthanasie in Galk-hausen, 1933–1945*, edited by Matthias Leipert, Rudolf Styrnal, and Winfried Schwarzer. Dokumente und Darstellungen zur Geschichte der Rheinischen Provinzialverwaltung und des Landschaftsverban-des Rheinland, vol. 1. Cologne, 1987.

Grauhan, A. "Berufsethische Normen in der Krankenpflege." *Deutsche Krankenpflegezeitschrift* (Stuttgart), no. 7 (1975).

Grubitzsch, Siegfried. "Revolutions- und Rätezeit 1918/19 aus der Sicht deutscher Psychiater." *Deutscher Psychiater, Psychologie und Gesell-schaftskritik* 33/34 (1985).

Güse, Hans-Georg, and Norbert Schmacke. *Psychiatrie zwischen bürgerlicher Revolution und Faschismus*. Kronberg, 1976.

Hamerow, Theodore. *On the Road to the Wolf's Lair: German Resistance to Hitler*. Cambridge, Mass., 1997.

Hertling, Marianne Elisabeth. *Die Provinzial Heil- und Pflegeanstalt Düren: Die Entwicklung einer großen psychiatrischen Anstalt der Rheinprovinz von ihrer Gründung, 1878 bis 1934.* Herzogenrath, 1985.

Hilberg, Raul. *The Destruction of the European Jews* Student edition. New York, 1985.

Höll, Thomas, and Paul-Otto Schmidt-Michel. *Irrenpflege im 19. Jahrhundert: Die Wärterfrage in der Diskussion der deutschen Psychiater.* Bonn, 1989.

Hoser, Cornelia, and Birgit Weber-Dickmann. "Zwangssterilisationen an Hadamarer Anstaltsinsassen." In *Psychiatrie im Faschismus: Die Anstalt Hadamar, 1933–1945,* edited by Dorothee Roer and Dieter Henkel. Bonn, 1986.

Hühn, Marianne. "Psychiatrie im Nationalsozialismus am Beispiel der Wittenauer Heilstätten." In *Aktion T4. 1939–1945: Die "Euthanasie"- Zentrale in der Tiergartenstrasse 4,* edited by Götz Aly. Berlin, 1989.

Hummel, Eva. *Krankenpflege im Umbruch (1876–1914): Ein Beitrag zum Problem der Berufsfindung "Krankenpflege."* Freiburger Forschungen zur Medizingeschichte, edited by Eduard Seidler and Barbro Kuhlo, vol. 14. Freiburg, 1986.

Jetter, Dieter. *Grundzüge der Geschichte des Irrenhauses.* Darmstadt, 1981.

Kaiser, Jochen-Christoph. "Kritische Anmerkungen zu Neuerscheinungen über die Geschichte von Heil- und Pflegeanstalten im Kontext von Eugenik—Sterilisation—'Euthanasie.' " *Westfälische Forschungen* 18 (1988).

Katscher, Liselotte. *Geschichte der Krankenpflege: Ein Leitfaden für den Unterricht an Krankenpflegeschulen.* Berlin, 1958.

———. *Krankenpflege und "Drittes Reich": Der Weg der Schwesternschaft des Evangelischen Diakonievereins, 1933–1939.* Stuttgart, 1990.

Kaul, F. K. *Die Psychiatrie im Strudel der Euthanasie: Ein Bericht über die erste industriemäßig durchgeführte Mordaktion des Naziregimes.* Frankfurt, 1979.

Kershaw, Ian. *Popular Opinion and Political Dissent in the Third Reich: Bavaria, 1933–1945.* Oxford, 1983.

Kersting, Franz-Werner, Karl Teppe, and Bernd Walter, eds. *Nach Hadamar: Zum Verhältnis von Psychiatrie und Gesellschaft im 20. Jahrhundert.* Paderborn, 1993.

Klee, Ernst. *"Euthanasie" im NS-Staat: Die "Vernichtung lebensunwerten Lebens."* Frankfurt, 1983.

———. *Was sie taten, was sie wurden.* Frankfurt, 1986.

Klee, Ernst, ed. *Dokumente zur Euthanasie.* Frankfurt, 1985.

Kleßmann, Christoph, ed. *Nicht nur Hitlers Krieg: Der Zweite Weltkrieg und die Deutschen.* Düsseldorf, 1989.

Klüppel, Manfred. *Euthanasie und Lebensvernichtung am Beispiel der Landesheilanstalten Haina und Merxhausen.* Kassel, 1984.

Koch, Franz. "Die Beteiligung von Krankenschwestern und Kranken-pflegern an Massenverbrechen im Nationalsozialismus." In *Kranken-pflege im Nationalsozialismus*, edited by Hilde Steppe, Franz Koch, and Herbert Weisbrod-Frey, 3d ed. Frankfurt, 1986.

Köhler, E. *Arme und Irre: Die liberale Fürsorgepolitik des Bürgertums*. Berlin, 1977.

Landeswohlfahrtsverband Hessen, ed. *Mensch achte den Menschen: Frühe Texte über die Euthanasieverbrechen der Nationalsozialisten in Hessen*. Kassel, 1985.

———, ed. *Euthanasie in Hadamar: Die nationalsozialistische Vernichtungs-politik in hessischen Anstalten*. Kassel, 1991.

Leipert, Matthias, Rudolf Styrnal, and Winfried Schwarzer, eds. *Verlegt nach unbekannt: Sterilisation und Euthanasie in Galkhausen, 1933–1945*. Dokumente und Darstellungen zur Geschichte der Rheinischen Pro-vinzialverwaltung und des Landschaftsverbandes Rheinland, vol. 1. Cologne, 1987.

Loos, Herbert. "Die psychiatrische Versorgung in Berlin im 19. und zum Beginn des 20. Jahrhunderts—Aspekte der sozialen Bewältigung des Irrenproblems in einer dynamischen Großstadtentwicklung." In *Geschichte der Psychiatrie im 19. Jahrhundert*, edited by Achim Thom. Berlin, 1984.

Lüdtke, Alf. "Funktionseliten: Täter, Mit-Täter, Opfer? Zu den Bedin-gungen des deutschen Faschismus." In *Herrschaft als soziale Praxis: Historische und sozial-anthropologische Studien*, edited by Alf Lüdtke. Göttingen, 1991.

Lutzius, Franz. *Die barmherzige Luge: Euthanasie im Dritten Reich*. Bochum, 1984.

Mader, Ernst T. *Das erzwungene Sterben von Patienten der Heil- und Pflegean-stalt Kaufbeuren-Irsee zwischen 1940 und 1945 nach Dokumenten und Be-richten von Augenzeugen*. Blöcktach, 1982.

McFarland-Icke, Bronwyn. "Moral Consciousness and the Politics of Ex-clusion: Nursing in German Psychiatry, 1918–1945." Ph.D. diss., Uni-versity of Chicago, 1997.

Meyer, J. E. " 'Die Freigabe der Vernichtung lebensunwerten Lebens' von Binding und Hoche im Spiegel der deutschen Psychiatrie vor 1933." *Der Nervenarzt* 59 (1988).

———. "Psychiatrie im Nationalsozialismus." In *Dienstbare Medizin: Ärzte betrachten ihr Fach im Nationalsozialismus*, edited by H. Friedrich and W. Matzow. Göttingen, 1992.

Mommsen, Hans. *Beamtentum im Dritten Reich*. Schriftenreihe der Viertel-jahreshefte für Zeitgeschichte, edited by Hans Rothfels and Theodor Eschenburg, no. 15. Stuttgart, 1966.

Mommsen, Hans. "Anti-Jewish Politics and the Implications of the Holocaust." In *The Challenge of the Third Reich: The Adam von Trotta Memorial Lectures,* edited by Hedley Bull. Oxford, 1986.

Moore, Barrington, Jr. *Injustice: The Social Bases of Obedience and Revolt.* White Plains, N.Y., 1978.

Morlok, Karl. *"Wo bringt ihr uns hin?"—Geheime Reichssache Grafeneck.* Stuttgart, 1985.

Müller-Hill, Benno. *Tödliche Wissenschaft.* Reinbek, 1984.

Niemand, Fritz. "Ich war in der Tötungsanstalt Meseritz-Obrawalde: Erinnerungen, Erfahrungen, Dokumente (zusammengestellt von Stefan Romey)." In *Krankenpflege im Nationalsozialismus,* edited by Hilde Steppe. 5th ed. Frankfurt, 1989.

Nowak, Kurt. *"Euthanasie" und Sterilisierung im "Dritten Reich": Die Konfrontation der evangelischen und katholischen Kirche mit dem "Gesetz zur Verhütung erbkranken Nachwuchses" und der "Euthanasie"-Aktion.* Göttingen, 1980.

Oliner, Samuel P. "The Unsung Heroes of Nazi Occupied Europe: The Antidote for Evil." *Nationalities Papers* 12, no. 1 (Spring 1984).

Orth, Linda. *Die Transportkinder aus Bonn: "Kindereuthanasie."* Dokumente und Darstellungen zur Geschichte der Rheinischen Provinzialverwaltung und des Landschaftsverbandes Rheinland, vol. 3. Cologne, 1989.

Panse, Friedrich. *Das psychiatrische Krankenhaus.* Stuttgart, 1964.

Peiffer, Jürgen, ed. *Menschenverachtung und Opportunismus: Zur Medizin im Dritten Reich.* Tübingen, 1992.

Peukert, Detlev. *Inside Nazi Germany: Conformity, Opposition, and Racism in Everyday Life.* Translated by Richard Deveson. New Haven, Conn., 1987.

Peukert, Detlev, and Jürgen Reulecke, eds. *Die Reihen fast geschlossen: Beiträge zur Geschichte des Alltags unterm Nationalsozialismus.* Wuppertal, 1981.

Platen-Hallermund, Alice. *Die Tötung Geisteskranker in Deutschland.* Frankfurt, 1947.

Prinz, Michael, and Rainer Zitelmann, eds. *Nationalsozialismus und Modernisierung.* Darmstadt, 1991.

Proctor, Robert. *Racial Hygiene: Medicine under the Nazis.* Cambridge, Mass., 1988.

Roer, Dorothee, and Dieter Henkel, eds. *Psychiatrie im Fascismus: Die Anstalt Hadamar, 1933–1945.* Bonn, 1986.

Rorty, Richard. *Contingency, Irony, and Solidarity.* Cambridge, 1989.

Roth, Karl Heinz, ed. *Erfassung zur Vernichtung: Von der Sozialhygiene zum "Gesetz über Sterbehilfe."* Berlin (West), 1984.

Rückleben, Hermann. *Deportation und Tötung von Geisteskranken aus den badischen Anstalten der Inneren Mission Kork und Mosbach.* Karlsruhe, 1981.

Sachße, Chistopher, and Florian Tennstedt. *Bettler, Gauner und Proleten.* Reinbeck, 1983.

Schaper, Hans-Peter. *Krankenwartung und Krankenpflege: Tendenzen der Verberuflichung in der ersten Hälfte des 19. Jahrhunderts.* Sozialwissenschaftliche Studien, vol. 22. Opladen, 1987.

Schmidt, Gerhard. *Selektion in der Heilanstalt, 1939–1945.* Stuttgart, 1965.

Schmuhl, Hans-Walter. *Rassenhygiene, Nationalsozialismus, Euthanasie: Von der Verhütung zur Vernichtung "lebensunwerten Lebens."* Göttingen, 1987.

———. " 'Euthanasie' im Nationalsozialismus: Ein Überblick." In *Euthanasie in Hadamar: Die nationalsozialistische Vernichtungspolitik in hessischen Anstalten,* edited by Landeswohlfahrtsverband Hessen. Kassel, 1991.

———. "Kontinuität oder Discontinuität? Zum epochalen Charakter der Psychiatrie im Nationalsozialismus." In *Nach Hadamar: Zum Verhältnis von Psychiatrie und Gesellschaft im 20. Jahrhundert,* edited by Franz-Werner Kersting, Karl Teppe, and Bernd Walter. Paderborn, 1993.

Schneider, Hugo. "Die ehemalige Heil- und Pflegeanstalt Illenau: Ihre Geschichte, ihre Bedeutung." *Die Ortenau* 61 (1981).

Schneider, Wolfgang, ed. *Vernichtungspolitik: Eine Debatte über den Zusammenhang von Sozialpolitik und Genozid im nationalsozialistischen Deutschland.* Hamburg, 1991.

Schrapper, Christian, and Dieter Sengling. *Die Idee der Bildbarkeit. 100 Jahre Sozialpädagogische Praxis in der Heilerziehungsanstalt Kalmenhof.* Weinheim-Munich, 1988.

Schröter, Sonja. "Psychiatrie in Waldheim/Sachsen von ihren Anfängen bis zum Ende des zweiten Weltkrieges (1716–1945): Ein Beitrag zur Geschichte der forensischen Psychiatrie in Deutschland." Med. diss., University of Leipzig, 1993.

Seidel, Ralf, and Wolfgang Franz Werner, eds. *Psychiatrie im Abgrund: Spurensuche und Standortbestimmung nach den NS-Psychiatrie-Verbrechen.* Dokumente und Darstellungen zur Geschichte der Rheinischen Provinzialverwaltung und des Landschaftsverbandes Rheinland, vol. 6. Cologne, 1991.

Seidler, Eduard. *Geschichte der Pflege des kranken Menschen.* 2d ed. Stuttgart, 1966.

———. "Die moderne Krankenpflege in ihrer historischen Entwicklung." *Hippokrates* 23 (1968).

Sick, Dorthea. *Euthanasie im Nationalsozialismus am Beispiel des Kalmenhofs in Idstein im Taunus.* Frankfurt, 1982.

Siemen, Hans Ludwig. *Das Grauen ist vorprogrammiert: Psychiatrie zwischen Faschismus und Atomkrieg*. Gießen, 1982.

———. *Menschen blieben auf der Strecke . . . : Psychiatrie zwischen Reform und Nationalsozialismus*. Gütersloh, 1987.

———. "Reform und Radikalisierung: Veränderungen der Psychiatrie in der Weltwirtschaftskrise." In *Medizin und Gesundheitspolitik in der NS-Zeit*, edited by Norbert Frei. Schriftenreihe der Vierteljahreshefte für Zeitgeschichte. Munich, 1991.

Sozialpsychiatrische Informationen ("Psychiatrie im deutschen Faschismus"), no. 2 (1983).

Sozialwissenschaftliche Informationen ("Zivilisation und Barbarei"), no. 2 (1996).

Steppe, Hilde. "Die historische Entwicklung der Krankenpflege als Beruf: Auswirkungen dieser Entwicklung auf heutige Strukturen." *Deutsche Krankenpflegezeitschrift*, no. 5 (Supplement) (1985).

———. "Dienen ohne Ende: Die historische Entwicklung der Arbeitszeit in der Krankenpflege in Deutschland." *Pflege* (Bern), no. 1 (1988).

———. "Das Dilemma der pflegerischen Ethik." *Sozialpsychiatrische Informationen*, no. 2 (1988).

———. "Mit Tränen in den Augen zogen wir dann die Spritzen auf. . . ." In *Krankenpflege im Nationalsozialismus*, edited by Hilde Steppe. 5th ed. Frankfurt, 1989.

———. "Pflege bis 1933." In *Krankenpflege im Nationalsozialismus*, edited by Hilde Steppe. 5th ed. Frankfurt, 1989.

———. "Das Selbstverständnis der Krankenpflege." *Deutsche Krankenpflegezeitschrift*, no. 5 (1990).

———, ed. *Krankenpflege im Nationalsozialismus*. 5th ed. Frankfurt, 1989.

Steppe, Hilde, Franz Koch, and Herbert Weisbrod-Frey, eds. *Krankenpflege im Nationalsozialismus*. 3d ed. Frankfurt, 1986.

Sticker, Anna, ed. *Die Entstehung der neuzeitlichen Krankenpflege: Deutsche Quellenstücke aus der ersten Hälfte des 19. Jahrhunderts*. Stuttgart, 1960.

Stoffels, Hans. "Die Gesundheitsutopie der Medizin im Nationalsozialismus." In *Sozialpsychiatrische Informationen* ("Psychiatrie im deutschen Faschismus"), no. 2 (1983).

———. "Utopie und Opfer: Sozialanthropologische Überlegungen zu den nationalsozialistischen Krankentötungen." In *Psychiatrie im Abgrund: Spurensuche und Standortbestimmung nach den NS-Psychiatrie-Verbrechen*, edited by Ralf Seidel and Wolfgang Franz Werner. Cologne, 1991.

Stolz, Peter. "Die Rolle der Irrenanstalten im Faschisierungsprozeß der deutschen Psychiatrie." *Recht und Psychiatrie* (Rehburg-Loccum), no. 2 (1983).

Storz, Dieter. "Politische Psychiatrie II." *Psychologie heute*, no. 3 (1976).

Tec, Nechama. *When Light Pierced the Darkness: Christian Rescue of Jews in Nazi Occupied Poland.* Oxford, 1986.

Teppe, Karl. *Massenmord auf dem Dienstweg: Hitlers "Euthanasie"-Erlaß und seine Durchführung in den westfälischen Provinzialheilanstalten.* Münster, 1989.

Thom, Achim. "Erscheinungsformen und Widersprüche des Weges der Psychiatrie zu einer medizinischen Disziplin im 19. Jahrhundert." In *Geschichte der Psychiatrie im 19. Jahrhundert*, edited by Achim Thom. Berlin, 1984.

―――. "Das Schicksal der Psychiatrie in der Zeit der faschistischen Diktatur." *Psychiatrie, Neurologie und medizinische Psychologie* 37 (1985).

―――. "Kriegsopfer der Psychiatrie: Das Beispiel der Heil- und Pflegeanstalten Sachsens." In *Medizin und Gesundheitspolitik in der NS-Zeit*, edited by Norbert Frei. Schriftenreihe der Vierteljahreshefte für Zeitgeschichte. Munich, 1991.

Thom, Achim, ed. *Geschichte der Psychiatrie im 19. Jahrhundert.* Berlin, 1984.

Thom, Achim, and G. Caregorodcev, eds. *Medizin unterm Hakenkreuz.* Berlin (East), 1989.

Thom, Achim, and Horst Spaar, eds. *Medizin im Faschismus.* Berlin, 1983.

Todorov, Tzvetan. *Facing the Extreme: Moral Life in the Concentration Camps.* Translated by Arthur Denner and Abigail Pollak. New York, 1996.

Tröster, Werner. *Suttrop-Dorpke: Zur Geschichte des Westfälischen Landeskrankenhauses Warstein.* Warstein, 1980.

Walter, Bernd. "Psychiatrie in Westfalen, 1918–1945: Soziale Fürsorge—Volksgesundheit—totaler Krieg." In *Selbstverwaltungsprinzip und Herrschaftsordnung: Bilanz und Perspektiven landschaftlicher Selbstverwaltung in Westfalen*, edited by Karl Teppe. Veröffentlichungen des Provinzialinstituts für westfälische Landes- und Volksforschung des Landschaftsverbandes Westfalen-Lippe, vol. 25. Münster, 1987.

―――. *Psychiatrie und Gesellschaft in der Moderne: Geisteskrankenfürsorge in der Provinz Westfalen zwischen Kaiserreich und NS-Regime.* Forschungen zur Regionalgeschichte, vol. 16, edited by Karl Teppe. Paderborn, 1996.

Weindling, Paul. *Health, Race, and German Politics between National Unification and Nazism, 1870–1945.* Cambridge, 1989.

Wettlaufer, Antje. "Die Beteiligung von Schwestern und Pflegern an den Morden in Hadamar." In *Psychiatrie im Fascismus: Die Anstalt Hadamar, 1933–1945*, edited by Dorothee Roer and Dieter Henkel. Bonn, 1986.

Zeller, Eberhard. *The Flame of Freedom: The German Struggle against Hitler.* London, 1967.

Index

NSDAP, 104–105, 115, 126, 172–176, 184–191, 194–196, 204, 244, 251, 299n.4, 302n.61; and patient abuse, 53, 59, 87–95, 136, 175–177, 181, 183–186, 215–216, 217–218, 230, 254, 260, 297n.122; and patient discipline, 143, 159–163; and patient killings in the East, 220–223; and patient restraint techniques, 48–50, 143, 259, 269n.7, 270n.24, 278n.64, 295nn. 73 and 74; and patient supervision, 17–18, 192–193, 203–204, 296–297n.109; and patient transports, 57, 144, 216, 219–226, 236, 278n.64, 311n.68, 312n.73; political fanaticism among, 181–189; preferred language technique of, 55–59, 144–146; prescribed ethical orientation of, 11, 21, 45–46, 58–59, 67–75, 141–142, 151–155, 163–171, 199–200, 259, 278n.71; private lives of, 18, 27–29, 51–52, 70–73, 189–191, 196–200, 207–208, 282nn. 8 and 16, 305nn. 94 and 97; professional organization of, 20–22, 26; refusals and conflicts of conscience among, during "euthanasia" measures, 216, 238–240, 246–250, 252–254; and shock therapy, 137; and the struggle for better working conditions and social benefits, 19–22, 25–32, 271n.31, 272nn. 57 and 58; suicide among, 122, 253; and the T4 program, 218–220, 311nn. 52 and 68; technical responsibilties of, 14, 17–18, 46–48, 166–167, 214, 227; training and certification of, 19, 25, 29–31, 131–133, 198–199, 273nn. 66 and 71; and unofficial "euthanasia," 226–256; and work therapy, 47–48, 145, 157–159, 259, 275n.21; during World War I, 22–25. *See also* attendants

occupational therapy. *See* work therapy
Oliner, Samuel P., 265n.2
outpatient care, 38–39, 130–131

patients: abuse of, 53, 59, 87–95, 136, 175–177, 181, 183–186, 215–216, 217–218, 230, 254, 260, 284n.64; criminals among, 44, 142–143, 158, 163–166, 177; discipline of, 143, 159–163, 298n.138; escape of, 55, 57, 83, 144, 167, 192–193; favorable influence of nurses on, 47–48, 55–59, 144–146, 258–259; moral status of, 34–38, 45–46, 58–63, 137–138, 140–143, 150–155, 163–171, 258–260, 296n.109,

298n.138; as objects of nurses' trust, 58–59, 83–84, 145; physical restraint of, 48–50, 143, 259, 269n.7, 270n.24, 278n.64, 295nn. 73 and 74; relatives of, 7, 11, 24, 52–53, 56, 58, 120, 123, 129, 134–135, 139–140, 146, 153, 155, 176, 188, 213–215, 220, 223, 234, 236, 280n.101; sterilization of, 130, 133–135, 209; suicide of, 46, 55, 57, 84–85, 120, 123, 131, 142, 144, 151–153, 166, 167; transport of, 57, 144, 219–226, 278n.64, 311n.68; during World War I, 22–25. *See also* shock therapy; T4 Program; unofficial "euthanasia"; work therapy
Pfannmüller, Hermann, 310n.46
Pinel, Philippe, 15
Poland, viii, 218
Pomerania, 213, 220, 244, 311n.68
Posen, 17
psychiatrists: as administrative mediators, 88–93, 297n.122; alienation of, from the public, 42, 129–130; compliance of, with National Socialist policies, 6, 129, 130–132, 133–135, 210; and the crisis of legitimacy, 33–41, 130, 258; on eugenics and sterilization, 44, 65–66, 130–133, 146–151; on euthanasia, 46, 65–66, 152, 277n.54, 297n.113; on the ideal nurse, 50–59, 144–146, 278n.73; and the implementation of the GVeN, 130–135, 147, 155, 292n.22; on the moral status of patients, 34–38, 45–46, 59–63, 137–138, 141–143, 150–155, 163–166; on the nature of mental illness, 43–45, 140–141; as nurses' hierarchical superiors, 18–19, 22, 54–55, 139–140, 155–157, 279nn. 89 and 96, 297n.122; on nurses' training and certification, 29–30, 131–132; on nurses' working conditions and social benefits, 19–21, 26; and patient abuse, 53, 59, 215, 230; on scarcity, 24, 34–38, 168–169; and shock therapy, 136–137, 143, 212, 260; on work therapy, 39–41, 47–48, 157–159, 259, 275n.21, 276nn. 29 and 30, 298nn. 138 and 147
psychiatry, advent of no-restraint treatment in, 14–15, 48–49, 278n.64; effects of sterilization law on, 138–139; historiography of, 5–7, 10–11; and humane intent, 11, 34, 48–49, 59–63, 128–129, 140–143, 146–151, 154, 210–211, 257–259;